Implants in the Aesthetic Zone

Todd R. Schoenbaum
Editor

Implants in the Aesthetic Zone

A Guide for Treatment of the Partially Edentulous Patient

Springer

Editor
Todd R. Schoenbaum
Division of Constitutive and Regenerative Sciences
University of California
Los Angeles, CA
USA

ISBN 978-3-319-72600-7   ISBN 978-3-319-72601-4 (eBook)
https://doi.org/10.1007/978-3-319-72601-4

Library of Congress Control Number: 2018954624

This Springer imprint is published by the registered company Springer Nature Switzerland AG
The registered company address is: Gewerbestrasse 11, 6330 Cham, Switzerland

I would like to thank my amazing wife Amy for her support and patience during this project. Through her, and with her, all things are possible. I would also like to extend my deepest gratitude to the amazing scientists, clinicians, and technicians who contributed to this book. They were selected because they are unsurpassed in their expertise in the profession. I am forever in their debt. Lastly, I would like to thank you, the reader, for taking the time to read this text. It is my sincere hope that it contributes to you, your practice, and your patients.

Foreword

Aesthetics is commensurate with health and well-being, and this is no more true than when considering teeth and oral health. The absence of teeth, through trauma, disease, or genetic disturbance, is considered by many patients a form of disability. With the advent of dental implants, we, the dental profession, have the means of resolving these issues and improving the quality of life for our patients.

Dr. Todd Schoenbaum has succeeded in bringing together some of the master scholars within the field of implant dentistry, both surgeons and restorative clinicians. The contributors to this text come from all over the world; all have unique abilities that lie not only in treating patients in their clinics, but also the desire to pass on their knowledge and expertise. The intention is to provide the reader with a foundation to further expand their own capabilities and ultimately improve the treatment of those under our care.

Chandur P. K. Wadhwani

Preface

This text is intended to serve as a clinical guide for treatment of implants in the aesthetic zone. This area and treatment modality is uniquely complex in dentistry, requiring skill and expertise from surgeons, restorative clinicians, and technicians. Success requires a team approach. Here you will see I have assembled an unmatched group of authorities from around the world to assist you in this process. Each brings their unique expertise and experience to their work here. You will find these experts are straightforward and generous with their knowledge.

I hope you enjoy reading this book as much as we did in creating it.

> Do you think that I count the days? There is only one day left, always starting over: it is given to us at dawn and taken away from us at dusk.—Sartre

Los Angeles, CA, USA — Todd R. Schoenbaum

Contents

Contributors

Tara Aghaloo Section of Oral and Maxillofacial Surgery, UCLA School of Dentistry, Los Angeles, CA, USA

Anirudha Agnihotry Arthur A Dugoni School of Dentistry, San Francisco, CA, USA

Sam Alawie Owner/Ceramist Beverly Hills Dental Lab, Beverly Hills, CA, USA

Luigi Canullo University of Valencia, Valencia, Spain

Mohammed A. Husain Section of Oral and Maxillofacial Radiology, UCLA School of Dentistry, Los Angeles, CA, USA

Hajime Igarashi Private Practice, Kyoto, Japan

Joseph Y. K. Kan Department of Restorative Dentistry, Loma Linda University School of Dentistry, Loma Linda, CA, USA

Perry R. Klokkevold Section of Periodontics, University of California, Los Angeles, CA, USA

Bach Le Department of Oral and Maxillofacial Surgery, Herman Ostrow School of Dentistry at USC, Los Angeles, CA, USA

Private Practice, Whittier, CA, USA

Rachel Lim Department of Oral and Maxillofacial Surgery, University of Washington, Seattle, WA, USA

Tomas Linkevicius Faculty of Medicine, Institute of Odontology, Vilnius University, Vilnius, Lithuania

Taichiro Morimoto Private Practice, Fukuoka, Japan

Alireza Moshaverinia Division of Advanced Prosthodontics, School of Dentistry, University of California, Los Angeles, CA, USA

Peter K. Moy Dental Implant Center, University of California, Los Angeles, CA, USA

Panos Papaspyridakos Division of Postgraduate Prosthodontics, Tufts University School of Dental Medicine, Boston, MA, USA

Joan Pi-Anfruns Division of Diagnostic and Surgical Sciences, Division of Regenerative and Constitutive Sciences, Dental Implant Center, UCLA School of Dentistry, Los Angeles, CA, USA

Algirdas Puisys Vilnius Implantology Center, Vilnius, Lithuania

Xavier Rodríguez Implantology Department, International University of Catalonia (UIC), Barcelona, Spain

Kitichai Rungcharassaeng Department of Orthodontics and Dentofacial Orthopedics, Loma Linda University School of Dentistry, Loma Linda, CA, USA

Akitoshi Sato Private Practice, Tokyo, Japan

Todd R. Schoenbaum Division of Constitutive and Regenerative Sciences, University of California, Los Angeles, CA, USA

Richard G. Stevenson III Stevenson Dental Solutions, Inc., San Dimas, CA, USA

Senichi Suzuki Private Practice, Ebina City, Japan

Sotirios Tetradis Section of Oral and Maxillofacial Radiology, UCLA School of Dentistry, Los Angeles, CA, USA

Xavier Vela Implantology Department, International University of Catalonia (UIC), Barcelona, Spain

Chandur P. K. Wadhwani Department of Restorative Dentistry, University of Washington, Seattle, WA, USA

Loma Linda University School of Dentistry, Loma Linda, CA, USA

Part I

Treatment Planning for Implants in the Aesthetic Zone

Treatment Planning for Implants in the Aesthetic Zone: Biological, Functional, and Aesthetic Considerations

1

Peter K. Moy, Todd R. Schoenbaum, and Sam Alawie

Abstract

Proper interdisciplinary treatment planning is the cornerstone of implant treatment in the aesthetic zone. It requires diligent and thoughtful consideration of surgical, prosthetic, and technical aspects of the care to be provided. Though some cases will present similar challenges, no two are identical. Patients will be best served when the clinicians and technicians involved on the case understand the challenges faced by the other team members. Additionally, depending on the severity of the defect, patient expectations may need to be tempered to accept the clinical realities of their case. The "team approach" is key here. Each member should know and be able to predict what the others are going to be doing during their treatment stage. Often an immediate load approach will be attempted in the aesthetic zone. This requires high-level coordination, collaboration, and communication.

1.1 Importance of Treatment Planning

The success with any dental implant treatment starts with an accurate and appropriately sequenced treatment plan. Brånemark (Fig. 1.1) first introduced osseointegration as a multidisciplinary effort and would only permit clinicians to train as a team

P. K. Moy (✉)
Dental Implant Center, University of California, Los Angeles, CA, USA
e-mail: pmoy@dentistry.ucla.edu

T. R. Schoenbaum
Division of Constitutive and Regenerative Sciences, University of California, Los Angeles, CA, USA
e-mail: tschoenb@ucla.edu

S. Alawie
Beverly Hills Dental Lab, Beverly Hills, CA, USA

Todd R. Schoenbaum (ed.), *Implants in the Aesthetic Zone*,
https://doi.org/10.1007/978-3-319-72601-4_1

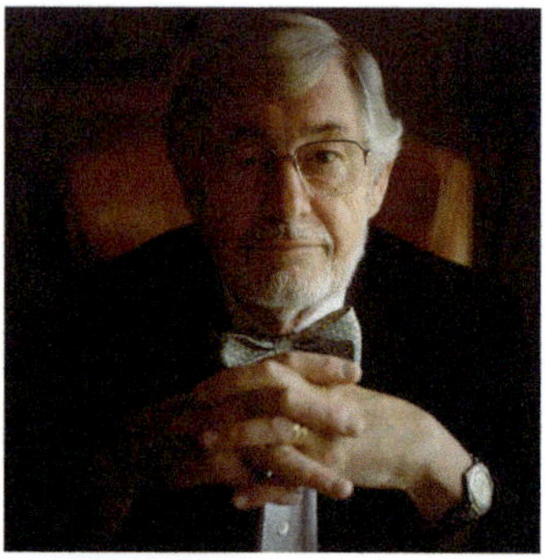

Fig. 1.1 Dr. P.I. Brånemark is the key innovator responsible for the modern approach to implant dentistry. His work in the field of osseointegration of titanium implants has revolutionized current dental treatment

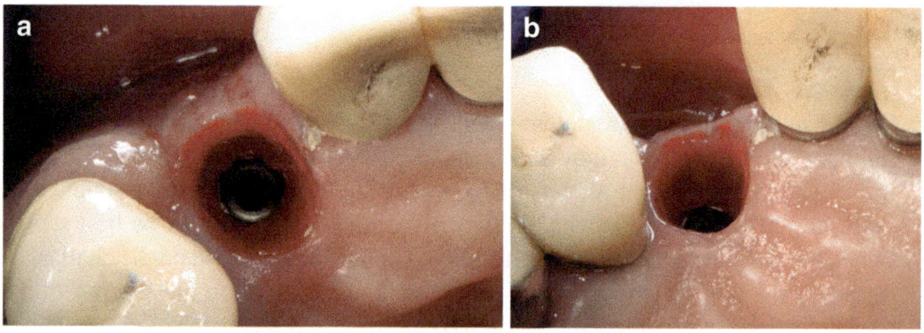

Fig. 1.2 (**a**, **b**) Peri-implant mucositis presents with various degrees of soft tissue pathologies, including inflammation, bleeding on probing, pus, fistula, and swelling

from both surgical and prosthodontic specialties. There are many factors to consider when treating the aesthetic zone with dental implants, even with a single missing tooth situation. Missing a single tooth in the aesthetic zone may often present as the most difficult and challenging to manage. The clinical assessment of the edentulous situation should be preceded by first identifying the cause of the edentulous state. If the cause for the loss of the tooth/teeth is not addressed first and corrected, once the implant is placed and has integrated, the alveolar defect that occurred and remains because of the tooth loss will lead to ongoing problems for the dental implant and implant-supported restoration. Ongoing problems such as inflammation of gingival tissues (better known as peri-implant mucositis) (Fig. 1.2a, b) leading to bone loss (peri-implantitis) (Fig. 1.3) will ultimately lead to the failure of the dental implant treatment. For example, if the tooth was lost due to trauma, there is often a concomitant loss of bone and/or soft tissues. If these deficiencies are present, an augmentation procedure or procedures should be performed first to restore lost tissues before placement of the dental implant. When the treatment is for the aesthetic zone, the best results occur when the alveolar ridges are ideally reconstructed to original contours and volume. This permits the ideal positioning of the implant during placement to best support the restoration. If the tooth was lost due to periodontal disease, not only must one worry about reconstructing lost hard and soft tissues but the periodontal status of the adjacent teeth and its effect on planned dental implant

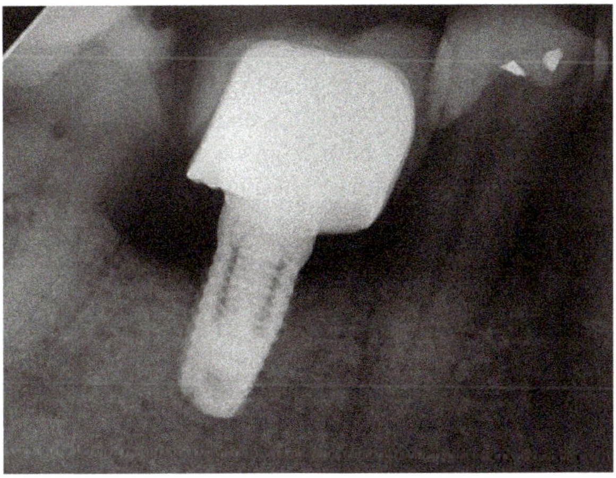

Fig. 1.3 Peri-implantitis is usually the result of untreated peri-implant mucositis. This results in a progression to atypical and aggressive bone loss around the implant. It may result in loss of the implant if unresolved

treatment must be accounted for. In a paper by Sgolastra et al. [1] using a systematic review of longitudinal prospective studies only, the authors identified strong evidence and with statistical significance that periodontitis is a risk factor for implant loss, moderate evidence and with statistical significance for periodontitis as a risk factor for peri-implantitis, and moderate evidence but not statistically significant for patients exhibiting periodontitis to experience greater peri-implant bone loss. For the aesthetic zone, the long-term outcome of implant treatment and maintenance of hard and soft tissue volume is extremely important in determining whether treatment was successful or not. A prosthetically driven, interdisciplinary, and systematic approach must be used if aesthetic risk factors are identified and managed accordingly [2].

1.2 Systematic and Interdisciplinary Approach

1.2.1 Medical Assessment

The implant patient's medical conditions will often affect the clinical outcomes of dental implant treatment, and the surgical specialist must be aware of these conditions so that preventative and/or corrective measures may be instituted to provide the implant patient with the best outcome. Several medical conditions are known to have negative effects on clinical outcomes with dental implant treatment [3]. Conditions such as diabetes, long-term steroid use, radiation therapy for oral-facial cancer, postmenopausal hormonal replacement therapy, and social habit (smoking) are associated with higher dental implant failure rates. The failures are due to delayed or poor healing of soft tissues typically related to poor vascularity resulting in exposure of the implant and surrounding bone structures. The 2005 article noted that although these medically related conditions present as relative contraindications for dental implant therapy, the overall failure rate of dental implants are low, and there are no absolute contraindications to implant placement. However, the medical conditions that present with increased risk for failure should be considered during treatment planning phase and included in the informed consent process. The implant patient with identified medical conditions that affect healing processes of hard and soft tissues must be made aware that their medical conditions should be stable or corrected prior to initiating implant treatment.

1.2.2 Dental Assessment

The dental assessment should include evaluation of the remaining dentition, how maintainable are the restorations, the periodontal status, and the volume of hard and soft tissues in the edentulous site and adjacent tooth structures. It is especially important to assess the dentition adjacent to the implant site. Residual infections from previous periapical abscess, periodontal disease, and/or soft tissue conditions where recession has exposed roots of adjacent teeth must be corrected.

1.2.3 Psychological (Patient MOTIVATION) Assessment

When the clinician is dealing with the aesthetic zone, the patient's expectations for treatment outcome must be understood. Once the clinician understands the patient's expectation, it is imperative that the clinician educate the patient on anticipated results and requirements for maintenance. Walia and coworkers [4] determined that a patient's seeking implant treatment (motivation) and their expectations (satisfaction at conclusion of treatment) with implant treatment differ. Patients today are more aware of dental implants as a viable treatment to replace missing teeth, thanks to large volume of available information on social media. However, the patients are not aware of the complications associated with implant treatment for the aesthetic zone, specifically the lack of hard and soft tissue volume as well as contours. There are varying reports on what patients are actually looking for when seeking implant treatment. Rustemeyer and Brernerich [5] identified 68% of women and 41% of men in their study felt aesthetics to be very important with their treatment results. In another study [6], the systematic review found the high cost of implant treatment often resulted in unrealistic expectations of the implant patient. Even with these concerns, Pjeteursson et al. [7] found in their 10-year prospective study that 90% of thc patients were completely satisfied with implant therapy, both from a functional and aesthetic standpoint. The use of dental implants to restore missing teeth in the aesthetic zone requires the treating clinician to have a thorough understanding of what motivates the patient and what their expectations are at the completion of treatment. The potential for poor aesthetic results due to loss of interproximal papilla or hard tissue contours must be explained to the patient and the likelihood of this risk occurring. Included in the discussion is the need to surgically correct the deficiencies prior to implant placement.

1.3 Restorative Considerations for Treatment Planning Implants in the Aesthetic Zone

Our three primary concerns restoratively are functional, biological, and aesthetic (Table 1.1).

1.3.1 Functional Concerns

We must understand the risks of abutment failure, crown or FDP (fixed dental prosthesis; aka "bridge") failure, and screw breakage/loosening. Titanium and cast alloy abutments will have the least risk of breakage. The primary disadvantage of metal abutments in the aesthetic zone is discoloration of the soft tissues. Full contour zirconia abutments will generally have the highest risk of breakage (Fig 1.4a, b). The zirconia abutment luted to a "Ti Base" seems promising

Table 1.1 Restorative considerations for implants in the aesthetic zone

Functional concerns	Biological concerns	Aesthetic concerns
Abutment fracture	Risk of retained cement	Discoloration of the gingiva
Crown fracture	Reactions to metal alloys	Shade match for the crown
Screw fracture	Loose screws	Margin reveal
Screw loosening	Gingival recession	Gingival recession
	Poor fitting components	Screw access showing
	Porosities in the metal or ceramic materials	

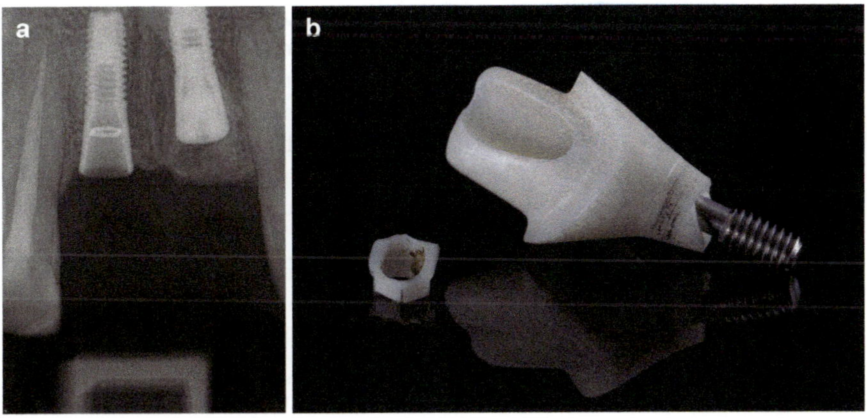

Fig. 1.4 (**a**, **b**) A full zirconia abutment has fractured inside the implant connection. The use of abutments without a Ti Base is risky due to this potential complication. The apical portion of the fractured zirconia abutment is visible on the radiograph as a radiopaque ring. Such fractures can be difficult to treat, as the remaining zirconia portion may be wedged in place requiring drilling to remove (courtesy of Dr. David Wagner)

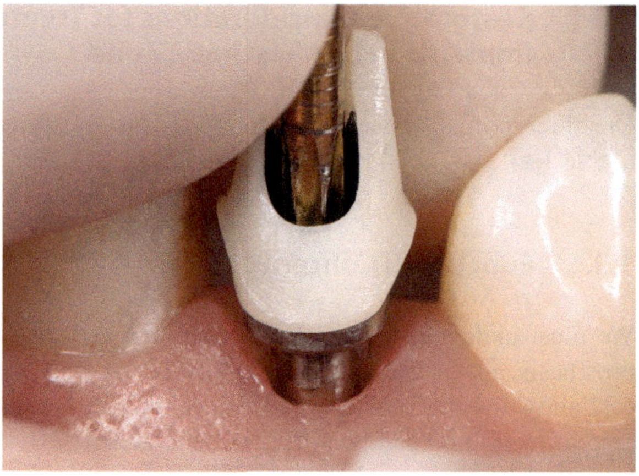

Fig. 1.5 When zirconia abutments are indicated (generally due to high smile line and thin gingival biotype), they should be fabricated with a Ti Base. This helps to increase strength and minimize the challenges of retreatment should the abutment break

(Fig. 1.5). At the current time, there has only been one study looking at the strength of the Zr/Ti Base abutments [8]. This design appears to decrease the risk of breakage during cyclic loading; however, this is dependent on the implant being used, the Ti Base, the cementation protocol, the thickness of the zirconia, and the lab used to manufacture them. The take-home point being that not all Zr/Ti abutments are created equal. There are also an increasing amount of anecdotal reports of the zirconia abutment debonding from the Ti Base. While obviously problematic, this is relatively easy to resolve by re-bonding. The laboratory technician must ensure that the cementation protocols are properly followed and that the Ti Base is as long as possible. Far too many of these restorations seem to have insufficient height of the Ti Base.

An additional advantage of the Zr/Ti abutment is that, should the zirconia break, retrieval and removal is simple and predictable. This is in stark contrast to the failure of full zirconia abutments, which usually occurs at the neck of the implant connection. This leaves a small ring of zirconia inside the implant, which can be difficult to remove, especially in some tapered connections. The remaining Zr piece may have to be drilled out if it cannot be pulled out. This can cause significant damage to the connection interface in the implant. As such, full contour Zr abutments (without the Ti Base) should be avoided.

For the crowns on implants in the aesthetic zone, most of the modern ceramic materials appear to be strong enough. However, for scenarios requiring an FDP with a pontic, the lithium disilicate materials are generally best avoided due to an increased possibility of fracture at the connector. PFM (porcelain fused to metal) or PFZ (porcelain fused to zirconia) would be preferable options.

Loose and broken screws (Fig. 1.6) used to be a common occurrence and frustration. Improved alloys (i.e., Ti alloys replacing Au alloys), widespread use of torque wrenches (Fig. 1.7), and improved coatings on the screws have decreased the incidence of loosening somewhat. However, the great reduction in loosening and breakage is due to improved implant—abutment connections. The early root form implants with an external hex were not designed to retain single-unit prostheses. In

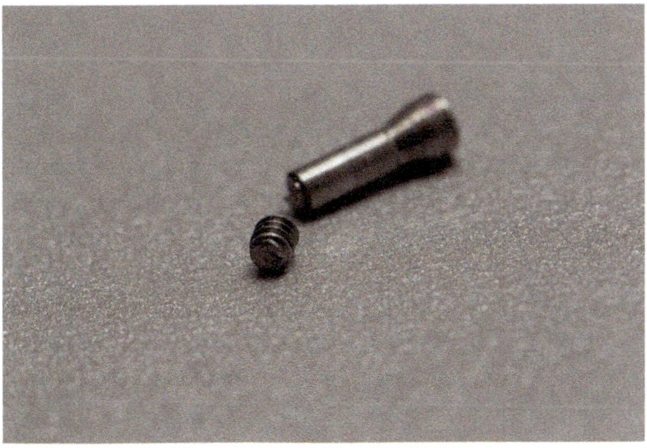

Fig. 1.6 Even modern titanium screws can fracture if they are improperly treated. Special care must be taken to ensure passive fit of the abutment and to not surpass the manufacturer torque values. The screw here was broken at delivery leaving the small threaded remnant to be carefully retrieved from inside the implant

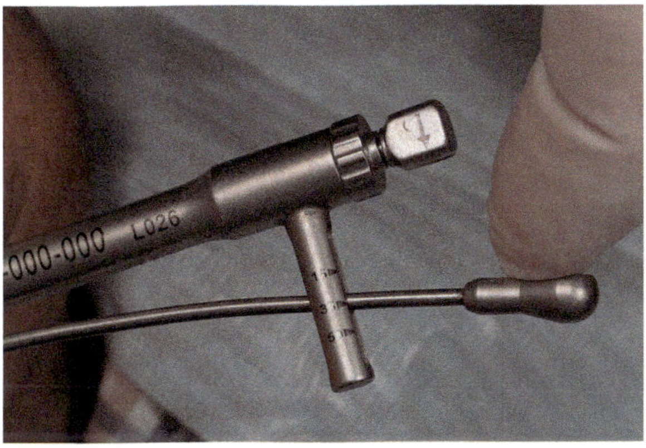

Fig. 1.7 The use of a torque wrench is essential for delivery of implant restorations. They help the clinician ensure that the screw creates the proper pre-load without fatiguing the screw or implant. Most (but not all) screws are designed to be torqued to 30–35 Ncm

fact, the external hex was primarily designed to interface with the available drivers, and retaining a prosthesis was its secondary job. The external hex is generally less than 1 mm in height. This provides very little resistance and retention, placing all the off-angle force vectors on the screw, thus resulting in screws coming loose or breaking over time. So much so that it is generally advisable that all external hex implants be restored with a screw-retained restoration to allow for ease of screw replacement and re-torqueing.

There are hundreds of variants of internal connections currently available. Although they vary greatly in their engineering, as a general rule, they have a much more intimate and robust connection. This results in significant reductions in screw loosening. Some of these connections are so well designed that abutments can be difficult to remove even after the screw has been taken out. For restoring implants in the aesthetic zone, internal connection implants should be used. Additionally, most (but not all) data [9–12] show that a platform switch design will aid in maintaining peri-implant bone and soft tissue levels.

Occlusal management of implants in the aesthetic zone is critical to long-term success. Dr. Stevenson covers this topic in depth in Chap. 18.

1.3.2 Biological Concerns

First and foremost, the restoration selected/designed should impose a minimal risk in inducing peri-implantitis or peri-implant mucositis. Residual cement on the abutment is the most frequently discussed cause of peri-implantitis. While this is undeniably true, implementation of some relatively common sense guidelines mitigate this risk. Chief among these guidelines is that all abutments for cemented restorations should be custom milled, such that the margins are clearly accessible (Fig. 1.8) when the crown/prosthesis is cemented. See Chap. 14 for more information on the proper use of cemented restorations. It is important for the restoring dentist to understand the low-risk cementation protocols, because it is inevitable that patients will present with implants that do not allow for a traditional screw-retained restoration (Fig. 1.9a, b). The use of lingual set screws may serve as an alternative solution

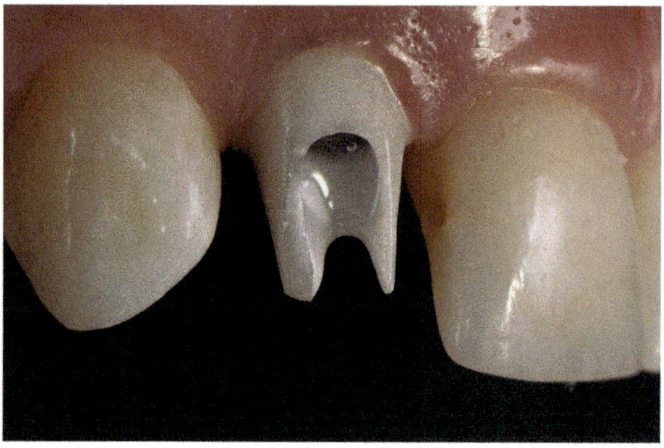

Fig. 1.8 Margin placement is the crucial factor for using cemented implant restorations with minimal risk of retained cement and peri-implantitis. Here the Zr/Ti Base abutment was prescribed to have margin at −0.5 mm on the distal, facial, and mesial and at 0 mm on the palatal. This ensures easy access for cement removal and evaluation with little risk of aesthetic concerns

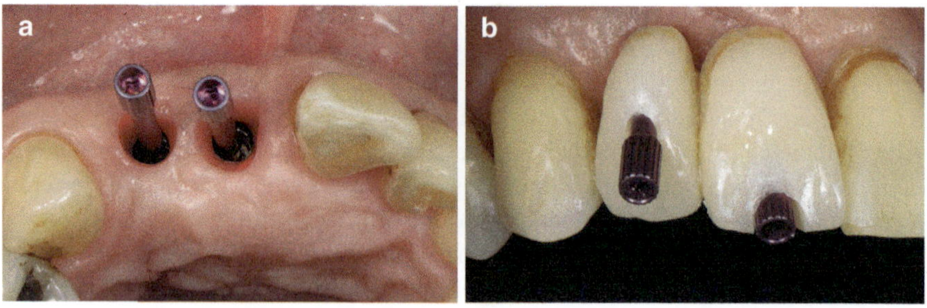

Fig. 1.9 (**a**, **b**) Unfortunately, not all implants are placed with access through the palatal, and not all manufacturers offer an angled screw channel option. Such cases are difficult to manage without a proper understanding of how to cement the restoration without the risk of retained cement on the abutment surface

to facially angled implants, but they are difficult to fabricate and have little to no evidence supporting their use. It should be well noted though that proper planning and surgical/restorative coordination *prior* to implant placement will minimize the frequency of such occurrences.

Additional prosthetic causes of peri-implantitis/mucositis include reactions to metal alloys, loose screws, poor fitting restorations and casted abutments (Fig. 1.10), poor fitting third party components, and porosities in the metal or ceramic materials. If left unresolved, peri-implant mucositis will lead to atypical bone loss around the implant.

The other area in which the restorative clinician affects the peri-implant biology is in the realm of abutment emergence profiles. The shape of the abutment where it joins the implant and as it emerges through the soft tissue will have significant effect on the health, cleansibility, and aesthetics of the peri-implant soft tissues. See Chap. 13 for more information on the design and effects of the abutment emergence profile.

Abutment cleanliness is also critical for the restorative clinician and technician to address prior to delivery of the prostheses. Most abutments and crowns regardless of design come out of the lab with significant amounts of particulate debris on their

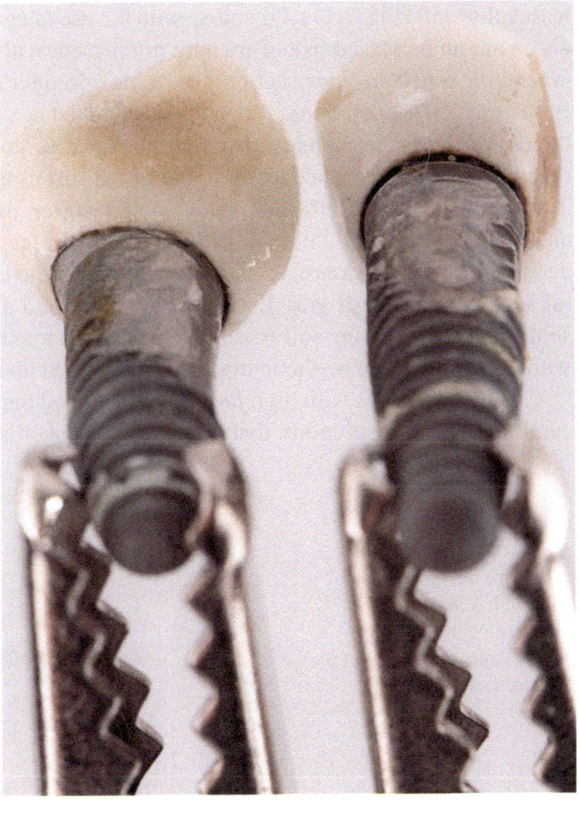

Fig. 1.10 Poorly designed abutments and poor fitting restorations allow for bacterial reservoirs that induce peri-implantitis. Here the margins of the crowns have a significant marginal gap unfilled by cement. Thus allowing plaque and bacterial to accumulate, ultimately resulting in loss of the implants

surface. Canullo et al. recently published a survey [13] on how and if clinicians clean and disinfect prosthetic implant components. Worldwide there is huge variation in how this is done (steam, chlorhexidine, autoclave), and for the most part, the components are being placed into surgical implant sites without sufficient cleanliness. Even when cleaned as described above, the components still retain a significant amount of particulate debris. Preliminary studies have shown that proper cleaning of the abutments (with plasma of Argon) prior to placement can significantly increase the levels of retained bone around the implant. At a bare minimum, implant abutments and prostheses should be thoroughly steam cleaned and disinfected.

1.3.3 Aesthetic Considerations

The restorative aesthetic considerations for implants in the aesthetic zone are soft tissue color, soft tissue contour, and crown/prosthesis shade. The various studies examining the effects of abutment material on the perceived color of the soft tissues have failed to reach uniform conclusions. Most show that silver-colored metals (i.e., gold alloys, titanium) produce the greatest amount of discoloration of the gingiva, while ceramic-type materials (i.e., zirconia, lithium disilicate, alumina) produce the least color shift (Fig. 1.11). Of course with the use of ceramic-type abutment materials comes an increased risk of fracture not present with metals. As described in the *functional considerations* section above, the zirconia abutments should have a Ti Base design. This *functional risk* must be weighed against the aesthetic demands of the case. As an intermediary material, anodized or coated titanium (pink or gold colors) (Fig. 1.12) produce less graying of the soft tissue than the uncoated metals. This process can be performed by the manufacturer, the laboratory, or in the clinician's office. Wadhwani et al. [14] have described the DIY anodization process in detail. Soft tissue thickness is also a key component to creating or maintaining natural soft tissue color. If gray tissue is present around an implant, the two possible solutions are increasing soft tissue thickness with a graft or replacing the abutment with one of the more aesthetic materials mentioned above.

Challenging cases with high *functional risks* and high *aesthetic demands* require carefully selected solutions that mitigate the potential for failure. When proper

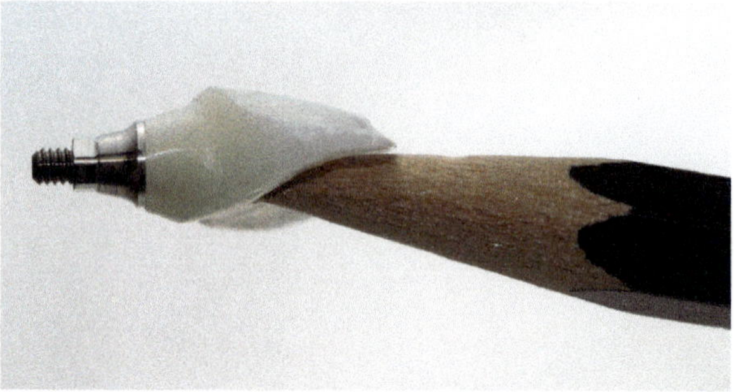

Fig. 1.11 The zirconia framework with Ti Base is an appropriate restoration design for the aesthetic zone with thin tissue biotypes and high smile lines. Here a screw-retained design was utilized

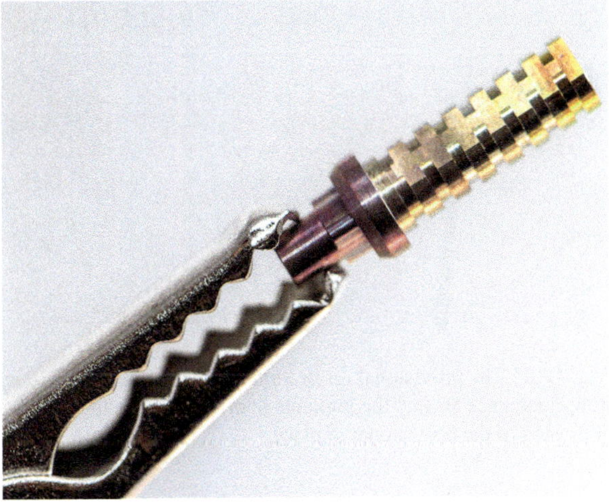

Fig. 1.12 Minor—moderate tissue discoloration can also be mitigated with the anodization of Ti abutments. Here a provisional abutment has to be anodized to have a pink hue in the emergence area and a gold hue in the crown area. This procedure can be easily accomplished in the office with simple materials (see [14])

planning and coordination has been performed prior to starting the treatment, implant selection and orientation can be determined prior to surgery to allow for management of these challenges. For the single-tooth implant in the aesthetic zone, the screw-retained zirconia/Ti Base crown + abutment may prove to be an ideal solution if the implant is able to be placed in an ideal position. See Chap. 15 for Linkevicius and Puisys' excellent review of this treatment option. It needs to be understood though that this restoration requires an attentive technician to ensure that the abutment is as long as possible and it is properly cemented.

Management of the soft tissue around the implant requires interdisciplinary coordination. The surgeon is responsible for creating/maintaining sufficient bone in which to place the implant(s), but also enough bone to properly support the peri-implant tissues. Patient factors (i.e., smoking, diabetes) will also affect the quantity and quality of the bone available. When bone is lost on the roots adjacent to the implant site, it can be very difficult to restore the bone to ideal positions. Soft tissues will generally represent the underlying bone architecture, although grafting procedures may be successful in masking bony defects with increased soft tissue thickness. Thicker soft tissue is less prone to atypical recession and remodeling, thus ensuring better long-term peri-implant aesthetics.

The restoring clinician is responsible for fine-tuning the contours of the soft tissues through the conscientious use of provisional restorations (Fig. 1.13a, b). The final form and position of the soft tissues can be moved (within a range) by changes in the shape of the provisional restoration. Generally, over-contouring of the emergence or pontic will move tissues apically, while flat or under-contoured shapes will allow tissue to move coronally. There are limitations and variables that will affect how much the tissues can be manipulated by the provisional restorations. As a general rule, the soft tissue architecture should be refined in the provisional stage, before making the definitive impression. It is much easier to perform additional surgeries or modify the prostheses in the provisional stage than it is to correct deficiencies after the definitive restoration has been delivered. See Chaps. 10 and 13 for

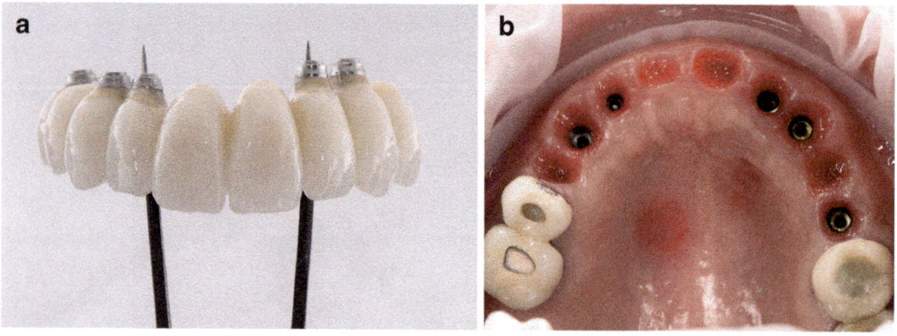

Fig. 1.13 The provisional restoration (**a**) has to be carefully designed with ovate pontics and narrow emergence around the implants in order to shape the soft tissues. (**b**) The tissue contours after 3 months of the provisional in place

more details on the process of fabricating provisional restorations and using them to modify the positions of the soft tissue.

1.4 Surgical Considerations for Treatment Planning Implants in the Aesthetic Zone

The surgical considerations to take into account during the treatment planning by the surgical specialist should mimic that of the restorative concerns and requirements of the restoration in order to provide the best surgical outcomes to support the planned restoration. Therefore, the restorative plan (type of implant restoration, emergence contours, and interproximal contacts) must be known. Otherwise, the surgeon will end up placing the implant where the best available bone dictates it to go rather than the implant restoration dictating the ideal implant position. The surgeon must know specific information concerning the restoration in order to place the implant in the ideal position. This includes the contours of the restoration, the emergence contours, the location of the central fossa, and the method of crown to implant connection.

1.5 Functional Concerns

1.5.1 Occlusion

Implants are designed to withstand heavy occlusal forces vertically. When there are excessive lateral forces, the distribution of forces is limited resulting in bone loss surrounding the implant (Fig. 1.14). Thus, the patient who exhibits grinding habits or bruxism must be placed into a night guard to compensate for the unnatural lateral movement of the jaw, preventing the excessive lateral forces and the excessive bone loss that occurs around the dental implant.

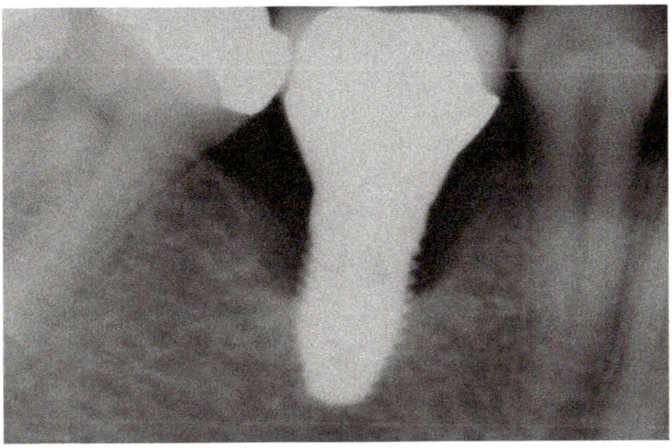

Fig. 1.14 Atypical bone loss around a posterior implant is illustrated in this radiograph. In the absence of any obvious factors, excessive occlusion should be considered as a possible etiology

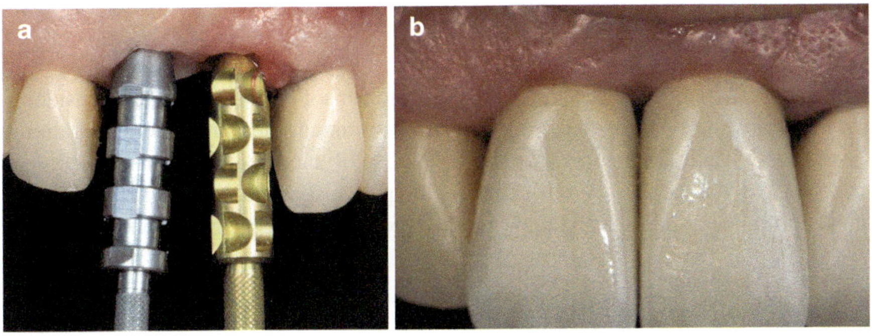

Fig. 1.15 (**a**, **b**) Special care must be used with adjacent implants in the aesthetic zone. These implants are slightly too close to each other and may have exacerbated the deficiency of the mesial papilla

1.5.2 One Versus Two Implants for Two-Teeth Edentulous Space

When the edentulous situation has two consecutively missing teeth, the length of the edentulous space is critical number to determine whether one or two implants will be used to replace the two missing teeth. This is especially critical in the incisor region.

Too close: no papilla
Too far : flat papilla

1.5.3 Spacing of Implants

The spacing between implants will be a determining factor for the shape, contours, and volume of the papilla. If implants are too close to each other or to the adjacent tooth, there will be a loss of the papilla (Fig. 1.15a, b). When the implants are too far from each other or the adjacent tooth, the papilla contour flattens (Fig. 1.16a, b). In the posterior quadrant, when this happens food impaction becomes a chronic issue for the patient.

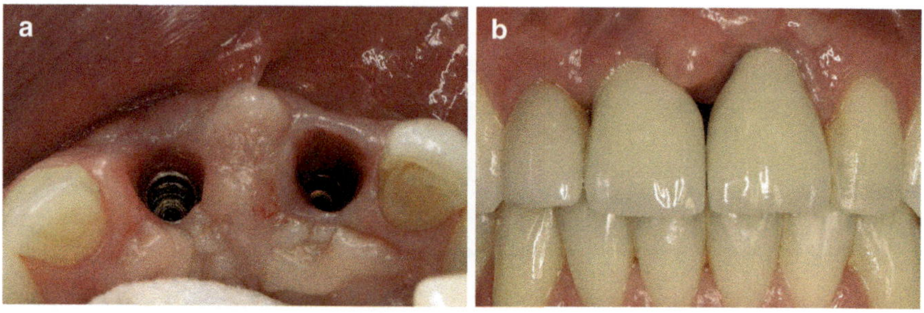

Fig. 1.16 At the other end of the spectrum, these implants (**a**, **b**) are placed too far apart, and this also makes creation of a reasonable papilla challenging at best

1.6 Biologic Concerns

1.6.1 Gingival Biotype [15, 16]

Thin biotype: use anodized Ti or Zr. for color mask

The thickness (real or perceived) of the peri-implant soft tissues should be considered prior to initiating implant treatment. Generally speaking, the thin tissue biotype must be carefully handled intraoperatively, and the use of anodized Ti or zirconia components will need to be considered. The thin biotype is also more susceptible to recession and appropriate remedies need to be planned for should this complication present.

1.6.2 Health of Periodontal Tissue

The periodontal status of the adjacent dentition will have a direct effect on the peri-implant soft tissue.

1.6.3 Future Health of Peri-implant Tissue

The maintenance of the peri-implant gingival tissue health is a concept implant patients must be educated on. The most common reason why the patient is missing a tooth or multiple teeth is due to periodontal disease. If the patient cannot maintain appropriate gingival health around natural dentition, they certainly will have problems maintaining gingival health around implants. This becomes more eminent as the patient ages and manual dexterity becomes an issue due to arthritic changes making it more difficult for the older patient to maintain hygiene around posterior implants. When the implant patient show signs of poor or inadequate oral hygiene home care, the conversion of the implant restoration from fixed to removable must be considered.

1.7 Aesthetic Concerns

1.7.1 Smile Line

The first inspection of the patient requiring an implant in the aesthetic zone is the smile line at rest or repose, half smile, and full smile. This assessment will help to determine facial asymmetries, the amount of gingival show during movements, in full smile, half smile, and at rest. This assessment will help the surgeon determine the critical nature of maintaining tissue volume and contours. Patients with high smile lines should be approached with caution. Any loss of tissue contours or volume with the surgical procedure will be clearly visible resulting in an extremely dissatisfied patient.

1.7.2 UCLA Aesthetic Implant Analysis

This is a simple, inexpensive method to identify deficiencies, discrepancies, and asymmetries with the patient's dentition as well as deficiencies of hard and soft tissues. The analysis requires a clinical photograph of the patient's maxillary anterior dentition with lips retracted. The photograph should show back to the bicuspids with the midline centered in the photograph. (Fig. 1.17) There are three horizontal lines drawn. The superior line, *gingival margin line*, connects the zenith of the gingival margin of the canine to the contralateral canine. The middle line, *mesial papilla line*, connects the mesial papilla of the canine to the contralateral mesial papilla. The inferior line (incisal edge line) is a line drawn from the incisal tip of the canine to the contralateral canine tip. Once the three lines are drawn, any asymmetries, irregularities, and deficiencies are easily detected. This analysis serves as documentation for the clinician to review with the implant patient and to record the clinical condition pre- and posttreatment (Fig. 1.17 and 1.18).

1.7.3 Implant Positioning

In the past, the description of implant positioning has always been stated as three-dimensional (3-D). This concept was formulated due to limited capabilities of the diagnostic tools that were available in the late 1980s and early 1990s with plane film radiography as well as using a freehand surgical approach as a standard to placement of dental implants. The three dimensions or positions that surgeons are

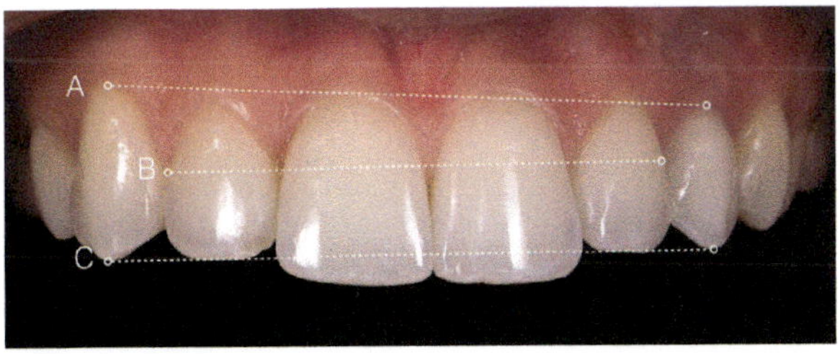

Fig. 1.17 This is the UCLA Aesthetic Implant analysis in use. A, is the *gingival margin line* connecting the gingival zeniths of the canines. B, the *mesial papilla line* connects the papilla mesial to the canines. C, The *incisal edge line* connects the cusp tip of the canines. Here, the UCLA Aesthetic Implant analysis is used to quickly gauge for symmetry and proportion following implant placement and restoration of the left canine, with reasonable (but not perfect) results

accustomed to identify when placing an implant are *mesial-distal*, *buccal-lingual/palatal* angulation (Fig. 1.19), and *apical-coronal* (depth) positions (Fig. 1.20). The modern use of digital technology, specifically the cone beam computed tomography (CBCT) scan, permitted the clinician to observe three-dimensional reconstructed views of the patient's hard tissue. Today the clinician may view the hard tissue structures in the axial, coronal, and sagittal views thus enhancing the ability for the surgeon to place the implant in the ideal three-dimensional position. The introduction of software programs to assist in treatment planning introduced a fourth

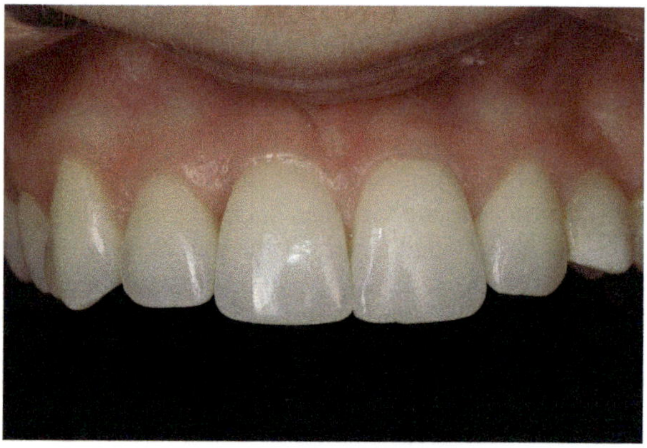

Fig. 1.18 The pretreatment view of the patient in Fig. 1.17, illustrating a buccal alveolar concavity and significant disproportion of the teeth and soft tissues due to the retained primary left canine

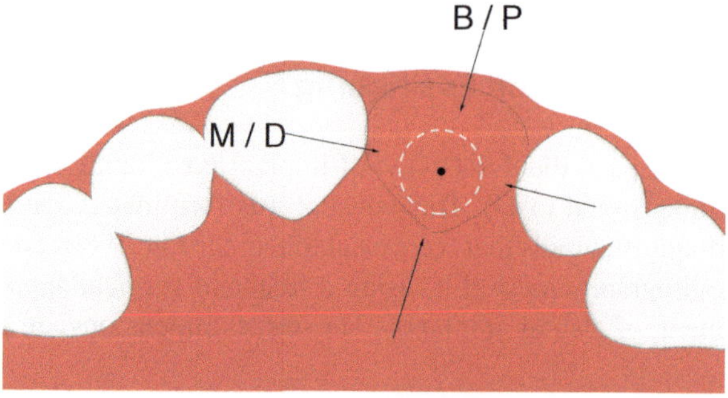

Fig. 1.19 The first two axes of the five-dimensional implant placement consideration. This figure represents both the mesial-distal and buccal-palatal position of the osteotomy

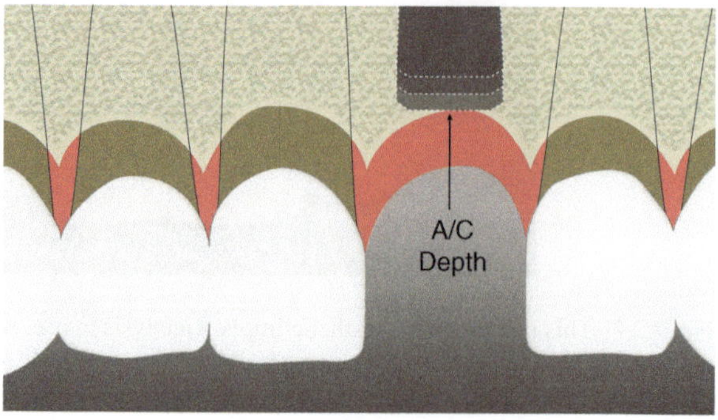

Fig. 1.20 The third axis is apical-coronal depth. This dimension is the depth to which the osteotomy is drilled and the implant placed relative to the planned gingival zenith

dimension to consider. This fourth dimension is known as "arch" position. Depending on the location of the implant in the arch and whether the arch is the maxilla or mandible, the tilt of the implant will differ. For example, an implant placed in the mandibular first molar position must be placed with the axis of the implant tilted slightly to the lingual. This differs from buccal-lingual angulation because accounting for this angulation is necessary to bring the access opening for a screw-retained restoration to come through the central fossa of the restoration. The arch position tilt accounts for the coronal shape of the restoration. The arch position assures the proper relationship of the working cusps of the maxillary and mandibular arches (Fig. 1.21). This fourth dimension becomes even more obvious when dealing with the fully edentulous arch. As the implant positions change from anterior to posterior in the mandible, the lingual tilt becomes more pronounced. If the surgeon attempt to place implants parallel to each other, the malposition of the posterior implants will be noticeable. As the surgical approaches for implant placement transitions from freehand to guided (CBCT planning programs) to navigation (dynamic guided), a fifth dimension became obvious. As the surgeon begins preparing the implant site using navigation approach, the focus is on placement of the drill tip on the cross hair image on the computer screen. Following this cross hair to depth represents the apical tip of the implant. Once the drill goes through the cortical layer on the crest of the ridge, the surgeon's focus is on the outer ring on the computer screen. This is seen as the angular deviation and represents the body of the implant and, ultimately, the neck of the implant located at the crest when the implant is completely seated (Fig. 1.22). This is called the "cone" position. The focus as the drilling preparation of the implant site proceeds, the surgeon attempts to keep the angular deviation as low as possible. Even with the deviation below one degree (1°), the neck position of the implant will have a variance that will change the access opening of the implant. As the technology and instrumentation improves, the surgeon must adapt to the use of the advancing technologies to ideally position the implants accounting for all five dimensions.

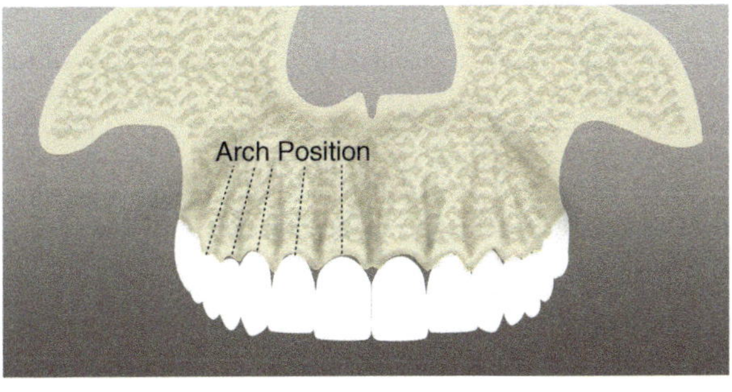

Fig. 1.21 The fourth axis is the *arch position*. This is to take into consideration the angulation of the jaw as we move around the arch. In the maxilla, it forms a somewhat cone shape, with the apical end of the implant being tipped palatally, while in the mandible it is generally the opposite due to the lingual concavity. Cross-sectional CBCT slices will aid the clinician in determining the appropriate angulation for the given patient

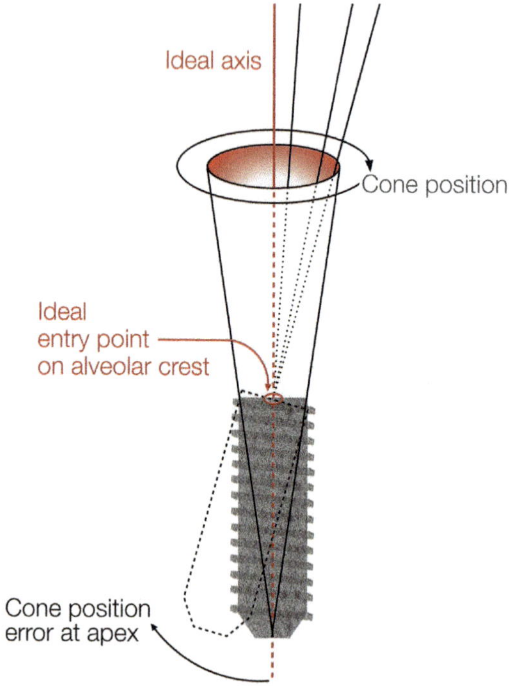

Fig. 1.22 The final axis is the *cone position*. This is to account for the rotational cone within which the surgeon is operating inside the guide or with the aid of navigation. Careful attention must be paid to this axis to ensure that the apical extent of the osteotomy/implant is properly positioned as well as having a significant effect on the exit of the screw channel within the prosthesis

References

1. Sgolastra F, Petrucci A, Severino M, et al. Periodontitis, implant loss and peri-implantitis. A meta-analysis. Clin Oral Implants Res. 2015;26(4):e8–16.
2. Levine RA, Nack G. Team treatment planning for the replacement of esthetic zone teeth with dental implants. Compendium. 2011;32(4):44–50.
3. Moy PK, Medina D, Shetty V, Aghaloo TL. Dental implant failure rates and associated risk factors. Int J Oral Maxillofac Implants. 2005;20:569–77.
4. Walia K, Belludi SA, Kulkarni P, Darak P, Swamy S. A comparative and a qualitative analysis of patient's motivations, expectations and satisfaction with dental implants. J Clin Diagn Res. 2016;10(4):ZC23.
5. Rustemeyer J, Bremerich A. Patients' knowledge and expectations regarding dental implants: assessment by questionnaire. Int J Oral Maxillofac Surg. 2007;36(9):814–7.
6. Yao J, Tang H, Gao XL, McGrath C, Mattheos N. Patients' expectations from dental implants: a systematic review of the literature. Health Qual Life Outcomes. 2014;12(1):153.
7. Pjetursson BE, Karoussis I, Bürgin W, Brägger U, Lang NP. Patients' satisfaction following implant therapy. Clin Oral Implants Res. 2005;16(2):185–93.
8. Kelly JR, Rungruanganunt P. Fatigue behavior of computer-aided design/computer-assisted manufacture ceramic abutments as a function of design and ceramics processing. Int J Oral Maxillofac Implants. 2016;31(3):601–9.

9. Al-Nsour MM, Chan HL, Wang HL. Effect of the platform-switching technique on preservation of peri-implant marginal bone: a systematic review. Int J Oral Maxillofac Implants. 2012;27(1):138–45.
10. Canullo L, Fedele GR, Iannello G, Jepsen S. Platform switching and marginal bone-level alterations: the results of a randomized-controlled trial. Clin Oral Implants Res. 2010;21(1):115–21.
11. Fickl S, Zuhr O, Stein JM, Hürzeler MB. Peri-implant bone level around implants with platform-switched abutments. Int J Oral Maxillofac Implants. 2010;25(3):577.
12. Lazzara RJ, Porter SS. Platform switching: a new concept in implant dentistry for controlling postrestorative crestal bone levels. Int J Perio Rest Dent. 2006;26:9–17.
13. Canullo L, Tallarico M, Chu S, Pennarocha D, Özcan M, Dent DM, Pesce P. Cleaning, disinfection, and sterilization protocols employed for customized implant abutments: an international survey of 100 universities worldwide. Int J Oral Maxillofac Implants. 2017;32(4):774–8.
14. Wadhwani CP, Schoenbaum T, King KE, Chung KH. Techniques to optimize color esthetics, bonding, and peri-implant tissue health with titanium implant abutments. Compendium. 2018;39(2):110–9.
15. Ferreira CF, Buttendorf AR, de Souza JG, Dalago H, Guenther SF, Bianchini MA. Prevalence of peri-implant diseases: analysis of associated factors. Eur J Prosthodont Restor Dent. 2015;23(4):199–206.
16. Goncalves Motta SH, Ferreira Camacho MP, Carvalho Quíntela D, Santana RB. Relationship between clinical and histologic periodontal biotypes in humans. Int J Periodontics Restorative Dent. 2017;37(5):737–41.

Radiographic Assessment for Implants in the Aesthetic Zone

2

Mohammed A. Husain and Sotirios Tetradis

Abstract

This chapter reviews the 2D and 3D imaging modalities available to the dental practitioner planning implants in the aesthetic zone while focusing on the unique advantages of cone-beam computed tomography (CBCT). An overview of the basic principles and technical parameters of CBCT technology is reviewed in order to offer guidelines for maximizing image quality. A systematic methodology for CBCT evaluation is then introduced to ensure comprehensive evaluation of the imaged volume while emphasizing the important anatomic considerations at the dental implant recipient site. The most common anatomic variants and osseous pathology encountered in the aesthetic zone are surveyed, with special regard to implications for dental implant therapy. Finally, in silico treatment planning and guided surgery are introduced as CBCT-based tools to enhance the likelihood of a successful surgical and prosthetic outcome.

2.1 Introduction

Radiography is an essential diagnostic tool in the pre- and postoperative assessment for implants in the aesthetic zone. Before the clinician proceeds with implant placement, information about the morphology, volume, and orientation of the alveolar ridge must be obtained. Additionally, the area must be evaluated for the proximity of vital structures, the presence of anatomic variants, and the absence of pathology. To this end, several imaging options are available to the clinician. These options include traditional plain-film radiography, such as periapical and panoramic

M. A. Husain (✉) · S. Tetradis
Section of Oral and Maxillofacial Radiology, UCLA School of Dentistry, Los Angeles, CA, USA
e-mail: mhusain@dentistry.ucla.edu; stetradis@dentistry.ucla.edu

Todd R. Schoenbaum (ed.), *Implants in the Aesthetic Zone*,
https://doi.org/10.1007/978-3-319-72601-4_2

radiographs, as well as advanced, cross-sectional, imaging modalities such as computed tomography (CT) and cone-beam computed tomography (CBCT). Each of these imaging modalities has strengths and limitations to be considered when prescribing appropriate imaging of the aesthetic zone. In many cases, combinations of plain-film and cross-sectional radiography are required for optimal assessment of the area of interest [1]. This chapter discusses common radiographic examinations, especially CBCT, for the preoperative planning and postoperative evaluation of implants in the aesthetic zone.

2.2 Periapical Radiographs

Periapical radiographs are a useful screening tool for the initial assessment of an edentulous site [2]. These radiographs are easy to acquire, deliver a low dose to the patient, and offer the highest resolution of any dental radiograph, higher even than 3D imaging modalities like CBCT [2, 3]. They provide a good overall assessment of the density and architecture of the alveolar bone at the edentulous site and depict adjacent teeth with exquisite detail (Fig. 2.1). Interpretation of these radiographs tends to be relatively straightforward, since the anatomy depicted is familiar to all dental practitioners. The relative absence of metallic artifacts on periapical radiographs makes them especially useful for intraoperative and postoperative implant evaluation.

Periapical radiographs, however, are limited in three key ways. The radiographs offer a small area of anatomic coverage, generally about the area of three teeth [4]. As a result, important vital structures outside the dentate area, such as the mandibular canal and sinus floor, may not be depicted. There is susceptibility to distortion (elongation or foreshortening) from changes in the angulation of the X-ray beam, thus limiting the reliability of linear measurements. This is especially pertinent for edentulous areas due to the difficulty in maintaining parallelism of the X-ray beam and detector in the absence of teeth [1]. Finally, periapical radiographs can at best be accurate 2D representations of the three-dimensional structures and therefore cannot offer diagnostic information regarding the buccolingual dimension of the alveolar ridge [5]. Additionally, the orientation of the alveolar ridge in 3D space and the possibility of buccal or lingual undercuts, for example, cannot be assessed.

2.3 Panoramic Radiographs

Panoramic radiography is among the most commonly used extraoral imaging modalities in dentistry and is useful in the initial diagnostic phase of implant planning. Probably the biggest strength of the panoramic radiograph is its broad area of anatomic coverage that includes both the maxilla and mandible in a single projectional image. The practitioner can relatively easily appreciate the relationship of the

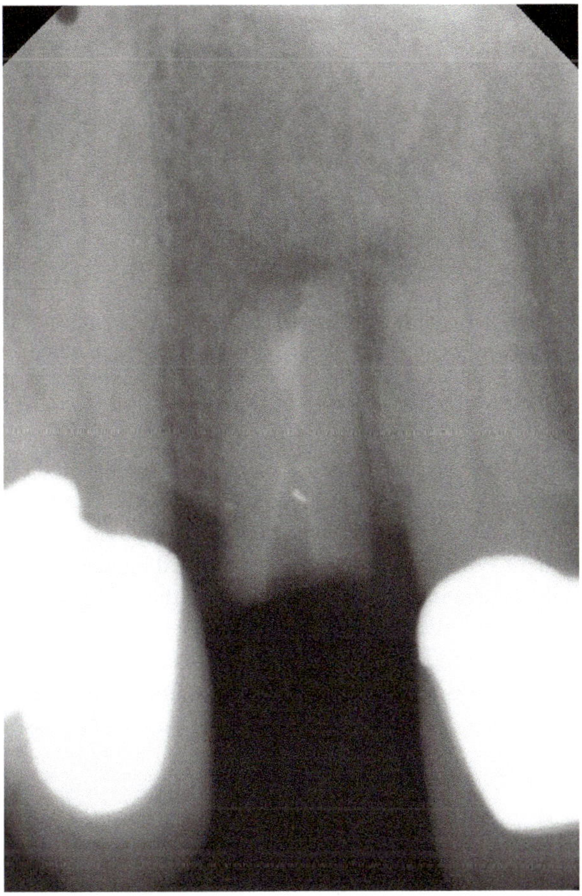

Fig. 2.1 Periapical radiograph at the area of the root tip of #7. The tooth demonstrates evidence of prior endodontic treatment and a widened apical PDL space. Note also the mild periodontal bone loss and generalized normal trabecular architecture

dental arches; the proximity of important anatomical structures such as the maxillary sinuses, nasopalatine, and mandibular canals; and the presence of pathology not readily apparent on intraoral radiographs. Additionally, the panoramic radiograph allows for quick assessment of maxillary sinus volume and the extent of pneumatization of the alveolar ridge. All of this information is obtained at a relatively low radiation dose to the patient.

There are a number of important limitations, however, of the panoramic radiograph. Most important perhaps is the variable magnification within the panoramic image that limits the accuracy and reliability of vertical and horizontal measurements [1, 2, 4, 6, 7]. Other limitations include the extent of anatomical superimposition that is present on the radiograph, and the limited resolution of the image. Like periapical radiographs, panoramic radiographs are 2D images in which buccolingual assessments of the alveolar ridge cannot be made. Unique to panoramic radiographs also is superimposition of a host of adjacent maxillofacial structures onto the dentoalveolar region. In the anterior maxilla, it is common to see superimposition of

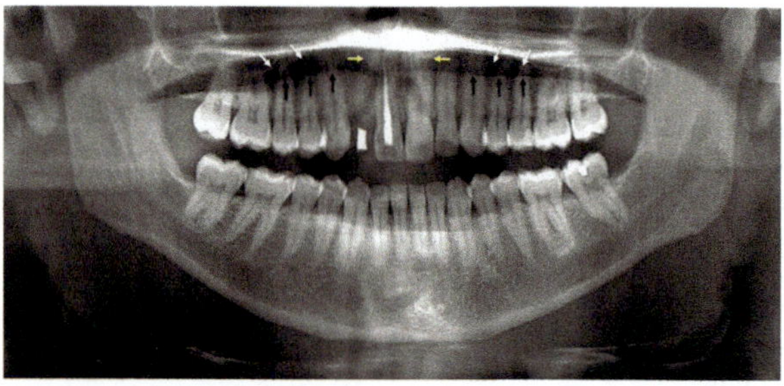

Fig. 2.2 Panoramic radiograph taken for the initial evaluation of the edentulous space at the site of missing tooth #7. Note the extent of superimposition of adjacent anatomic structures. Superimposition of the soft tissue of the nose (*colored arrows*), dorsum of the tongue (*black arrows*), and the oral airway space (*white arrows*) are indicated

the soft tissue of the nose, dorsum of the tongue, and upper cervical spine (Fig. 2.2). In some cases, the oral airway space is superimposed and may be observed as a broad radiolucent area over the roots of the maxillary teeth. This occurs when the patient's tongue is not raised to the hard palate during scanning acquisition. In the anterior mandible, superimposition of the cervical vertebrae can complicate assessment of the alveolar bone. An additional challenge during panoramic radiography is the narrow focal trough in the anterior region, since anatomic structures falling outside of it are distorted. These inherent limitations of panoramic radiography make it insufficient for comprehensive dental implant site assessment [1, 2].

2.4 Cross-Sectional Imaging

Cross-sectional imaging refers to those imaging modalities which produce multiple, thin, contiguous sectional images in axial, coronal, or sagittal planes (Fig. 2.3). Computed tomography (CT) and cone-beam computed tomography (CBCT) are examples of cross-sectional imaging modalities used to varying degrees in dentistry. The main advantages of cross-sectional imaging, and in particular CT imaging, are direct 3D visualization of anatomic structures free of superimposition and the reliability of linear measurements made from CT-generated cross sections [8]. These features allow for optimal assessment of the alveolar ridge for the purposes of implant planning [1]. It is for these reasons that cross-sectional imaging is recommended by the American Academy of Oral and Maxillofacial Radiology (AAOMR) prior to implant placement anywhere in the jaws, including the aesthetic zone [1]. Of the cross-sectional imaging modalities available, CBCT is generally acknowledged to be best adapted for dental imaging due to its relatively low radiation dose, high spatial resolution, and adjustable field of view (FOV) [9]. For a broad comparative evaluation of dental implant imaging modalities, see Table 2.1.

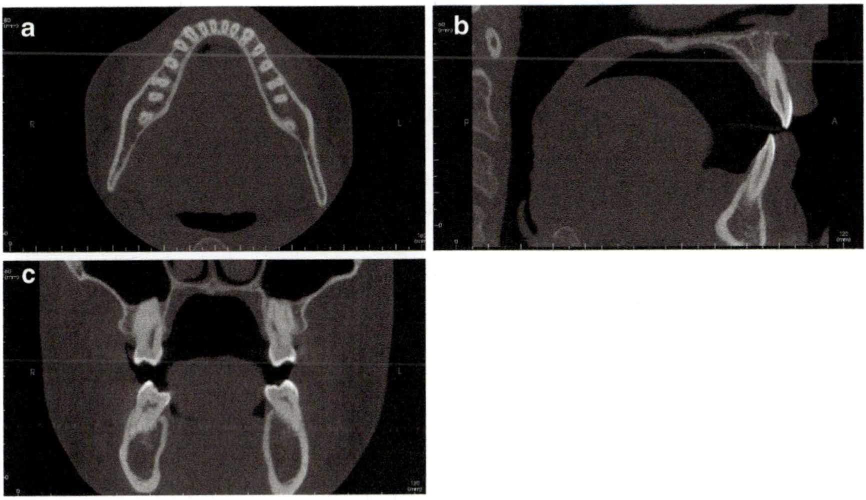

Fig. 2.3 Cone-beam computed tomography images in the multiplanar view (MPR), obtained using a medium field of view. (**a**) Axial view showing the mandibular arch. (**b**) Sagittal view showing the central incisors. (**c**) Coronal view in the area of the molar teeth

Table 2.1 Comparison of radiographic modalities for implant imaging

Imaging modality	Advantages	Disadvantages
Periapical radiography	High resolution, accessible, low radiation exposure, inexpensive	Limited anatomic coverage, 2D, susceptibility to distortion
Panoramic radiography	Broad anatomic coverage, low radiation exposure, inexpensive	2D representation of anatomy, unequal and unpredictable magnification, low resolution
Cone beam computed tomography	Accurate 3D representation of anatomy, reliable linear measurements, good resolution	Less accessible, expensive, higher radiation dose than 2D

2.5 Principles of CBCT Imaging

At their core, CBCT machines consist of an X-ray source and detector mounted on a rotating gantry. During the scanning acquisition process, the X-ray source and receptor rotate around the object of interest (patient's head, or a specific area of the dental arch), making a partial or full revolution (180–360° arc). The X-ray source emits a pulsatile cone-shaped beam of radiation toward the patient as it rotates. The beam is attenuated by the patient's tissues and is recorded by the detector. Given the pulsatile nature of the cone beam, what is recorded by the detector is in fact a series of 2D projectional images, known as basis images. A typical CBCT scan may expose approximately 300 basis images, each of which may be likened to an oblique skull projection obtained at a slightly different angulation [10]. After the scan has been completed, a reconstructive process ensues in which the raw data of these images are transformed using elaborate computer algorithms to create a three-dimensional map or volume of the region of interest (ROI) [11]. The volume created by this iterative reconstructive process can then be visualized in a variety of ways to assess the area of interest. Scrolling through individual slices in three orthogonal planes, the axial, coronal, and sagittal, is the simplest approach. Curved "panoramic" sections, cross sections, and multiple ways for 3D renderings offer a variety of options to optimally evaluate the various structures. This interaction and manipulation of the 3D volume is typically done in the manufacturer's proprietary viewing software or any other third-party DICOM viewing software.

2.6 CBCT Scanners

There are currently several CBCT scanners on the market manufactured by at least 20 companies [12]. The CBCT machines are distinguished primarily by fields of view (FOV) available, minimum voxel size (similar to a 3D pixel), and patient positioning. The fields of view available for the various CBCT machines vary widely, and although categorizations are made into small, medium, and large fields of view, there is considerable overlap among these three categories. It is generally understood that small FOV scans capture a portion of the dental arch (<8 cm), medium FOV scans capture both dentoalveolar arches in their entirety (8–15 cm), and large FOV scans (>15 cm) capture the maxillofacial structures in addition to the jaws [9]. Some CBCT machines offer a single fixed field of view, while others offer a limited or more expansive range. Those that offer a wider range are generally more expensive. For the purposes of implant planning, units that offer small and/or medium FOV are generally adequate.

Voxel size is another consideration when comparing CBCT units, since smaller voxel sizes contribute to higher resolution images. It is important to note that higher resolution does not necessarily mean a better image, since the small voxel size reduces the signal-to-noise ratio during scan acquisition. A method to improve signal-to-noise ratio is to increase the patient's exposure. While higher-resolution images are generally advantageous, implant planning is not a high-resolution task, so selecting a CBCT unit with the absolute lowest voxel size is not the most important factor.

Patient positioning in different CBCT units can vary significantly. Patients may be imaged standing, sitting, or supine. These variations have implications for handicap accessibility, which may be an important consideration in clinical practice.

2.7 Radiation Dose

Radiation doses from CBCT scans are typically a fraction of conventional MDCT scans, but higher than most 2D radiographic exams, such as lateral cephalometric radiographs, panoramic radiographs, and bitewing examinations [13]. The radiation dose from a CBCT exam can vary considerably, based on the field of view of the scan being acquired and on the specific CBCT unit being used. An approximate median value for a small FOV CBCT scan is approximately 47 microSieverts (μSv); a medium FOV CBCT scan, 98 μSv; and a large CBCT scan, 117 μSv. These values are well within the range of a full mouth set of intraoral radiographs, which deliver approximately 170 μSv of radiation [14]. For a list of effective doses from common radiographic examinations, see Table 2.2.

2.8 Protocol Optimization

Most CBCT units have a number of technical parameters that can be altered by the user. These include parameters related to X-ray exposure, FOV, and the number of basis projections. Optimizing these technical parameters is important to minimize patient radiation exposure and to maximize image quality (Table 2.3). The most important technical parameter that should be adjusted for each CBCT exam is the FOV. Small FOV CBCT scans, in general, yield higher-resolution images and deliver a lower radiation dose to the patient compared to larger FOV scans [9]. For this reason, smaller FOV scans should be preferred when they provide adequate anatomic coverage of the region of interest. For imaging in the aesthetic zone, small FOV (<8 cm) scans generally provide optimal anatomic coverage, although medium FOV scans may be used (8–15 cm) if visualization of both alveolar arches is desired.

X-ray exposure parameters may also be altered from patient to patient and relate to the X-ray tube voltage (kVp) and tube current (mA). Adjusting these parameters

Table 2.2 Effective radiation dose from common dental and medical radiographic exams[a]

Radiographic exam	Effective dose (uSv)	Equivalent days of background radiation
Panoramic	20	2
Full mouth series	177	21
Lateral cephalometric	5	1
CBCT (small FOV <8 cm)	47	6
CBCT (medium FOV 8–15 cm)	98	12
CBCT (large FOV >15 cm)	117	14
Chest X-rays (PA and lateral views)[b]	100	12
MDCT, maxillofacial w/o contrast	913	109
MDCT, abdomen[b]	8000	958

[a]Note: Adapted from Mallya, SM (2016) Principles of cone beam computed tomography. In: Fayad, M Johnson, B (eds) 3D Imaging in Endodontics. Springer

[b]Source*:* Mettler, F., et al. (2008) Effective doses in radiology and diagnostic nuclear medicine: a catalog. Radiology

Table 2.3 Three ways to optimize CBCT imaging protocol

1. Choose the smallest FOV appropriate for the imaging task
2. Adjust X-ray exposure parameters for children and large adults
3. Consider high-speed modes for patients prone to movement

is important given the variation in size and density of patients, particularly for pediatric patients who are most sensitive to the effects of ionizing radiation. However, not every CBCT unit allows for the user to alter these parameters. Most often, the parameters are indirectly altered by selecting preset pediatric, adult, or large adult settings prior to exposure.

Most CBCT units offer high-speed ("quick-scan") and high-res modes. Both modes operate by adjusting the number of basis projections obtained during scanning acquisition [9]. High-speed modes take fewer basis projections, while high-res modes take additional basis projections relative to the standard mode. Obtaining fewer basis projections, in high-speed mode, results in a faster scan, with a lower radiation dose but with inferior image quality. The opposite is true for a high-res scan. The additional basis projections result in a longer scan, with a higher radiation dose and superior image quality. High-speed mode should be considered for patients who are prone to movement and young children. High-res modes are generally unnecessary for implant imaging and further increase the probability of patient movement, often nullifying any gain in image quality.

2.9 CBCT Interpretation

The practitioner who has obtained the CBCT scan has the responsibility to review the entire imaged volume to confirm the presence or absence of disease [15]. Alternatively, the scan can be sent to an oral and maxillofacial radiologist for evaluation. Assessment of CBCT scans should follow a systematic approach to maximize the diagnostic yield from the radiographic examination and to ensure that abnormalities outside the immediate area of interest are not overlooked (Table 2.4). This is best accomplished by beginning the CBCT evaluation in the multiplanar (MPR) view. In this view, one will see cross-sectional images in three orthogonal planes: axial, coronal, and sagittal. The axial slices represent a series of transverse or horizontal sections through the imaged volume, the coronal a series of contiguous frontal sections, and the sagittal a series of lateral sections. It is best practice not to begin in the area of immediate interest, to reduce the likelihood of missing incidental pathology. Rather, one should begin at the superior edge of the imaged volume in the axial view and scroll to the inferior edge. Next, move through the sagittal slices from lateral edge to lateral edge, and finally in the coronal slices from the anterior

Table 2.4 Key steps in CBCT interpretation

1. Scroll through all axial, coronal, and sagittal slices
2. Note any abnormal findings, using natural anatomic symmetry as a guide
3. Observe suspected areas in all cross-sectional planes
4. Categorize finding as anatomic variant, physiologic calcification, or potential pathology
5. Determine whether finding will require follow-up, and if so, with radiographs, referral, or biopsy
6. Document
7. Proceed to area of immediate clinical interest

end of the volume to the posterior. While scrolling through the volume, a good understanding of the anatomy of the imaged field is necessary to detect abnormalities. Nonetheless, the natural anatomic symmetry of the patient, in many instances, can be used as a guide for this purpose. When an abnormality is identified, it should be viewed in all three planes to best assess its radiographic features. Additional reconstructions could be made to further visualize the area. After thorough visualization of the abnormal area has been performed, the abnormality should be categorized as an anatomic variant, clinically insignificant finding, or potential pathology. Suspected pathologic findings should be documented, differentially diagnosed, and addressed by radiographic follow-up, referral, and/or biopsy. If questions regarding the proper interpretation of the CBCT scan arise, referral to an oral and maxillofacial radiologist should be considered. After reviewing the entire volume, it is then appropriate to focus on the area of immediate interest.

The 3D volume rendering view is an attractive feature of CBCT imaging, sometimes present on the multiplanar view or elsewhere within the viewing software. Caution should be exercised when making diagnostic conclusions from the 3D rendering, since the rendering depicted is generated from an alterable thresholding function. All diagnoses should be based on the planar CBCT cross sections. The 3D views can be used as adjunctive radiographic evidence and are most useful for a broad evaluation of the patient's anatomy. Asymmetries, fractures, and growth alterations of the maxillofacial bones are more easily visualized on the 3D rendering.

2.10 Normal Anatomy of the Aesthetic Zone

Small FOV CBCT scans of the aesthetic zone will generally encompass the alveolar bone in the anterior maxilla and mandible, as well as a portion of the nasal cavity and maxillary sinuses. The alveolar bone in in these areas should demonstrate intact cortices of regular thickness. The trabecular bone should be lacy and relatively uniform in density. The primary vital structure in the anterior maxilla that can influence implant placement is the nasopalatine canal. This canal should be relatively symmetric in shape and houses the nasopalatine nerve, which exits the incisive foramen and supplies the mucosa of the anterior hard palate. In the anterior mandible, the lingual foramen and lingual canal are frequently observed and represent terminal branches of the lingual artery entering the anterior mandible. The diameter of the lingual canal should be noted, as it is a reflection of the blood-carrying capacity of the vessel and, if wide enough, may result in significant bleeding if violated during surgery [16].

Within the area of the nasal cavity and maxillary sinuses, dark airway spaces should be observed. These air spaces can vary significantly between right and left sides, as an anatomic variant. The nasal turbinates will be seen at the inferior aspect of the nasal cavity as soft-tissue density structures and may present quite asymmetrically. This is a normal finding and represents the physiologic process of nasal cycling.

2.11 Five Common Anatomic Variants in the Aesthetic Zone

One of the most common anatomic variants noted in the jaws, which also presents in the aesthetic zone, are areas of idiopathic osteosclerosis (Fig. 2.4a). The prevalence of this finding in the maxilla and mandible is approximately 6%, although there are reports of frequencies as high as 30% [17]. Areas of idiopathic osteosclerosis represent sites of high bone density and present on radiographs as localized, relatively uniform radiopacities and are incidentally detected. Unless extensive, the finding of osteosclerosis would not adversely affect implant placement. However, a resistance to drilling might be expected if the implant is placed through one of these areas due to increased bone density.

Variations in alveolar morphology are a frequent and important anatomic variation for treatment planning of implants in the aesthetic zone. The morphology and volume of the alveolar ridge can vary dramatically among patients. In particular, the

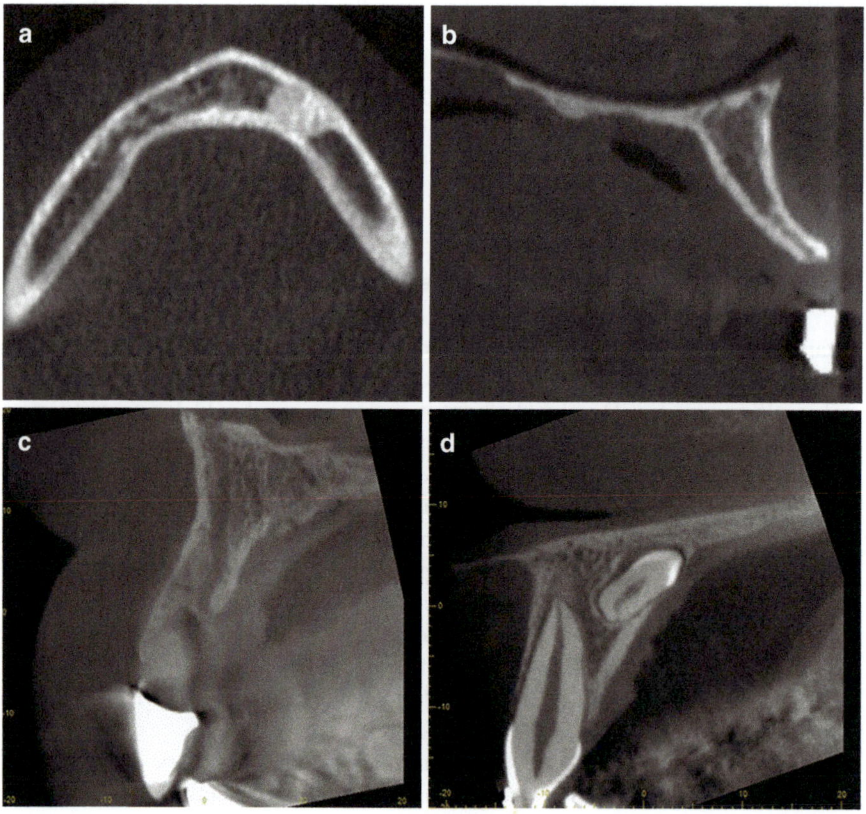

Fig. 2.4 CBCT images of common anatomic variants in the aesthetic zone. (**a**) Osteosclerosis of the left mandible at the canine area. (**b**) A marked buccal concavity at the area of missing tooth #7. (**c**) The canalis sinuosus running through the alveolus palatal tooth #9. (**d**) A mesiodens engaging the hard palate palatal to tooth #8

presence and depth of the buccal undercut, and the angulation of the alveolar ridge, can limit or alter the treatment approach (Fig. 2.4b). In the fully dentate maxillary arch, the buccal undercut tends to be most severe in the area of the maxillary lateral incisors [18]. This is an important anatomic variation to consider to avoid perforation of the buccal cortex, and an unacceptable aesthetic result. Moderate to severe defects of the alveolar ridge are to be expected with previous loss of teeth, previous loss of implants, severe periodontal disease, or trauma. A history of orthodontic treatment has the potential to adversely or positively affect the alveolar dimensions as well.

A neurovascular anatomic variation commonly seen in the aesthetic zone of the maxilla is the canalis sinuosus. This neurovascular canal contains accessory branches of the anterior superior alveolar nerve and artery. On radiographs, it is typically seen originating from the lateral aspect of the nasal fossa, coursing inferiorly through the alveolar ridge palatal to the maxillary lateral incisor and canine (Fig. 2.4c). Presence of canalis sinuosus should be noted during treatment planning, due to the likelihood of increased intraoperative bleeding upon canal violation [19].

Hyperdontia, or the presence of supernumerary teeth, is a relatively common finding in the jaws. Among supernumerary teeth, the mesiodens is most likely to occur in the anterior maxilla. The overall prevalence of the mesiodens is 0.15–1.9% [20]. These teeth are typically microdontic, commonly inverted, and located at the maxillary midline palatal to the roots of the central incisors (Fig. 2.4d). They may interfere with implant placement and are associated with benign pathological conditions, such as dentigerous cysts. Thus, their assessment prior to implant placement is important and may alter the selection and location of implants.

In the anterior mandible, one of the most important anatomic variations to consider during treatment planning is the anterior loop of the mandibular canal. Merely positioning the implant osteotomy site mesial to the mental foramen is not sufficient to avoid mandibular nerve damage during surgery. This is because the mandibular canal commonly courses in an anterior loop before exiting through the mental foramen. The length of the anterior loop is on average 2 mm but can reach lengths of 6 mm or more [21]. The exact location and shape of the anterior loop should be noted prior to surgery in the area.

2.12 Five Common Pathologies in the Aesthetic Zone

Excluding dental caries and periodontal disease, the most common osseous pathology of the jaws is apical periodontitis. Radiographically, this presents as a loss of bone density at the apex of a tooth (PARL) in response to pulpal infection and necrosis. These lesions, while they are small in size, may histologically represent a periapical granuloma or radicular cyst. However, larger lesions of over 1 cm in diameter, demonstrating corticated borders, are more likely to be radicular cysts [22]. Radicular cysts are the most common cystic lesions of the jaws and most frequently located in the anterior maxilla in association with the lateral incisor or

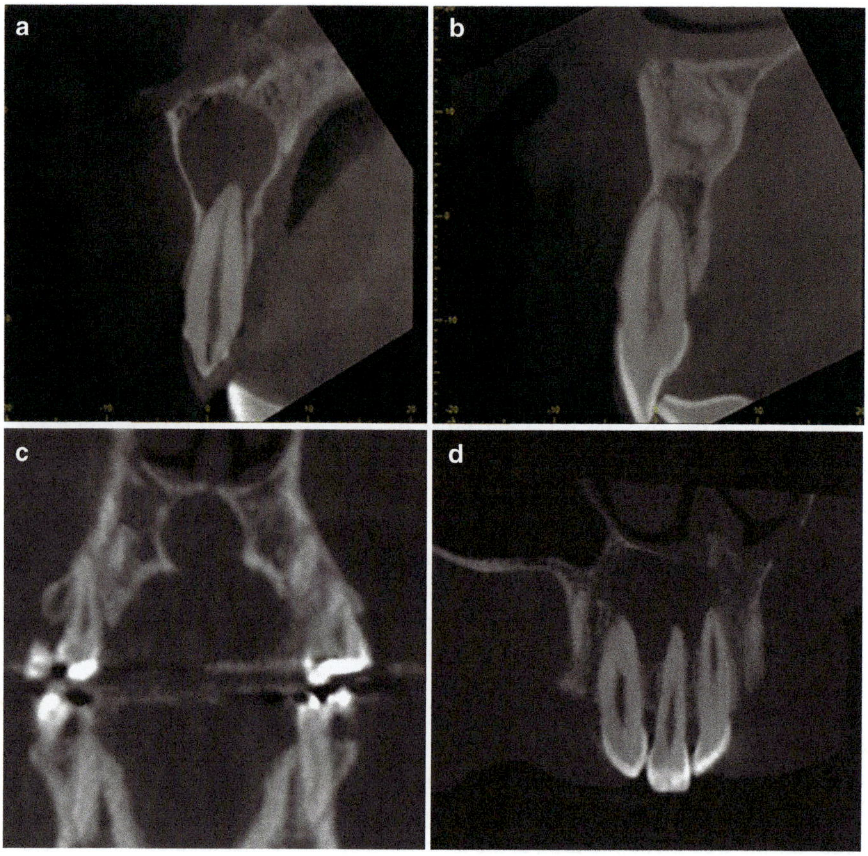

Fig. 2.5 CBCT images of pathologies involving the aesthetic zone. (**a**) Radicular cyst associated with the apex of tooth #7. (**b**) Mixed density periapical cemento-osseous dysplasia superior to the apex of tooth #9. (**c**) Nasopalatine canal duct cyst causing marked expansion of the nasopalatine canal. (**d**) Keratocystic odontogenic tumor scalloping around the apices of teeth #6–8

canine (Fig. 2.5a). Like other benign cysts, they may cause tooth displacement, root resorption, and cortical expansion. Treatment of the radicular cyst typically entails some combination of endodontic therapy, apical surgery, or extraction.

Periapical cemento-osseous dysplasia (PCD) represents the most common dysplasia of the jaws, characterized by a localized change of normal bone architecture. In localized areas, the normal trabecular bone is replaced by a disorganized mixture of fibrous tissue and cementum. This presents radiographically as mixed density areas in close association with the apices of teeth. Most commonly PCD occurs in association with the mandibular incisors, although it can also occur in the anterior maxilla (Fig. 2.5b). Lesions tend to undergo a maturation process over time, from mostly radiolucent to mostly radiopaque. The diagnosis of this entity is radiographically established, and no specific treatment is necessary. From the point of view of dental implants, areas of the jaws affected by PCD have reduced vascularity and therefore thought to have greater susceptibility to infection [23].

The odontoma is a benign, tumor-like malformation, characterized by the production of mature dental tissues: enamel, dentin, and pulp. The odontoma may present as a well-organized bundle of malformed denticles within a soft-tissue capsule (compound odontoma) or, alternatively, as a disorganized mass of dental tissues (complex odontoma.) The compound odontoma most frequently occurs in the anterior maxilla and may cause impaction or malpositioning of the adjacent teeth. The lesions develop during the growth phase, are self-limiting in size, are asymptomatic, and are treated by simple excision [24]. Removal of the odontoma and augmentation prior to implant placement is advised.

The nasopalatine canal duct cyst is a common cystic lesion occurring exclusively in the anterior maxilla and accounts for approximately 10% of the cysts of the jaws [25]. Embryonic epithelial remnants within the nasopalatine canal duct undergo proliferation and cystic degeneration to form the nasopalatine canal cyst. Lesions are very slow-growing and present radiographically as a round- or oval shaped expansile lesion within the nasopalatine canal (Fig. 2.5c). The lesion may cause tooth displacement or resorption of the maxillary incisors. Patients are typically asymptomatic, although swelling of the anterior hard palate and/or drainage of cystic fluid may occur. If a large incisive canal is seen during radiographic assessment of the anterior maxilla, radiographic follow-up is usually recommended to detect interval growth within the nasopalatine canal, thereby establishing the diagnosis. However, if a definite hydraulic enlargement of the canal, frequently asymmetric, is observed, excisional biopsy of the lesion is recommended.

Benign neoplasms may occur in the aesthetic zone of the maxilla and mandible, though they are most frequent in the posterior mandible. The two most common benign neoplasms of the jaws are the keratocystic odontogenic tumor (KOT) and ameloblastoma. Radiographically, both are corticated, scalloping, radiolucent lesions that can cause significant expansion, tooth displacement, and resorption (Fig. 2.5d). These lesions are distinguished from most other odontogenic cysts of the jaws, by not having an epicenter associated with the crown or apex of a tooth. Incisional or excisional biopsy of suspected neoplastic lesions is recommended. Treatment can range from enucleation to resection of the jaws.

2.13 Radiographic Assessment of the Recipient Site

While the initial pathology review of the CBCT study should be done in the multiplanar (MPR) view, the evaluation of the recipient site is better accomplished on reformatted alveolar cross sections through the area of interest. Most CBCT software has a designated tab or module for the purpose of preoperative implant evaluation (Fig. 2.6). This tab typically consists of a "panoramic" reconstruction, an axial scout slice, and a series of alveolar cross sections. The "panoramic" reconstruction depicted will be derived from an alterable focal trough that is usually depicted on the axial slice. One should ensure that the focal trough follows the maxillary and/or mandibular curvature, in order for the individual cross sections to be perpendicular to the alveolus. This will ensure that the 2D measurements made on the individual

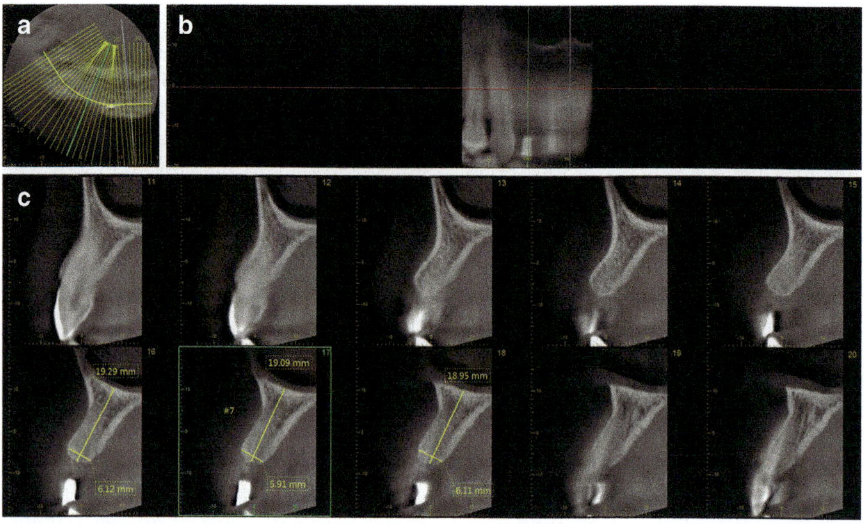

Fig. 2.6 Reformatted CBCT images for implant planning. (**a**) Axial view depicting the focal trough through the maxillary ridge and locations of the orthogonal alveolar cross sections. (**b**) Panoramic reconstruction of the anterior maxilla. (**c**) Alveolar cross sections through the area of teeth #6–8, displaying measurement at the sites of missing tooth #7

cross sections truly reflect intended anatomic assessment. Frequently, a series of lines will be observed perpendicular to the focal trough, designating the locations of the alveolar cross sections. A marking or series of markings may also be seen on the panoramic reconstruction correlating the origin of a selected alveolar cross section to a site on the maxilla or mandible. Users have the option to vary the interval and thickness between successive alveolar cross sections. The interval should be adjusted such that cross sections are visualized through the entire area of interest. Increasing the thickness of the individual slices is a useful strategy to mitigate noise on an image and can allow for better visualization of the mandibular canal. However, the thickness of the slices should generally not exceed 2 mm; otherwise the accuracy of the measurements may be compromised.

One of the primary goals of preoperative implant imaging is a quantitative evaluation of alveolar bone volume in order to choose an appropriately sized implant. Implant selection should maintain adequate space between adjacent implants (3–4 mm), teeth (1.5–2 mm), and buccal and palatal cortical margins (>1 mm) to prevent peri-implant bone loss and cortical dehiscence [26, 27]. When measuring the maxillary alveolus, measurements should extend from the alveolar crest to the base of the alveolus, in the absence of vital structures. Mandibular alveolar measurements begin from the alveolar crest and extend to the superior cortical border of the mandibular canal. The alveolar measurements should be made on successive interval cross sections through the edentulous area. In order to properly orient the alveolar measurements to the position of the final prosthesis, it is imperative that the patient wear a radiographic guide during the CBCT scan. Radiographic guides are typically made of acrylic and formed from diagnostic casts of pre-prosthetic wax-ups at the proposed implant sites. The guide should indicate the proposed angulation of the implant through the crown and the external contours of the crown. The former is important in determining available bone volume at the proposed angulation. The crown contours (in particular the gingival margin of the prosthesis) are critical in determining the ideal depth of the proposed implant. The angulation should be noted with a highly radiopaque material (i.e., barium mixed into composite) placed into the tooth at the proposed implant angulation. The external contours of the tooth can be noted with lead foil applied to the facial surface of the guide. Use of the radiographic guide aids in the localization of linear and angular measurements, increasing precision and alignment of the alveolar ridge with the position of the final prosthesis. The radiographic guide is then converted to a surgical template to guide the osteotomy.

Quantitative measurements of the alveolar bone at the recipient site help to characterize the type and extent of alveolar deficiency. This will guide the decision-making process regarding the necessity and type of bone augmentation procedure required for successful implant placement. Cases with significant alveolar defects will require ridge augmentation as discussed in Part II of this text. When performing ridge augmentation in a delayed approach, additional CBCT imaging after ridge augmentation but prior to implant placement allows the clinician to evaluate the success of the augmentation. The clinician can measure the improved dimensions of the alveolar ridge and confirm successful osseointegration of grafting material (Fig. 2.7). Radiographically, the grafting material should appear to blend in with the adjacent bone, although some types of material may retain a density higher than native bone. If the grafting material is disconnected from the surrounding alveolar bone, failure of integration should be expected. Obtaining this information prior to the implant surgery minimizes intraoperative surprises.

Radiographic evaluation of the recipient site should not simply be limited to measurements of alveolar volume. Several other factors play an important role in predicting the likelihood of a successful outcome. This is especially the case in the presence of an existing tooth. The thickness of the labial cortex adjacent to an existing tooth should be visualized and measured on the CBCT volume, as it is an important prognostic factor of the extent of vertical bone loss and remodeling after extraction. Teeth that are facially positioned in the maxillary alveolus tend to have thin or nonexistent labial cortices (Fig. 2.8) and undergo significantly more vertical and horizontal bone loss upon extraction. For such cases, two-stage implant placement and/or ridge augmentation prior to implant placement should be considered [27]. Dental pathology associated with existing teeth should also be closely assessed on CBCT for its tendency to compromise the adjacent labial cortex. Periapical lesions or periradicular bone loss around the roots of teeth commonly extend to and perforate the labial cortex (Fig. 2.9), increasing the likelihood of vertical bone loss and collapse of gingival architecture upon extraction.

The proximity of adjacent teeth and their levels of bony attachment are important considerations in the predictability of a favorable aesthetic outcome. Both of these features should be closely evaluated on the CBCT volume. Malpositioned adjacent

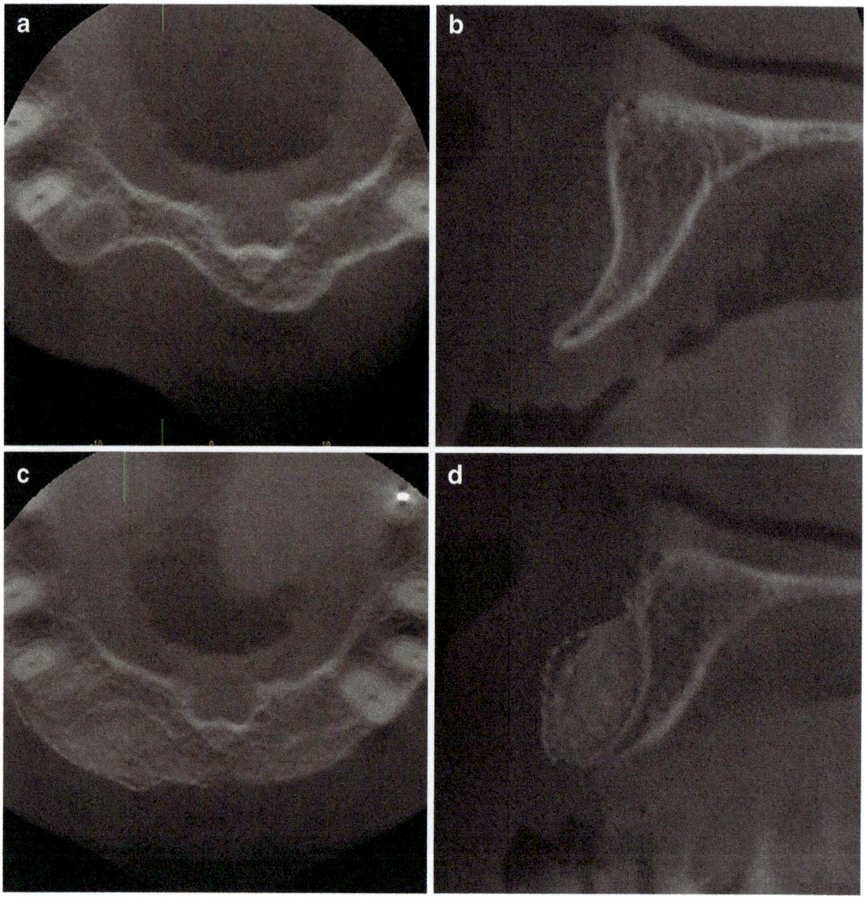

Fig. 2.7 CBCT images pre- and post-lateral ridge augmentation. (**a**, **b**) Axial and sagittal images showing horizontal alveolar deficiency due to a pronounced buccal undercut in the lateral incisor area. (**c**, **d**) Axial and sagittal images after ridge augmentation showing well-adapted grafting material at the buccal aspect of the alveolar ridge supported by a non-resorbable membrane

teeth or teeth with dilacerated roots extending into the edentulous area can compromise ideal implant positioning. In the event that an implant is positioned in close proximity to adjacent roots, there is an increased risk of a lateral resorption and peri-implant bone loss [26, 27]. In such cases, orthodontic repositioning of the malpositioned roots [27], selection of tapered/shortened implants, or alternative implant sites should be considered. Coronal and sagittal cross-sectional CBCT images of the adjacent teeth should also be reconstructed to assess their level of bony attachment (Fig. 2.10). This is because the presence or absence of peri-implant papillae, a critical factor in a successful aesthetic outcome, is directly related to the interproximal bone height of the adjacent teeth [26, 28].

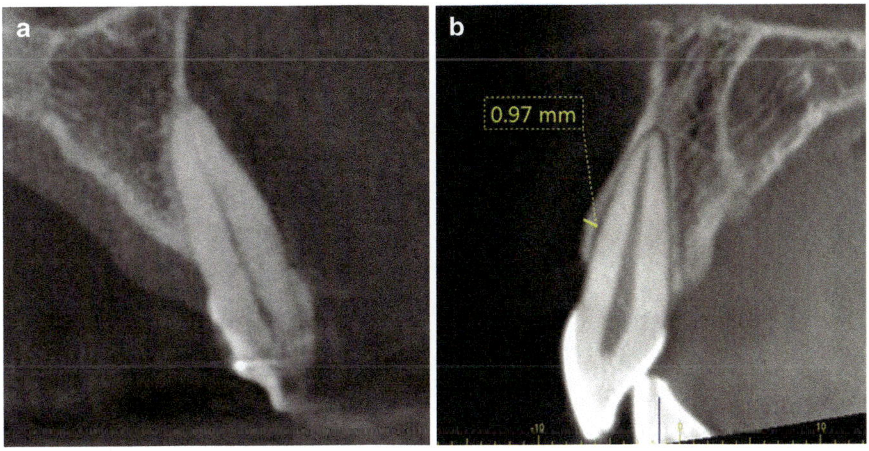

Fig. 2.8 Cross-sectional CBCT images showing marked variation in labial cortical thickness. (**a**) A likely dehiscent labial cortex along the root of tooth #7. (**b**) A thicker labial cortex along the root of tooth #9 measuring approximately 1 mm in the cervical area

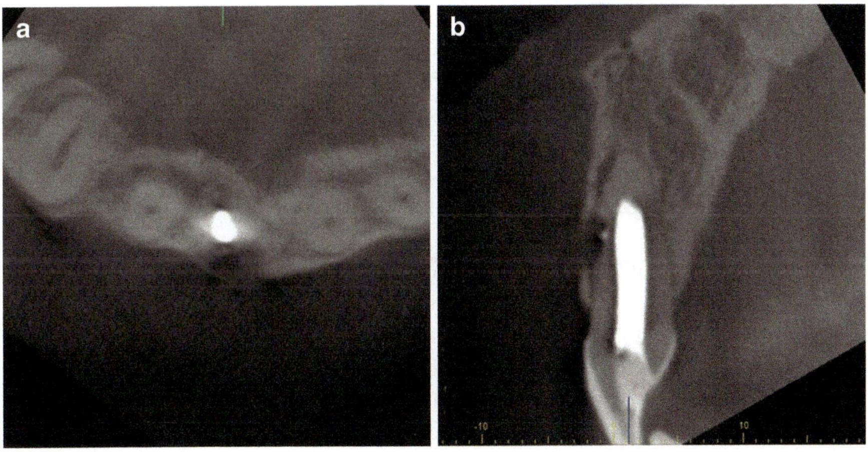

Fig. 2.9 CBCT images depicting external resorption and periradicular bone loss associated with tooth #8 causing a labial cortical defect. (**a**) Axial view and (**b**) cross-sectional view

The quality of trabecular bone at the proposed implant sites should be evaluated on the CBCT volume. At present, this entails a subjective visual evaluation of bone density. For most patients this will be in the average to good range, which indicates a likelihood of successful osseointegration [13]. In some cases, areas of significant trabecular porosity may be visualized, and the absence of a distinct cortication of the mandibular canal. These findings may alter the clinician's treatment approach, especially to avoid potential damage to the mandibular nerve. Quantitative means of

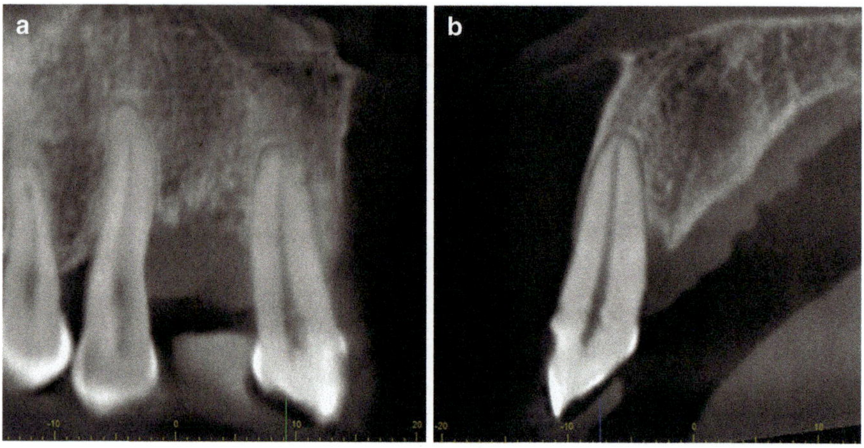

Fig. 2.10 CBCT images of teeth adjacent to the edentulous site of #7 demonstrating marked loss of bony attachment. (**a**) Oblique coronal view and (**b**) cross-sectional view of tooth #8

assessing alveolar bone density, using Hounsfield units, have been explored [29]. In principle, this method seeks to correlate gray values from the CBCT images to relative bone density. However, the variable influence of factors other than object density on the depiction of gray value [9] renders this approach unreliable with dental CBCT units. This is particularly true for small FOV scans [30, 31].

2.14 Virtual Implant Placement

An added advantage of CBCT imaging for preoperative implant planning is the ability to simulate implant placement in silico. Within most CBCT software, the clinician has the ability to select an implant; specify its manufacturer, design, and dimensions; and virtually place it at the desired location in the CBCT volume. The user can manipulate the location of the implant in all three dimensions (M-D, B-L, and S-I), as well as its orientation in space. The implant can be visualized in a 3D rendering view, in addition to standard axial, coronal, and sagittal cross sections. Seeing the implant directly on the reconstructed CBCT volume in full dimensions more easily reveals areas of bone deficiency, as well as the spatial relationships of the implant to the proposed prosthesis and adjacent anatomic structures (Fig. 2.11). This is a useful exercise to confirm the adequacy of the alveolar bone for the proposed implant or can help in determining the need/type of bone grafting, custom abutments, or other alterations to the surgical/restorative plan.

Third-party CBCT software generally have more sophisticated modules for implant simulation. These software are designed to enable the clinician to perform guided implant surgery by faithfully translating an in silico surgical plan to the

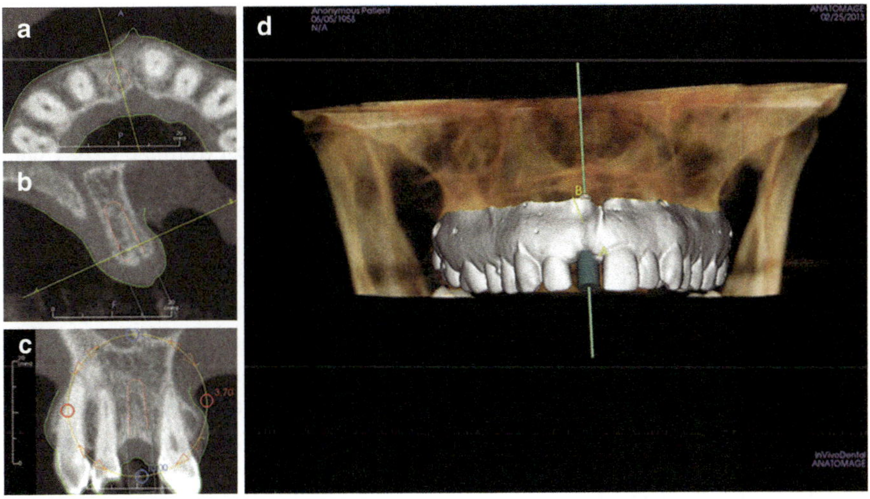

Fig. 2.11 In silico implant placement at the area of missing tooth #8. (**a**–**c**) Axial, sagittal, and cross-sectional views showing the outline of the implant superimposed on the alveolar ridge. (**d**) 3D view showing the orientation of virtual implant #8 relative to the adjacent teeth and maxillofacial structures. Note the fusion of optical scan data with the CBCT volume. (Images courtesy of *Anatomage, Inc.*)

patient via the use of a custom-fabricated surgical template. In order to use such software, one must first export the patient's CBCT data into DICOM format. Every manufacturer's proprietary software has a slightly different method of doing this. DICOM is a universal file format and is the standard for transmitting imaging data in medicine and dentistry. It is distinguished from other file formats in the way that patient identifiers are embedded into the imaging data. Once exported, the DICOM data can then be uploaded into a variety of third-party 3D imaging software for virtual treatment planning.

Guided implant surgery offers the possibility of greater precision and predictability in translating the in silico surgical plan to the patient. In order to successfully create a custom surgical template, additional information regarding the teeth and the mucosa are required. This information can be obtained from an optical scan of a diagnostic cast or directly of the patient. The data from the optical scan is fused with the CBCT volume, which then more precisely depicts the mucosa and contours of teeth, otherwise obscured by artifact. This is an important step because the custom surgical template needs to fit snugly around the teeth and mucosa in order to be effective. Once the virtual treatment plan has been completed, the surgical plan is exported and serves as the basis for the fabrication of the custom surgical template. The guided surgical template is shaped like an orthodontic splint and contains metal sleeves at the proposed implant sites. These sleeves guide the drilling and direction of the implant fixture into the preplanned location and orientation.

2.15 3D Modeling

Dimensionally accurate stereolithographic anatomical models of the mandible or maxilla can be produced from cross-sectional imaging data, including from CBCT scans. This is done by segmenting the bony surfaces of interest from the CBCT data set into a digital 3D surface rendering. The rendering is exported as an STL file printable by a 3D printer. The anatomical models allow for an accurate reproduction of the patient's anatomy, including the course of the mandibular canal, into an object that can be held and directly observed by both clinician and patient (Fig. 2.12). This hands-on inspection of the printed edentulous alveolus can offer a deeper appreciation of the patient's anatomy in challenging cases. For such complex cases, the model can also offer the clinician an opportunity to perform a mock surgery or fabricate custom graft scaffolds prior to actual implant placement. Additionally, patient communication can be facilitated using such a model, in regard to the nature of the implant procedure, the unique challenges presented by the patient's anatomy, and the goals of treatment.

2.16 Intraoperative and Postoperative Assessment

Intraoperative imaging may be utilized to verify proper implant angulation and placement. There also may be a need to visualize the proximity of important anatomic structures. For these purposes, periapical radiographs are preferred, due to their high resolution, ease of acquisition, and low radiation dose. Digital radiographs are particularly advantageous for this purpose due to their near instantaneous display.

Postoperatively, periapical radiographs are the preferred choice for assessment of implant position, peri-implant bone levels, and degree of osseointegration. In asymptomatic patients, a cone-beam CT is generally not required for evaluating

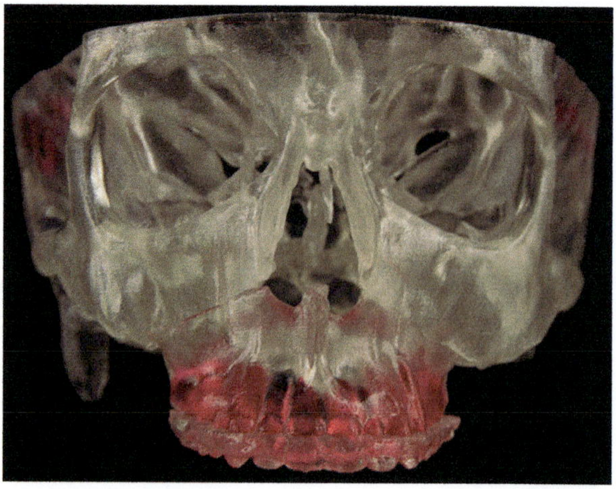

Fig. 2.12 Frontal view of a translucent stereolithographic anatomical model of the maxilla. Note the red coloration of the crowns and roots of the dentition. (Image courtesy of *3D Systems*)

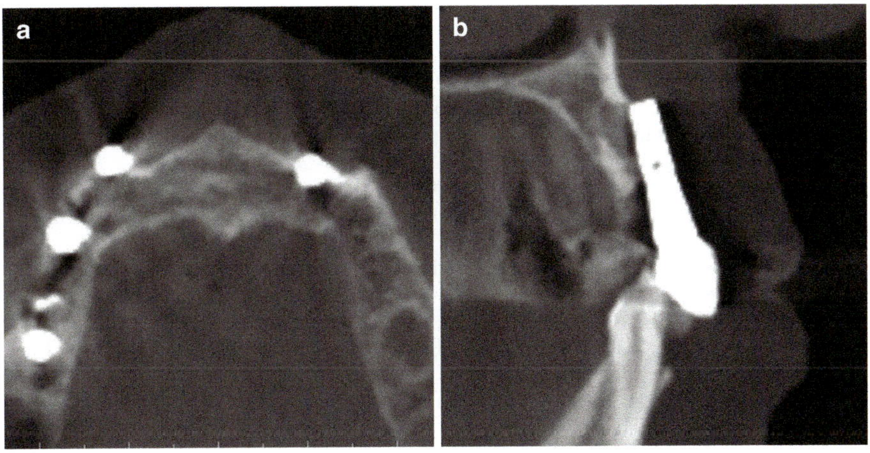

Fig. 2.13 Buccally positioned implants #7 and 10 on CBCT imaging. (**a**) Axial view showing loss of the labial cortex adjacent to both implants. (**b**) Cross-sectional view of implant #7 showing marked buccal positioning and complete dehiscence of the labial cortex

dental implants, due to the pervasiveness of artifacts which obscure peri-implant bone [1]. Of note, radiographic artifacts related to the implant tend to be most evident mesial and distal to the implant fixture. Assessment of the buccal and lingual bone adjacent to the implant is generally more reliable. Atypical loss of peri-implant bone and indistinct osseous contact along the implant are radiographic signs suggestive of failed osseointegration or peri-implantitis.

In cases of postsurgical implant complications, CBCT is an invaluable tool and tends to add important diagnostic information not seen on 2D radiographs. For patients reporting altered sensation postsurgically, CBCT can establish whether an implant is impinging on a neurovascular canal, an important determinant in the decision regarding implant removal. For implants demonstrating immediate postoperative mobility, cone-beam CT imaging can provide information regarding the implant position and, importantly, whether perforation of the cortical plates has occurred (Fig. 2.13) [13].

Conclusion

Radiography is an indispensable diagnostic tool for successful implant planning and treatment. Selecting the appropriate radiographic modality at different stages in the therapeutic process will maximize the diagnostic yield while minimizing radiation dose. CBCT is unique as a dental imaging modality for its ability to offer direct 3D visualization of patient anatomy and precise linear measurements of the recipient site. A disciplined approach to CBCT interpretation and an understanding of normal anatomy are essential to maximizing the diagnostic yield from these radiographs. Virtual implant simulation tools are also available within most CBCT software to allow for a more predictable surgical and prosthetic outcome.

References

1. Tyndall DA, Price JB, Tetradis S, Ganz SD, Hildebolt C, Scarfe WC. Position statement of the American Academy of Oral and Maxillofacial Radiology on selection criteria for the use of radiology in dental implantology with emphasis on cone beam computed tomography. Oral Surg Oral Med Oral Pathol Oral Radiol. 2012;113(6):817–26.
2. Mupparapu M, Singer SR. Implant imaging for the dentist. J Can Dent Assoc. 2004;70(1):32.
3. Nair MK, Nair UP. Digital and advanced imaging in endodontics: a review. J Endod. 2007;33(1):1–6.
4. Chan HL, Misch K, Wang HL. Dental imaging in implant treatment planning. Implant Dent. 2010;19(4):288–98.
5. Benavides E, Rios HF, Ganz SD, et al. Use of cone beam computed tomography in implant dentistry: the International Congress of Oral Implantologists consensus report. Implant Dent. 2012;21(2):78–86.
6. Guerrero ME, Noriega J, Castro C, Jacobs R. Does cone-beam CT alter treatment plans? Comparison of preoperative implant planning using panoramic versus cone-beam CT images. Imaging Sci Dent. 2014;44(2):121–8.
7. Yim JH, Ryu DM, Lee BS, Kwon YD. Analysis of digitalized panorama and cone beam computed tomographic image distortion for the diagnosis of dental implant surgery. J Craniofac Surg. 2011;22(2):669–73.
8. Suomalainen A, Vehmas T, Kortesniemi M, Robinson S, Peltola J. Accuracy of linear measurements using dental cone beam and conventional multislice computed tomography. Dentomaxillofac Radiol. 2008;37(1):10–7.
9. Mallya SM. Evidence and professional guidelines for appropriate use of cone beam computed tomography. J Calif Dent Assoc. 2015;43(9):512–20.
10. Scarfe WC, Farman AG. What is cone-beam CT and how does it work? Dent Clin N Am. 2008;52(4):707–730, v.
11. De Vos W, Casselman J, Swennen GR. Cone-beam computerized tomography (CBCT) imaging of the oral and maxillofacial region: a systematic review of the literature. Int J Oral Maxillofac Surg. 2009;38(6):609–25.
12. Nemtoi A, Czink C, Haba D, Gahleitner A. Cone beam CT: a current overview of devices. Dentomaxillofac Radiol. 2013;42(8):20120443.
13. Klokkevold PR. Cone beam computed tomography for the dental implant patient. J Calif Dent Assoc. 2015;43(9):521–30.
14. Mallya SM. Principles of cone beam computed tomography. 3D imaging in endodontics. Berlin: Springer; 2016. p. 1–14.
15. Carter L, Farman AG, Geist J, et al. American Academy of Oral and Maxillofacial Radiology executive opinion statement on performing and interpreting diagnostic cone beam computed tomography. Oral Surg Oral Med Oral Pathol Oral Radiol Endod. 2008;106(4):561–2.
16. Loukas M, Kinsella CR Jr, Kapos T, Tubbs RS, Ramachandra S. Anatomical variation in arterial supply of the mandible with special regard to implant placement. Int J Oral Maxillofac Surg. 2008;37(4):367–71.
17. Yonetsu K, Yuasa K, Kanda S. Idiopathic osteosclerosis of the jaws: panoramic radiographic and computed tomographic findings. Oral Surg Oral Med Oral Pathol Oral Radiol Endod. 1997;83(4):517–21.
18. Zhang W, Skrypczak A, Weltman R. Anterior maxilla alveolar ridge dimension and morphology measurement by cone beam computerized tomography (CBCT) for immediate implant treatment planning. BMC Oral Health. 2015;15:65.
19. Oliveira-Santos C, Rubira-Bullen IR, Monteiro SA, León JE, Jacobs R. Neurovascular anatomical variations in the anterior palate observed on CBCT images. Clin Oral Implants Res. 2013;24(9):1044–8.
20. Russell KA, Folwarczna MA. Mesiodens-diagnosis and management of a common supernumerary tooth. J Can Dent Assoc. 2003;69(6):362–7.

21. Uchida Y, Noguchi N, Goto M, et al. Measurement of anterior loop length for the mandibular canal and diameter of the mandibular incisive canal to avoid nerve damage when installing endosseous implants in the interforaminal region: a second attempt introducing cone beam computed tomography. J Oral Maxillofac Surg. 2009;67(4):744–50.
22. Gahleitner A, Watzek G, Imhof H. Dental CT: imaging technique, anatomy, and pathologic conditions of the jaws. Eur Radiol. 2003;13(2):366–76.
23. Alsufyani NA, Lam E. Osseous (cemento-osseous) dysplasia of the jaws: clinical and radiographic analysis. J Can Dent Assoc. 2011;77:b70.
24. de Oliveira BH. Compound odontoma-diagnosis and treatment: three case reports. Pediatr Dent. 2001;23(2):151–7.
25. White SC, Pharoah MJ. Oral radiology: principles and interpretation. New York: Elsevier; 2014.
26. Al-Sabbagh M. Implants in the esthetic zone. Dent Clin. 2006;50(3):391–407.
27. Jivraj S, Chee W. Treatment planning of implants in the aesthetic zone. Br Dent J. 2006;201(2):77–89.
28. Kan JY, Rungcharassaeng K, Umezu K, Kois JC. Dimensions of peri-implant mucosa: an evaluation of maxillary anterior single implants in humans. J Periodontol. 2003;74(4):557–62.
29. Oliveira ML, Tosoni GM, Lindsey DH, Mendoza K, Tetradis S, Mallya SM. Influence of anatomical location on CT numbers in cone beam computed tomography. Oral Surg Oral Med Oral Pathol Oral Radiol. 2013;115(4):558–64.
30. Pauwels R, Jacobs R, Singer SR, Mupparapu M. CBCT-based bone quality assessment: are Hounsfield units applicable? Dentomaxillofac Radiol. 2015;44(1):20140238.
31. Pauwels R, Nackaerts O, Bellaiche N, et al. Variability of dental cone beam CT grey values for density estimations. Br J Radiol. 2013;86(1021):20120135.

Part II

Site Preparation: Hard and Soft Tissue Augmentation

Indications for Augmentation Prior to/at Implant Placement

3

Senichi Suzuki, Taichiro Morimoto, Akitoshi Sato, and Hajime Igarashi

Abstract

Site preparation for ideal implant placement in the aesthetic zone is an important concept to achieve successful aesthetic results and patient satisfaction. Several procedures have been applied by many clinicians. In order to perform ideal site preparations, we should understand biologic, anatomic, surgical, and prosthetic principles so that we could select the optimal procedure for a particular case at the optimum timing. The sites should be prepared for also long-term predictable peri-implant aesthetic outcomes. Although generally bone and/or soft tissue augmentation are performed for implant site preparation, high technique-sensitive procedures are sometimes required to reconstruct compromised site for future optimal implant placements. Considering a risk of surgical failure and trauma, we should know alternative approach for site preparation with risk assessment. Procedures and concepts for ideal site preparation in three different timings (pre-extraction, at extraction, healed sites) would be described in this chapter.

S. Suzuki (✉)
Private Practice, Ebina City, Japan
e-mail: lion@kd5.so-net.ne.jp

T. Morimoto
Private Practice, Fukuoka, Japan
e-mail: t.morimoto@morimotodental.com

A. Sato
Private Practice, Tokyo, Japan
e-mail: mic-sato@topaz.plala.or.jp

H. Igarashi
Private Practice, Kyoto, Japan
e-mail: info@igarashi-dent.com

Todd R. Schoenbaum (ed.), *Implants in the Aesthetic Zone*,
https://doi.org/10.1007/978-3-319-72601-4_3

3.1 Introduction

When patients present with dental problems and need dental implants, they may have insufficient bone and soft tissue to support dental implants, for example, cases with narrow alveolar crest, vertical and horizontal bone resorption, facial undercut of alveolar bone, and lack of keratinized mucosa and papillae [1, 2].

Alveolar ridge defects have various causes:

- Tooth extraction
- Root fracture
- Internal and external root resorption
- Periapical lesion
- Endodontic failures
- Decay
- Periodontal disease
- Trauma
- Congenitally missing teeth

In order to enhance the predictability of the treatment and achieve long-term implant stability, it is important to perform implant site preparation. Especially for the success of implant treatment in the aesthetic zone, the quality and quantity of alveolar bone and keratinized mucosa are important [3]. If implants are placed without site preparation, we may encounter aesthetic, biological, or functional problems. To avoid implant aesthetic failures, it is important to understand the concept of site preparation and understand the biology around implants [4]. This chapter describes the basic principles of hard and soft tissue management for implant placement in the aesthetic zone in conjunction with the following treatment modalities.

1. Pre-extraction: minor tooth movement (MTM)
2. At extraction: immediate implant placement, alveolar ridge preservation
3. Healed sites: ridge augmentation only, or implant placement and augmentation simultaneously

3.2 Pre-extraction: Minor Tooth Movement (MTM)

When performing implant site preparation before placing implants, it is common to perform hard and soft tissue augmentation. There is, however, another way using a nonsurgical approach with orthodontic minor tooth movement (MTM). There have been reports on its benefits, showing good results for challenging cases in the aesthetic zone [5]. Especially single-implant immediate loading cases have a great advantage from the tooth extrusion using orthopedic device before extraction [6, 7].

Due to the facial bone resorption after tooth extraction and simultaneous implant placement and temporization, the margin line of the implant restoration may move

2–3 mm apically [8]. This cannot be avoided because the facial bone of the anterior teeth is always thin and very sensitive to extraction trauma.

Of course we can provide bone and soft tissue grafting facially to the extraction socket at the time of implant placement to avoid facial bone resorption and changes in the gingival margin, but it is difficult to prevent completely [9].

Orthodontic extrusion can be a treatment option to increase the vertical bone height and volume and to establish more favorable soft tissue characteristics prior to implant placement.

Its advantages are:

1. Avoids additional surgical trauma
2. Reduced risk of surgical failure
3. Relatively easy technique
4. Minimal invasiveness
5. Predictability
6. Low cost

3.3 Implant Site Development Using Orthodontic Extrusion

1. Use of Orthodontic Appliance with Wire and Bracket

This procedure can provide extrusion of the tooth or teeth to an ideal position for implant site preparation [10]. It is relatively easy and predictable to control the gingival margin position. However, an increase in the treatment time can be a disadvantage for this procedure.

2. Root Extrusion Using Hook and Elastic

In the case of a remaining root without its clinical crown, a small hook is cemented on the root, and the root is pulled up with elastic using a Maryland bridge. This is a widely known conventional approach to extrude a root, and it is easy to manage the procedure [5].

3.4 Extrusion Period

Typically it takes about 2–3 weeks to reach the intended position for tooth extrusion. New periodontal tissue is formed along with the alveolar bone and soft tissue moved with the tooth approximately 8 weeks after extrusion (Figs. 3.1 and 3.2).

After finishing extrusion, the tooth should be held in that state in order to stabilize the optimal position. The advantages of this are:

1. Prevention of relapse. We should wait as long as possible in order to prevent the periodontal ligament from pulling the extruded tooth back.

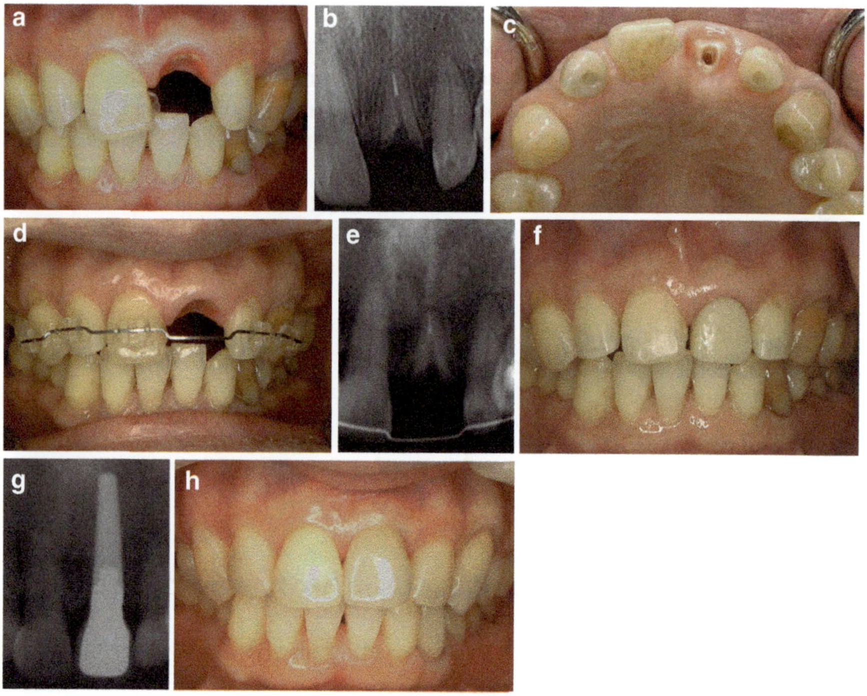

Fig. 3.1 Use of orthodontic appliance with a wire and brackets. (**a**) Upper left central incisor with horizontal root fracture caused by a traumatic injury. (**b**) Initial radiograph. (**c**) Due to the mobility and poor prognosis, it was necessary to extract. (**d**) Minor tooth movement (MTM) by orthodontic extrusion of the upper left central incisor with a wire and brackets was performed to gain a sufficient amount of soft tissue and bone around implant and to improve the compromised anterior aesthetics. (**e**) Post-extrusion radiograph. The tooth was held in position for 8 weeks after extrusion was completed to ensure soft tissue stability. (**f**) Post-extrusion, a sufficient amount of soft and hard tissue was obtained around the tooth. Subsequent to the extraction, the implant was placed and provisionalized. (**g**) Radiograph of the definitive restoration. (**h**) A 9-year post-op of the definitive implant restoration. The gingival margin position has receded apically but still in an aesthetically acceptable range

2. Retention of the new soft tissue and bone which were moved with the extruded tooth. Compared to the regular orthodontic treatment (full band) which takes considerably more time and cost, MTM can be performed relatively easily, safely, and economically.

3.5 At Extraction: Immediate Implant Placement and Alveolar Ridge Preservation

3.5.1 Facial Bone for Implants in the Aesthetic Zone

Much of the literature regarding implants in the aesthetic zone describe several methods for replacing a failing tooth [11–14]. Most of these studies analyze interproximal bone level mesially and distally to evaluate the hard tissue resorption after

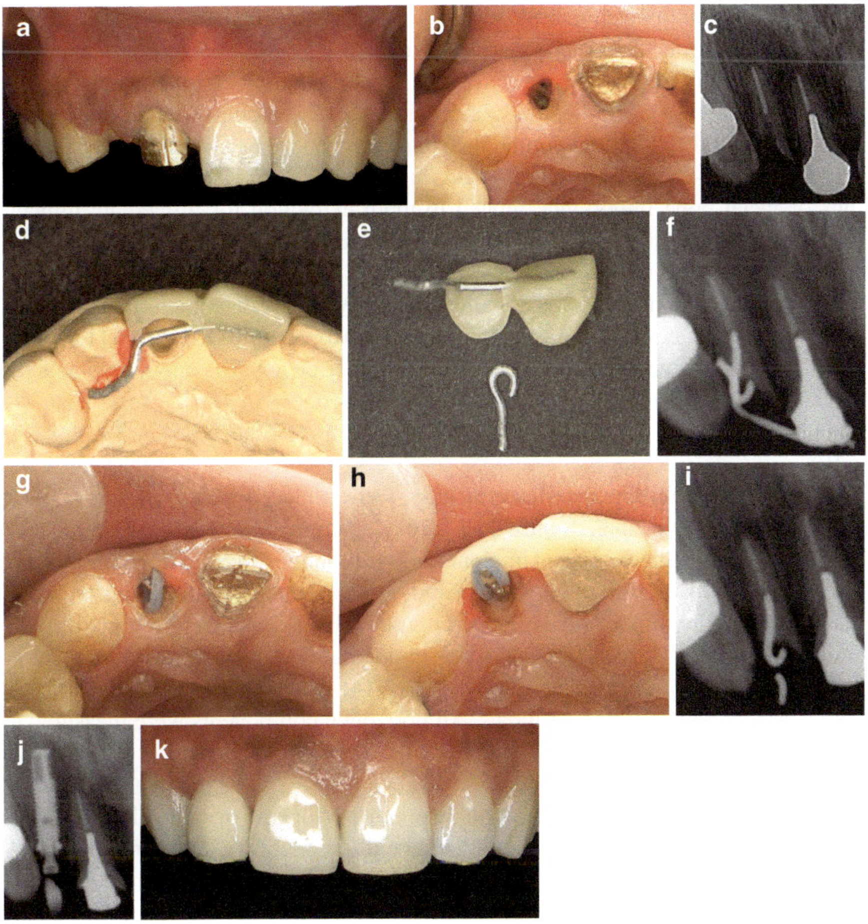

Fig. 3.2 Root extrusion using a hook and an elastic. (**a**) Frontal view of upper right lateral incisor. (**b**) Labial tissue was lost due to root fracture. (**c**) Initial radiograph. (**d**, **e**) Fabrication of an orthodontic appliance with a hook and elastic. (**f**) Radiograph of extrusion in process. (**g**) After the root was extruded to a certain degree, the exposed portion of the root was cut, and a new hook was attached to the remaining root. Then, the direction of the extrusion was adjusted with a new hook and an elastic. Upon the completion of extrusion, the position of the root was fixed and retained for over 8 weeks. (**h**) A temporary prosthesis used for a second stage orthodontic extrusion. The position of the hook has been adjusted. (**i**) Radiograph following completion of the second stage extrusion. (**j**) Radiograph of the implant placement and provisionalization. (**k**) Clinical photograph 9 years after the final implant restoration was delivered. Bone and soft tissue around the implant are stable and healthy

implant placement. The use of CBCT (cone-beam computed tomography) could also facilitate clinicians' ability to analyze the facial and palatal bone [15].

Optimal aesthetic outcome with dental implants requires proper facial bone quantity and quality to achieve proper gingival tissue architecture. It is meaningful to focus on the facial bone especially in aesthetic zone. A recent systematic review described buccal horizontal and vertical bone dimensional reductions following immediate implant placement into extraction socket [16]. Only a few previous articles regarding immediate placement and provisionalization of single implants also reported both horizontal and vertical facial bone resorptions around 1 mm or less after about 1 year or less healing period [17–19]. Therefore, the long-term facial hard tissue stability following immediate placement and provisionalization of single implants has not been well documented, nor has short-term stability. Recent findings of facial bone importance related to tooth extraction for immediate implant placement will be discussed in this following section.

Analysis of "Facial bone alterations on maxillary anterior single implants for immediate placement and provisionalization following tooth extraction: a superimposed cone beam computed tomography study" (Morimoto COIR 2015) [18].

This retrospective study described the facial bone changes on single implants for immediate placement and provisionalization procedures in the aesthetic zone via cone-beam computed tomography (CBCT) (Figs. 3.3, 3.4, 3.5, 3.6, 3.7, 3.8, 3.9, and 3.10).

A total of 12 failing maxillary incisors were replaced with a single implant attached to a provisional. Synthetic hydroxylapatite (HA) was used in the gap between the immediately placed implants and surrounding alveolar bone (Figs. 3.11, 3.12, and 3.13). Approximately 1-year radiographic outcomes focusing on facial hard tissue on the implants using superimposed CBCT scans were reported in this study. Facio-palatal cross-sectional scans of another case were shown as a demonstration for parameter measurements (Fig. 3.14). The results using Spearman's analysis from this data are as follows. All horizontal components were measured at the implant platform level (IPL) (Fig. 3.15 and Table 3.1).

1. Statistically significant correlation between postoperative bone thickness (C) and DOBI (distance between outer surface of preoperative bone to implant surface) (E) ($rs = 0.839$, $P = 0.001$) was found. Statistically significant correlation between postoperative bone thickness (C) and horizontal gap distance (E–A) ($rs = 0.620$, $P = 0.032$) was also found.
2. Horizontal gap distance (E–A) did not influence the amount of facial bone resorptions (E–C, B–D).

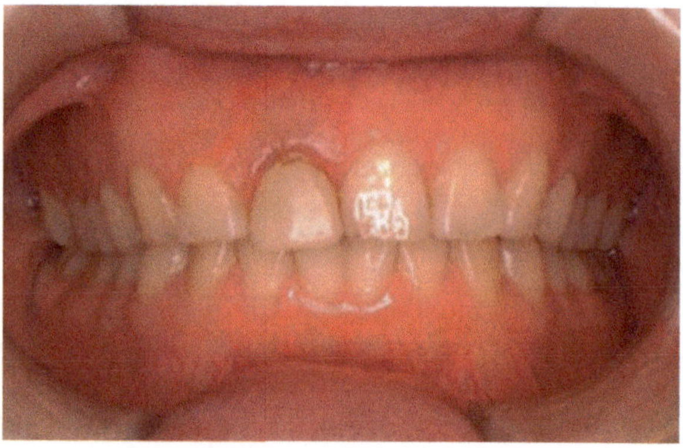

Fig. 3.3 Preoperative frontal view and periapical radiograph. Maxillary right central tooth was failing

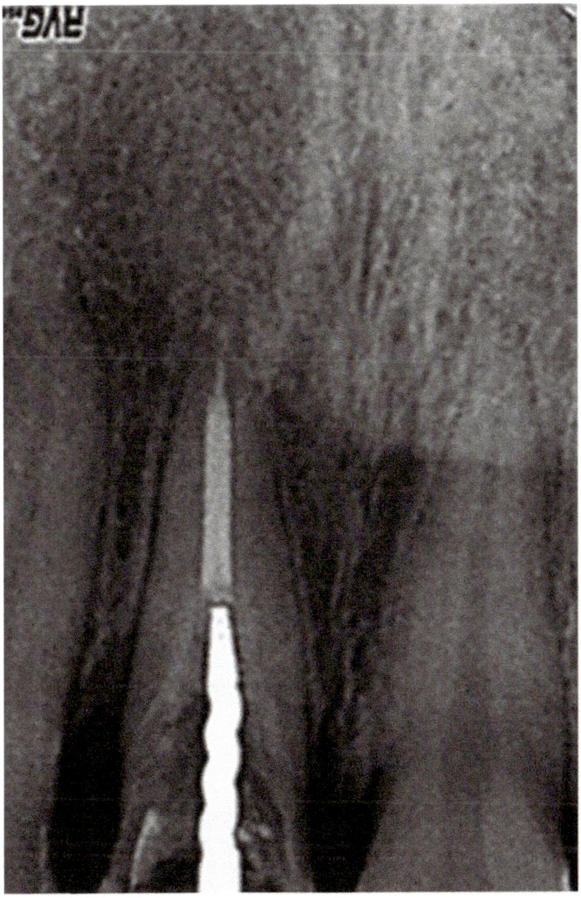

Fig. 3.4 Preoperative frontal view and periapical radiograph. Maxillary right central tooth was failing

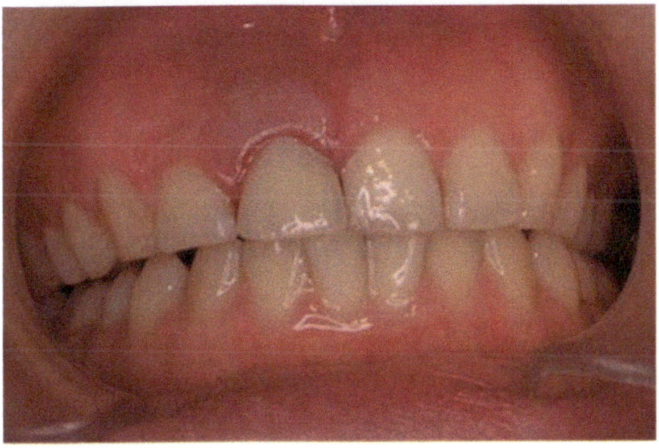

Fig. 3.5 Immediate postoperative frontal view and periapical radiograph. Maxillary right central tooth was replaced with immediate implant and provisional

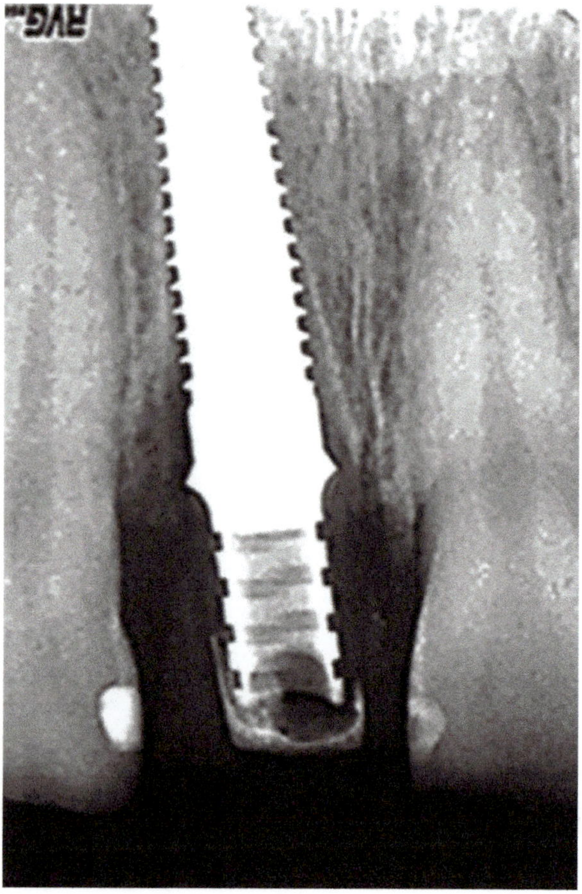

Fig. 3.6 Immediate postoperative frontal view and periapical radiograph. Maxillary right central tooth was replaced with immediate implant and provisional

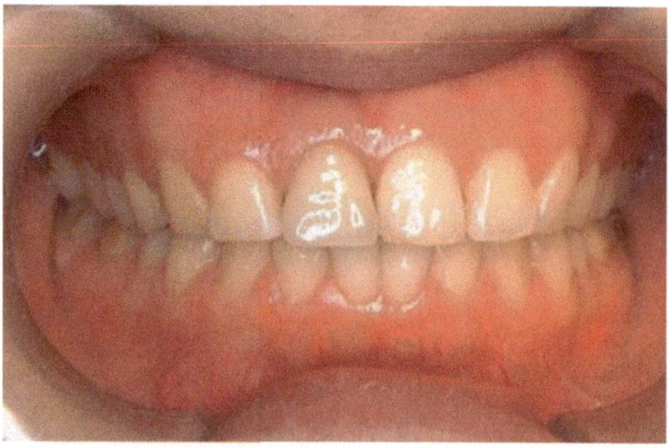

Fig. 3.7 Frontal view and periapical radiograph at 1 year. Maxillary right central tooth was replaced with immediately placed single implant and metal ceramic crown

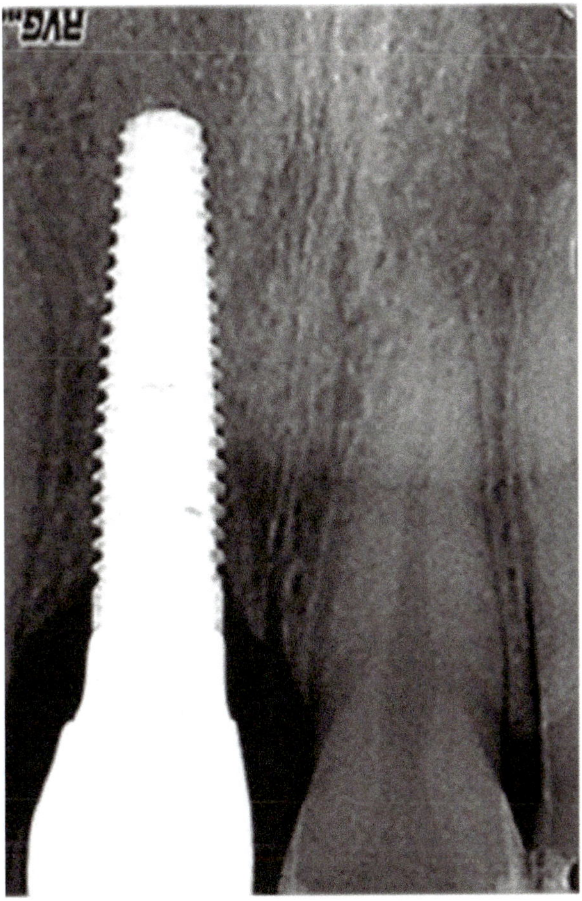

Fig. 3.8 Frontal view and periapical radiograph at 1 year. Maxillary right central tooth was replaced with immediately placed single implant and metal ceramic crown

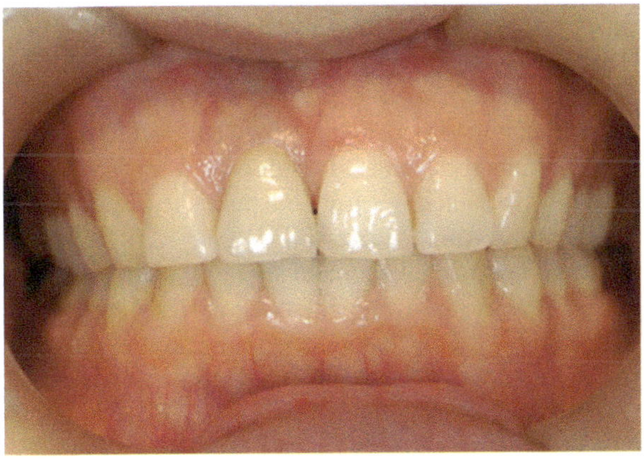

Fig. 3.9 Frontal view and periapical radiograph at 4 year

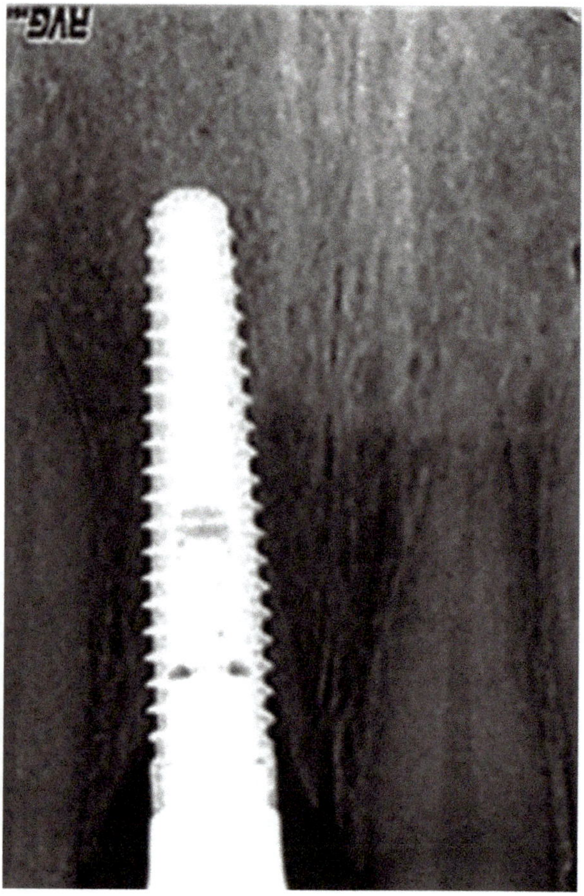

Fig. 3.10 Frontal view and periapical radiograph at 4 year

3. Preoperative facial bone thickness (A) did not correlate with the vertical or horizontal facial bone resorptions (E–C, B–D).

The healing of peri-implant hard and soft tissue for long-term alterations has not been thoroughly evaluated, with only a few longitudinal clinical studies [20–22]. However, the outcomes from the published data seem to be stable and satisfied aesthetic results. Another case is shown in Fig. 3.16, as an example of immediate placement and provisionalization of single-implant procedure at 12 months. It also shows decent 4 years and 1 month passed postoperatively result of cross-sectional CBCT image on Fig. 3.17. Stable facial bone around the implant has not been visibly lost for about 4 years. The implant site also has not experienced significant prosthetic complications during the follow-up period.

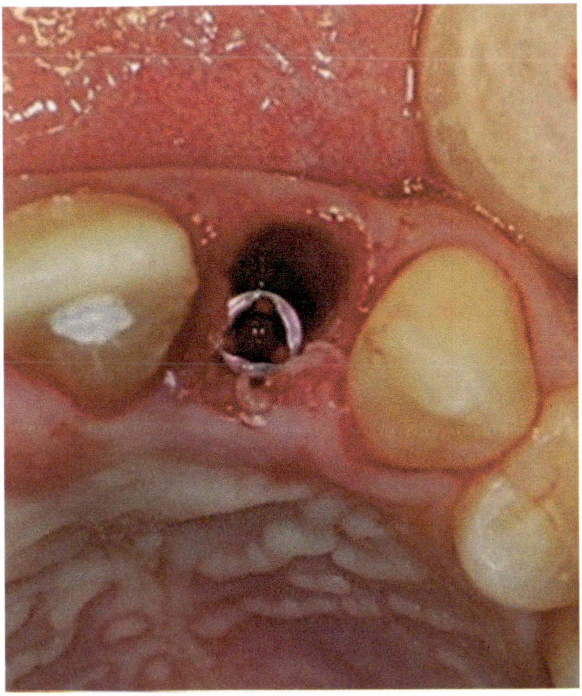

Fig. 3.11 Immediate implant was placed

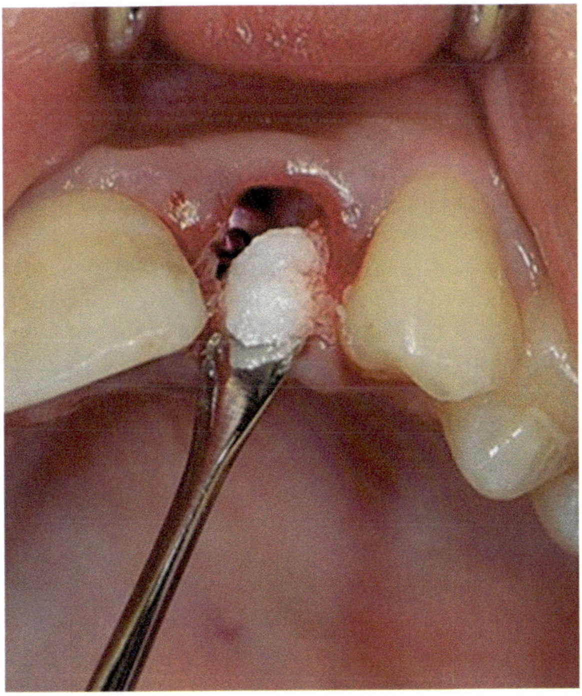

Fig. 3.12 Synthetic hydroxylapatite (HA) used to fill the gap between immediately placed implants and surrounding alveolar bone

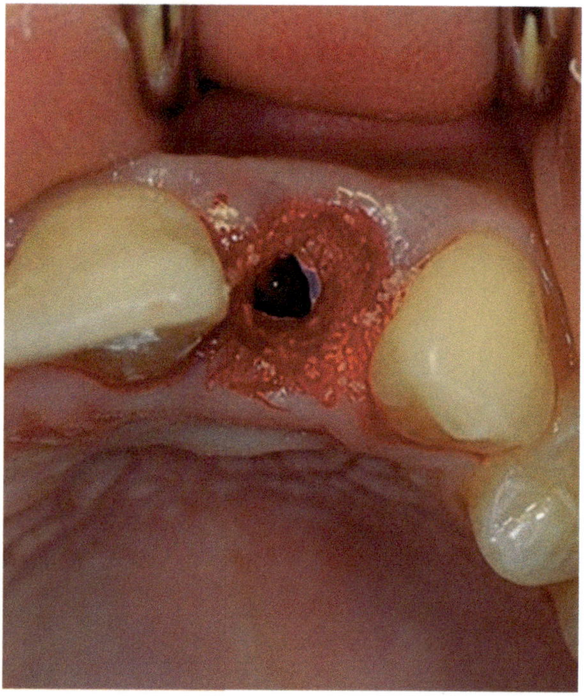

Fig. 3.13 HA has filled in the space and provisional would be delivered on the implant

3.5.2 The Role of Preoperative Facial Bone Through Extraction for Immediate Implant Placement

It is inevitable that failing tooth sites encounter bundle bone issues after extraction. Some animal studies have shown compromised bone postoperatively [23, 24]. Alveolar ridge models and remodels after tooth extraction [25]. Since immediate implant placement procedures always include tooth extraction, the prime concern emerges at aesthetic area.

It is necessary to place bone graft material in the gap between the facial bone and implant to prevent the subsequent bone resorption even when the gap is very small. The purpose of the grafting is to maintain the peri-implant hard and soft tissue condition, especially for the facial bone. However, the marginal bone resorption still occurs, and the bone material does not completely prevent facial bone loss [26, 27]. It may help to retain postoperative facial bone thickness after preoperative original bone has lost [19]. Therefore, the original facial bone may be able to act as a slow resorbable membrane to maintain the space for bone regeneration. If the facial bone thickness is wide enough to possess cortical bone and cancellous bone, the thickness may remain after extraction.

Unfortunately, facial bone thickness in the anterior maxilla is not as great as that in the molar area. It is natural to develop different approaches to treat aesthetic zone and posterior area. The average facial bone thickness in the aesthetic zone is usually reported as less than 1.0 mm [28–30]. The so-called thick facial bone in the anterior

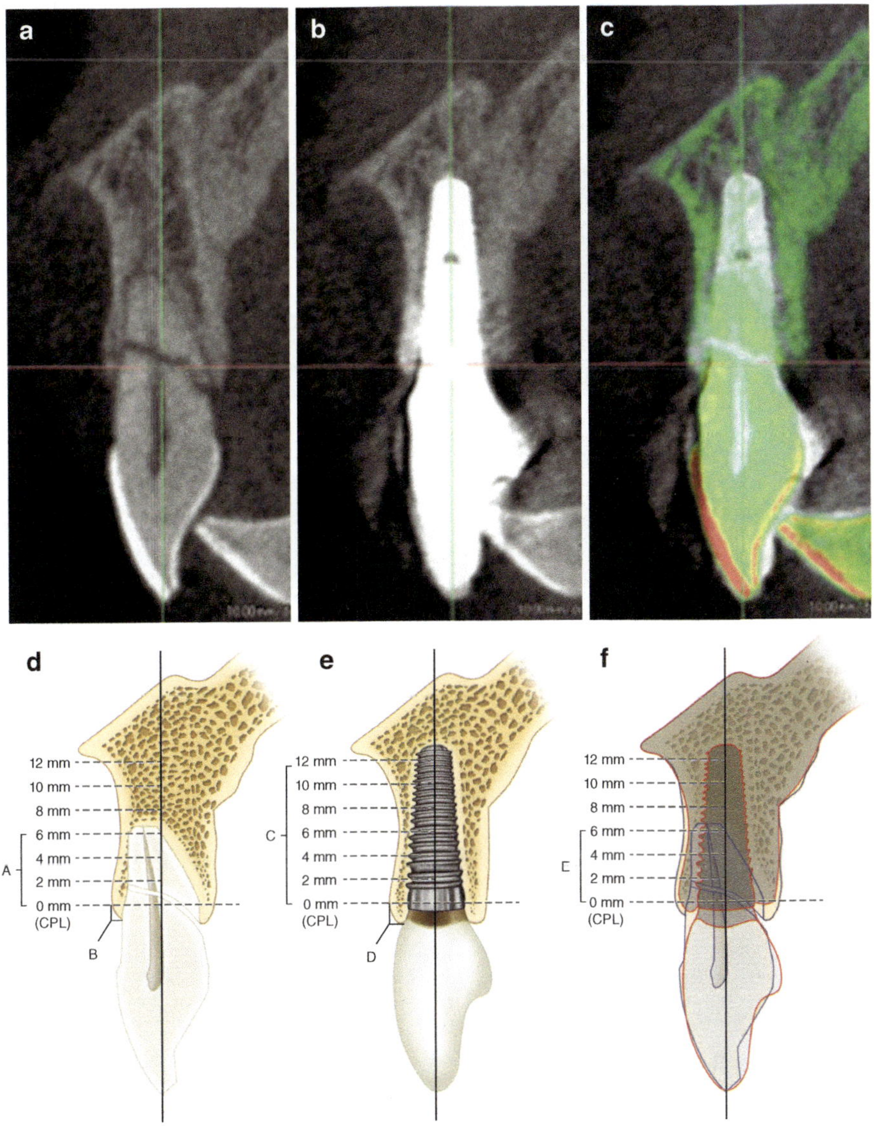

Fig. 3.14 The first case. Facio-palatal cross-sectional scans of implant placement site. Preoperative image of natural tooth before extraction (left image) and postoperative image of immediately placed and provisionalized single implant (middle image) at 14 months were superimposed facio-palatally (right image): (**a**) Preoperative facio-palatal. (**b**) Postoperative facio-palatal. (**c**) Superimposed facio-palatal. (**d**) Preoperative illustration. (**e**) Postoperative illustration. (**f**) Superimposed illustration. Postoperative image was displayed in gray scale on the superimposed illustration. A. Facial initial bone thickness measurements and B. facial vertical bone level measurement compared to the superimposed postoperative implant platform level (IPL). C. Facial residual bone thickness measurements and D. facial vertical bone level measurement compared to the IPL. E. DOBI (distance between outer surface of preoperative bone to implant surface) measurements

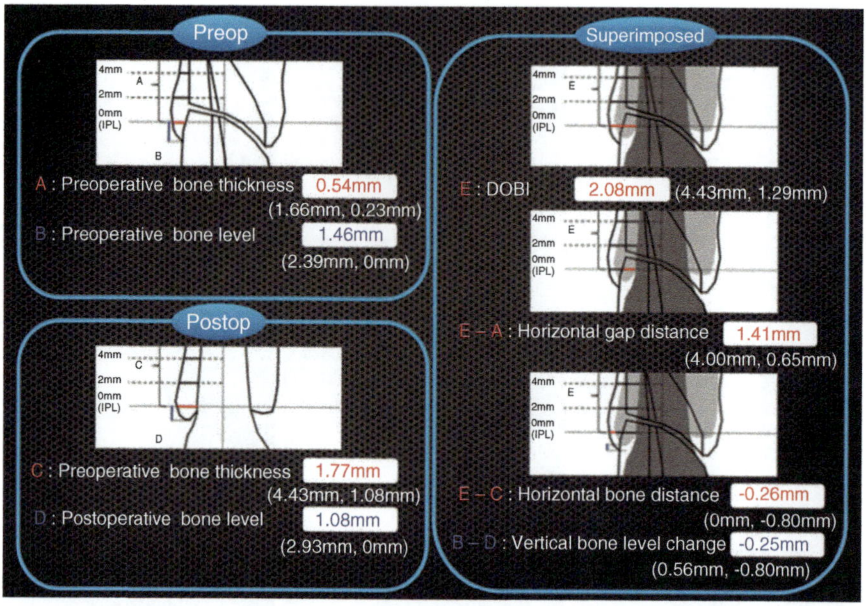

Fig. 3.15 Horizontal and vertical facial bone measurements: median (max, min) (mm). Horizontal measurements were performed at IPL. DOBI (distance between outer surface of preoperative bone to implant surface)

Table 3.1 Spearman's rank correlation coefficient analysis was used to evaluate relationship between the parameters as nonparametric statistics

	A Preoperative bone thickness	C Postoperative bone thickness	E DOBI	E-A Horizontal gap distance	E-C Horizontal bone change	B Preoperative bone level	D Postoperative bone level	B-D Vertical bone level change
A Preoperative bone thickness								
C Postoperative bone thickness			.839** .001	.620* .032		.685* .014	.627* .029	
E DOBI		.839** .001		.813** .001				
E-A Horizontal gap distance		.620* .032	.813** .001					
E-C Horizontal bone change						.756** .004		
B Preoperative bone level		.685* .014			.756** .004		.911** .000	
D Postoperative bone level		.627* .029				.911** .000		
B-D Vertical bone level change								

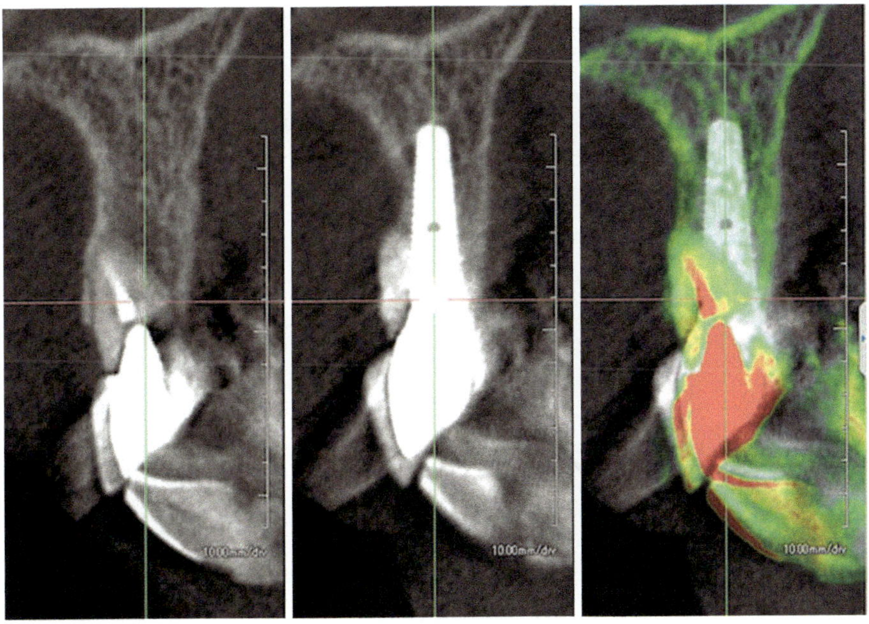

Fig. 3.16 The second case. Facio-palatal cross-sectional scans of implant placement site. Preoperative image of natural tooth before extraction (left image) and postoperative image of immediately placed and provisionalized single implant (middle image) at 12 months were superimposed facio-palatally (right image)

maxilla is not actually thick enough to keep the bone structure completely as it is at preoperative status and starts resorbing after extraction no matter what we apply in the socket only. Preoperative facial bone thickness had no significant correlation with horizontal or vertical facial bone resorption [18]. A study showed a similar result of no significant correlation between maxillary anterior preoperative buccal bone width and the soft tissue and aesthetic results after immediate implant placement and restoration [31]. Overlay bone graft around the socket in combination with the intra-socket bone graft procedure might be helpful to overcome the situation. On the other hand, a recent study found a correlation between hard tissue changes and preoperative bone thickness and gap distance after immediate implant placement in between maxillary premolars sites [32]. But since more than half of the implants were placed at the premolar sites and bone width was measured at 1 mm apically from alveolar crest at the surgery, it is hard to compare the results to our study.

3.5.3 Gap Consideration for Immediate Implant

It had been said that it is not necessary to place any bone materials in horizontal gap when the gap size is smaller than 1.0 mm. It is currently seen to receive bone grafting in the gap around implants no matter how small the gap size is.

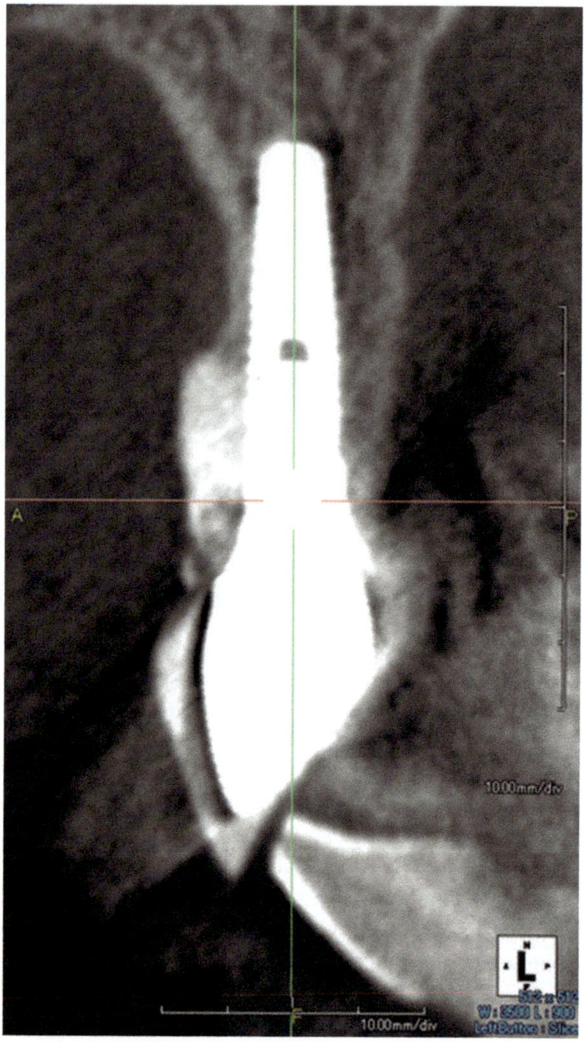

Fig. 3.17 A period of 4 years and 1 month passed since the immediate tooth replacement: CBCT cross-sectional result

The aim for the bone grafting in the gap is not only to minimize facial bone resorption but also to increase the postoperative facial bone thickness. Types of bone materials would be obviously influencing the outcome [11]. The bone filled in the space around immediately placed implant should be resorbing at slow speed relatively. Scaffold property of the grafting bone is necessary to maintain the space at healing period [33]. It has been reported that at least 2 mm buccal bone thickness is ideal to restore single implant in the aesthetic zone [34, 35]. The requisite buccal bone thickness should be determined from the perspective of anatomic [36], surgical [37], and prosthetic [38] limitations for each individual patient.

Leaving a certain horizontal gap distance would not prevent horizontal bone resorption completely but has a merit to retain proper remaining bone thickness following inevitable bone resorption after extraction. Horizontal gap distance is correlated with postoperative facial bone thickness. In addition, horizontal gap distance plus preoperative facial bone thickness is strongly correlated with postoperative facial bone thickness [18]. Therefore, it is able to predict remaining facial bone width reasonably by calculating the two components (horizontal gap distance plus preoperative facial bone thickness) compared to total alveolar ridge width and implant diameter and position determination on the facio-palatal cross-sectional CBCT image at case planning before even extracting a failing tooth. Appropriate implant diameter has been assessed from facio-palatal socket dimension in also other studies [39, 40].

3.5.4 Advantage of Immediate Implant Placement with Non-submerged Approach

The ultimate goal to achieve optimal aesthetics for dental implants is to prepare stable healthy gingival tissue around implants in harmony with surrounding natural teeth. Gingival stability is linked to underlying hard tissue situation. It is necessary to achieve appropriate stable hard tissue in order to maintain appropriate soft tissue condition [41, 42]. Five diagnostic keys for predictable single-tooth peri-implant aesthetics at immediate implant placement implants were introduced [43]. They are relative tooth position, form of the periodontium, biotype of the periodontium, tooth shape, and position of the osseous crest [37, 38, 44–48].

Timing of single-implant placement related to bone loss was analyzed by literature review [49]. Marginal bone loss around immediate, early, and delayed implant placement was found to be comparable in long-term observation [20, 50].

Immediate single-tooth implants should be provisionalized for optimal aesthetics facially if primary implant stability is acquired [51]. The reason is that immediate implant placement may produce an advantage to preserve original ridge contour. Maintaining the grafted bone for postoperative facial bone thickness is linked to gingival management. Proper sealing by marginal gingival tissue is requisite to hold the grafted bone in the space. Immediately placed implant enables to place an abutment over as either immediate provisional or healing abutment [52–54]. The abutment could be a provisional using temporary abutment or a customized healing abutment for one-stage approach. The critical point is to place root-shaped customized abutment that could support the preoperative gingiva around implant. The customized healing abutment has been used also for edentulous site [55]. Tarnow et al. explained contoured healing abutment or provisional with bone grafted material results in better marginal bone condition around immediately placed implants [56]. The group also showed an advantage for soft tissue volume after immediate tooth replacement with using bone graft and provisional [57]. Interproximal papilla tissue support is also effectively affected by the method. However, we can't take the advantage of alveolar ridge preservation in this approach.

When only preserving preoperative hard and soft tissue is adequate enough for future definitive restorations, immediate implant placement could be recommended for optimal results. It should overcome anatomical limitations to achieve implant primary stability and possess appropriate original facial bone configurations for bone grafting [37]. As finding of peri-implant tissue being deficient in this procedure, soft and/or hard tissue ridge augmentation would be needed in conjunction with implant placement. Cases should be diagnosed, selected, and planned carefully for immediate implant placement to achieve predictable peri-implant aesthetic outcomes [58].

3.5.5 Soft Tissue Management at Immediate Implant Placement

For ultimate outcome to accomplish predictable aesthetics, adequate amount and quality of soft tissue characteristics are essential factors. Immediate implant placement procedure including bone grafting in the gap is not usually enough to achieve the ideal outcome for anterior maxilla. Connective tissue graft inserted around the implant abutment is necessary to augment the existing gingival tissue [59–61]. In other words, it is also useful to cover open extraction space around implant abutment when applied at the time of immediate implant placement. However, it should not be expected to prevent further marginal bone resorption. Soft tissue graft is often recommended for optimal outcome if possible for implant placement in the aesthetic zone. The long-term tissue stability after surgical procedures is still needed to clarify with enough literature support.

3.5.6 Alveolar Ridge Preservation

Alveolar ridge preservation has been applied to maintain existing hard tissue and soft tissue around the extraction sites by preventing alveolar bone loss and to facilitate implant placement in a prosthetically driven position [62–65].

Previous literature showed horizontal and vertical bone changes even after ridge augmentation and described that reduction of alveolar ridge width is the most significant concern from this method [66, 67]. That might be due to less gingival support at alveolar ridge preservation procedure compared to, at immediate implant placement using an abutment, preoperative facial bone and gingival volume that may compromise after healing.

Ridge atrophy before implant placement does not provide an acceptable foundation for aesthetic zone. There are some situations that immediate implant placement could not be performed, for instance, active infection, large bone defect, and implant primary instability. Delayed or early placement approach would be a substitute modality for the undesirable sites. Advanced surgical technique or different bone substitute may improve the outcome of alveolar ridge augmentation in the future.

3.6 Healed Sites: Only Augmentation or Augmentation with Simultaneous Implant Placement

For healed extraction sites, many cases have insufficient hard and soft tissue at the alveolar ridge. Especially in the anterior region, the facial bone is very thin, and the bone is resorbed after tooth extraction. Furthermore, in multiple missing teeth cases, a huge volume of vertical and horizontal alveolar bone resorption occurs along with the loss of soft tissue and papilla [68].

It is difficult to achieve implant success in aesthetic zone if we do not improve such negative situations utilizing site development techniques because there are multiple numbers of aesthetic problems which exist for these patients including papilla loss, uneven gum line, long implant tooth, and so on.

It is important to properly diagnosis and treatment plan before performing implant site preparation. How much bone and soft tissue necessary? Which surgical procedure we should perform? And the amount of vertical and horizontal augmentation required is related to the five dimensions of implant placement which is documented in Chap. 3. These should be decided based on the design of definitive restoration, and after all it should be based on an ideal diagnosis and treatment plan using smile line, dentofacial evaluation, intraoral conditions, study model, X-rays, and CT [69].

3.6.1 Optimal Diagnosis and Treatment Planning for Site Preparation

1. Extraoral

Dentofacial evaluation for diagnosis.

Check the balance of smile line, midline, teeth position, gum line, etc.

Based on the concept of smile design, a treatment plan is made considering aesthetic factors. For the planning, digital simulation is useful.

2. Intraoral Examination

Conditions of extraction site, tooth position/form, occlusion, gingival conditions, and biotype are examined.

3. Study Model and Diagnostic Wax-Up

Conditions of extraction site, tooth position/form, occlusion, etc. are examined.

4. X-ray and CT Evaluation

3D diagnosis of alveolar bone height and width, etc. is examined.

In order to make a good treatment planning in the aesthetic zone, it is quite important to involve the dental technicians, and they should be reflected in the plan to achieve a proper implant restoration [70].

On top of these requirements, patients' concerns, and agreement with the treatment options are of the utmost importance. Consideration must be given to patient treatment desires, age, gender, occupation, illness, financial concerns, etc.

After determining the ideal five-dimensional implant position and the ideal restoration based on the comprehensive diagnosis and treatment planning with smile design, the hard and soft tissue augmentation necessary to support implants must be decided before starting surgery.

Even when patients do not accept our ideal treatment plans and options based on smile design and only desire to have their missing tooth to be replaced with an implant without improving the surrounding tissue, we should attempt to provide these patients with all possible options to improve their conditions based on the available evidence and inform them of what ideal implant treatment would be for them. It is significantly important and also useful for avoiding any risks and troubles (Figs. 3.18, 3.19, 3.20, 3.21, 3.22, 3.23, and 3.24).

3.7 Timing of Implant Site Preparation

Implant site preparation with and without simultaneous implant placement

1. Augmentation only (before implant placement)
2. Augmentation with simultaneous implant placement

Notice: It is possible to perform hard and soft tissue augmentations as site preparation *after* implantation, at second stage surgery, and at the delivery of the restoration; however, it is quite difficult to succeed in the bone grafting after implant placement. Therefore, such treatment should occur before or during the implant placement.

1. Augmentation only (before implant placement)

Building up the peri-implant site with hard and soft tissue before implant placement is important for the long-term predictability of implant aesthetics, health, and function. For the hard tissue augmentation, techniques like GBR (guided bone regeneration; see Chap. 5), ridge expansion, and sinus augmentation are widely known. There are a variety of materials used for these techniques such as autograft, xenograft, allograft, and growth factors including rh-BMP2.

For soft tissue augmentation, in addition to the frequently practiced soft tissue grafts such as CTG and FGG, procedures using AlloDerm, PRP, PRF, and CGF are often reported.

Please refer to Chaps. 5, 6, and 7 of this book for the details of these procedures and the selection of materials.

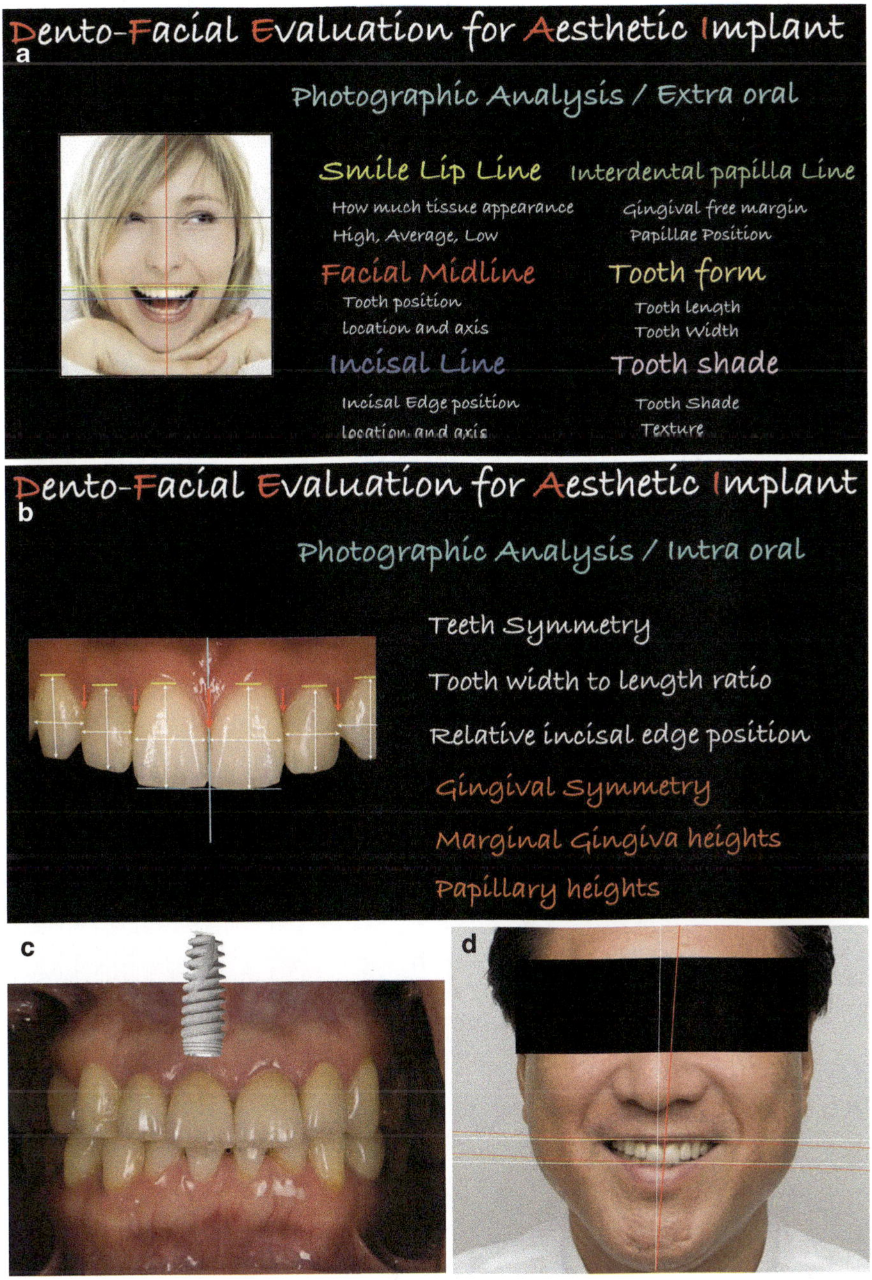

Fig. 3.18 Dentofacial evaluation extraoral and intraoral for diagnoses. (**a**, **b**) The whole symmetrical dentofacial balance must be checked and problems identified. (**c**, **d**) For example, this is an implant case for #8 due to a root fracture. The intraoral examination alone may not be sufficient for us to make an accurate diagnosis. It is necessary to make a treatment plan based on a comprehensive examination including a facial diagnosis and to give a thorough explanation of the plan to the patient

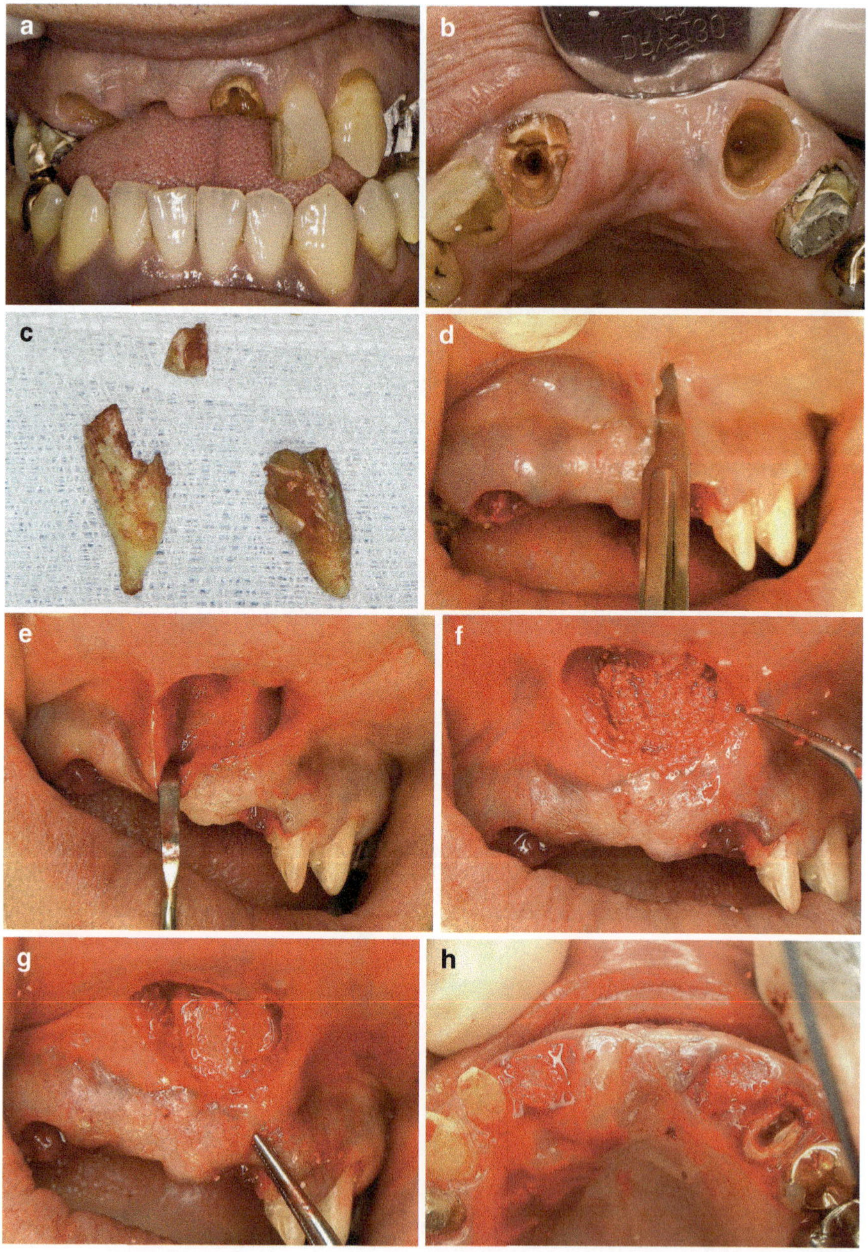

Fig. 3.19 Augmentation-only case (bone graft). (**a**–**c**) Clinical photographs maxillary canine and central incisor with vertical root fractures and extracted roots. (**d**–**g**) For this patient, access to the facial undercut of alveolar bone was from the vestibule to allow grafting of bovine bone particles and a resorbable membrane. (**h**) Socket augmentation using bovine bone during the same surgery. (**i**, **j**) Achieving horizontal tissue volume for proper implant position and hard tissue maintenance

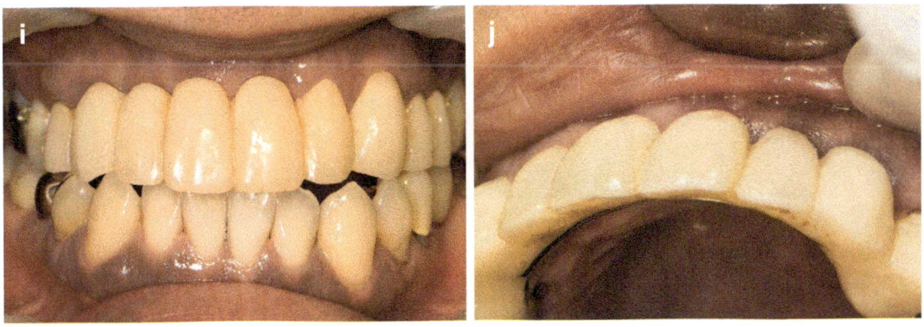

Fig. 3.19 (continued)

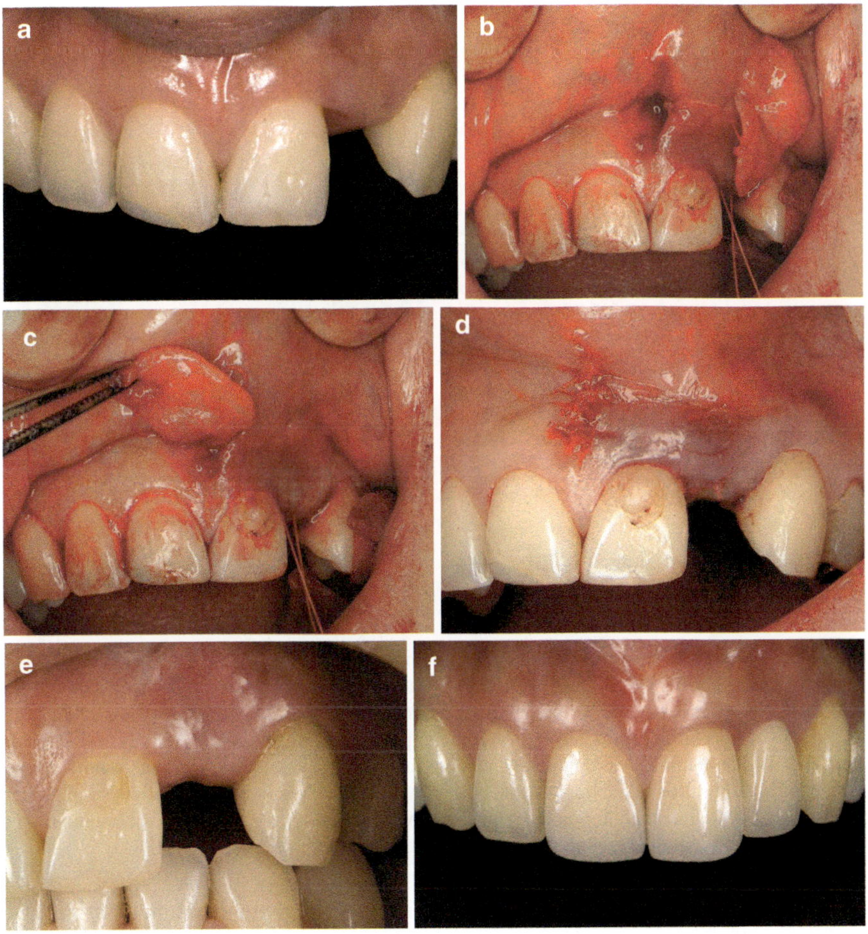

Fig. 3.20 Augmentation-only case (soft tissue graft). (**a**) Frontal view, lack of papillae distal to maxillary left central incisor unfavorable conditions for implantation at #10. (**b**–**d**) Palatal CTG to #10 using VISTA technique. (VISTA (vestibular incision subperiosteal tunnel access)) [71]. (**e**) After CTG papillae reconstruction and improvement of biotype. (**f**) Final implant restoration delivered on maxillary left lateral incisor with good soft tissue and bone support

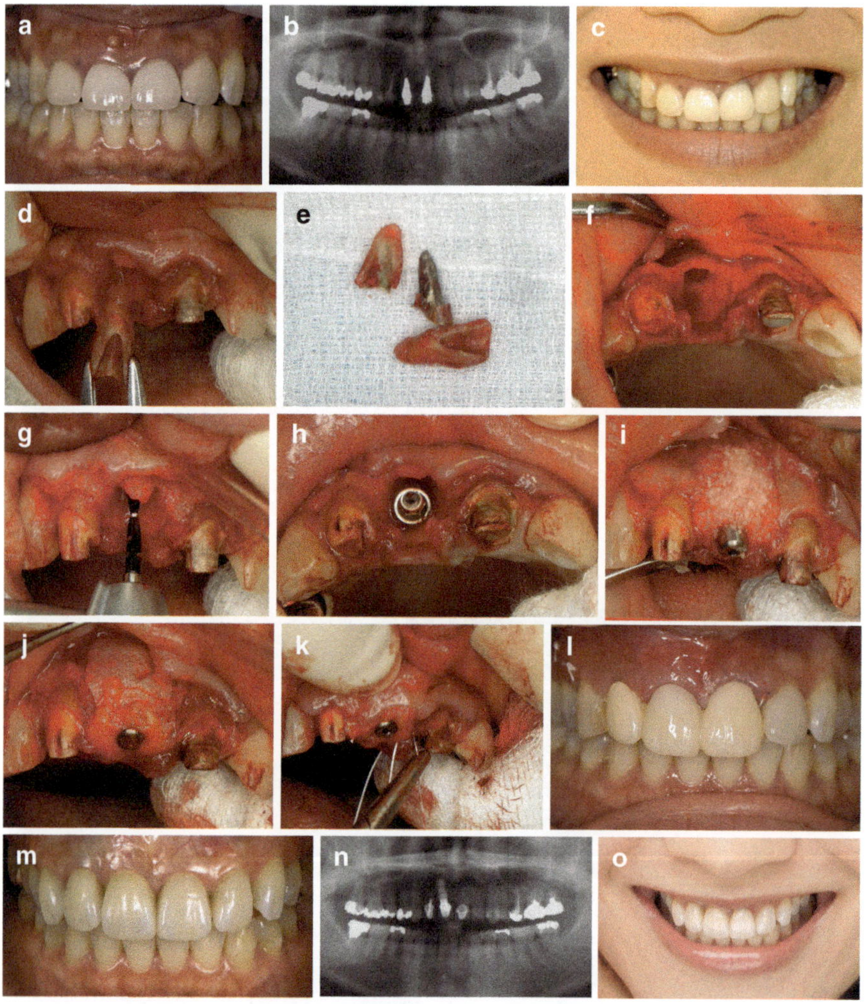

Fig. 3.21 Augmentation with simultaneous implant placement (bone and soft tissue graft). (**a–c**) Frontal view: Maxillary right central incisor had a vertical root fracture and was needed to be extracted. (**d, e**) The tooth was extracted using a conventional method. (**f**) There was a labial bone defect due to a vertical root fracture. (**g, h**) Implant placed in the three-dimensionally correct position. (**i**) The alveolar bone was augmented with bovine bone. (**j, k**) Connective tissue was harvested from palate and grafted to the implant site. (**l**) Frontal view, provisional restoration delivered after the surgery. (**m**) Clinical photograph of the definitive restoration fabricated. (**n**) Panoramic radiograph showing the implant position. (**o**) A 3-year post-op smile

On one hand, building an ideal implant site environment with augmentation procedures will give us an advantage for implant surgery especially for the major reconstruction cases, but on the other hand, there are issues such as a prolonged treatment duration, multiple invasive surgeries may be necessary, and increased financial burden.

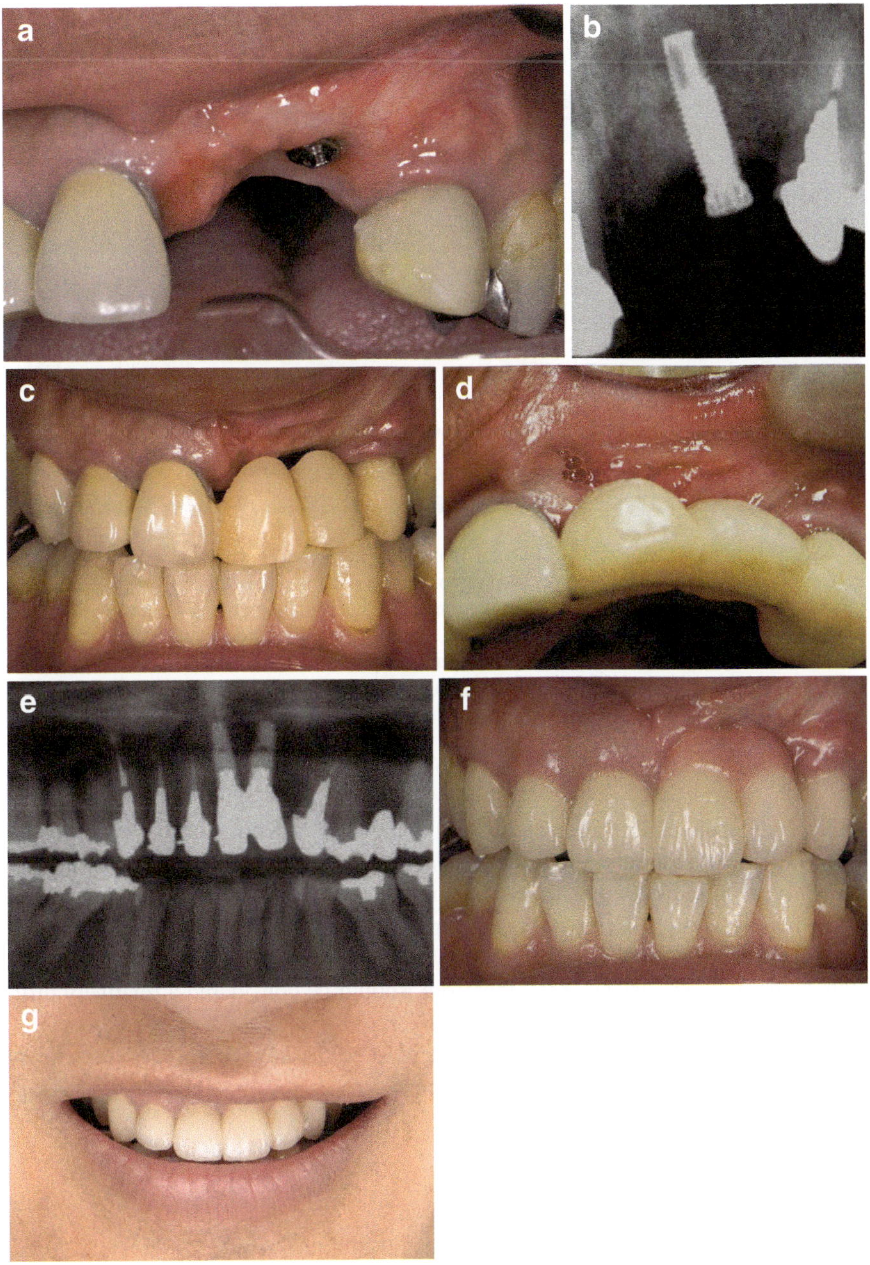

Fig. 3.22 Treatment of a large bone defect with failure of previous implant. (**a**) Malpositioned implant and mucogingival problem at #10. (**b**) Initial radiograph. Bone loss around implant, and the implant had to be removed. (**c**, **d**) After implant removal, there was a significant vertical and horizontal bone defect and deficient keratinized tissue. The patient declined further augmentation surgeries. (**e**) Bone reduction to prepare a flat bone table where two implants were placed. (**f**) Clinical photograph of final ceramic restoration with prosthetic soft tissue. (**g**) A 6-year post-op smile. Screw-retained restoration delivered

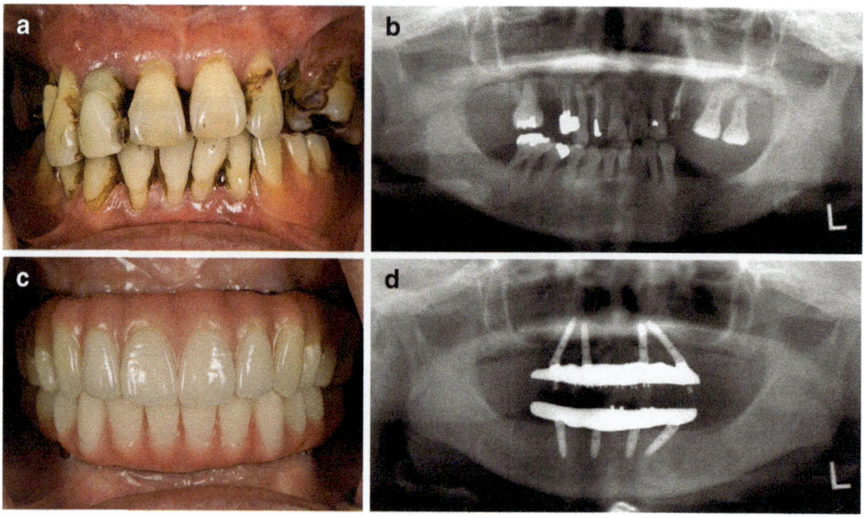

Fig. 3.23 Full-arch treatment. (**a**, **b**) A 53-year-old female patient with severe periodontal disease; most teeth with poor—hopeless—prognosis. The patient had difficulty eating because of mobility and pain. She requested full-arch treatment. All the remaining upper teeth were extracted, and four implants were placed to deliver a fixed implant restoration. The same treatment was provided for the mandible [72, 73]. (**c**) Clinical photograph of the definitive prostheses, with prosthetic soft tissue. (**d**) A 5-year post-surgery radiograph

2. Augmentation with Simultaneous Implant Placement

The biggest benefit of placing implant at the time of augmentation is the reduction of the treatment duration. With the conventional sequential method, we have to wait for 4–8 months for the grafted site to mature before implant placement.

Although this approach will give us a potential benefit of shorter treatment time, there is a risk of graft infection that may involve the implant and lead to the infection of the implant surface. This, therefore, should be considered a relatively difficult procedure.

The authors believe the following factors to be the keys to success for implant placement with simultaneous augmentation.

1. Case selection
2. Proper flap design
3. Releasing incisions
4. Primary closure with appropriate suturing techniques
5. Perioperative management

3.8 Resective Concept for Implant Site Preparation

There is also a way to performing implant site preparation by resecting bone and gingiva rather than augmenting them. This technique requires the use of a superstructure with prosthetic soft tissues. This may be necessary for the following reasons:

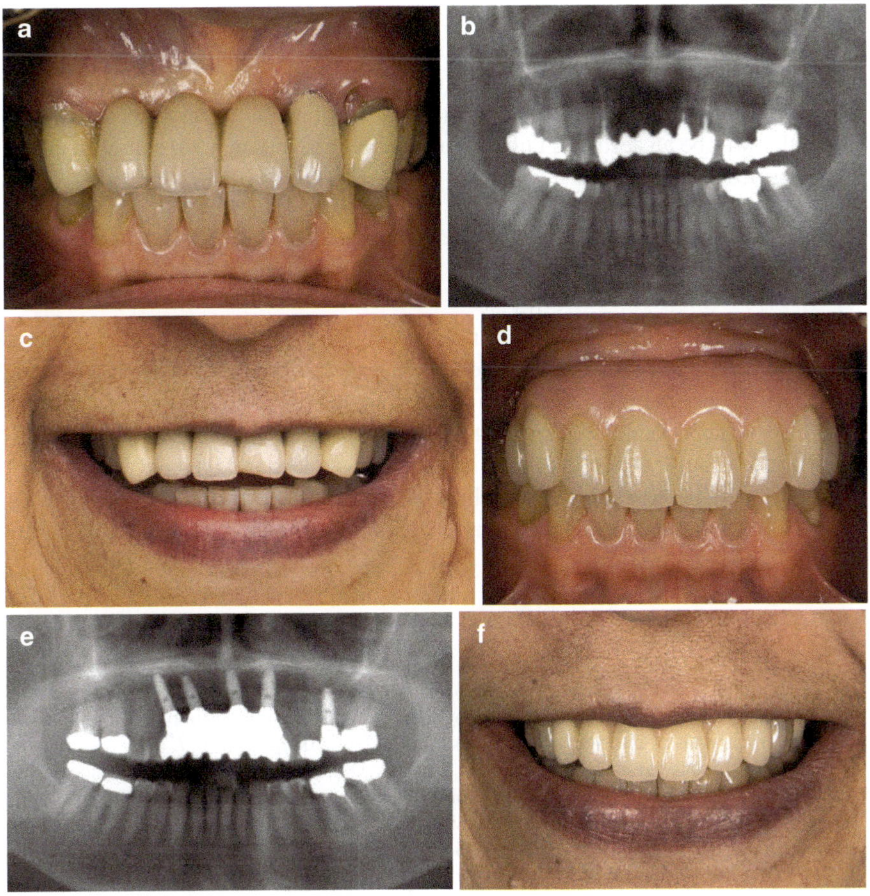

Fig. 3.24 Treatment with minimal surgical trauma. (**a**) A 78-year-old female patient. Her maxillary anterior bridge has failed due to root fractures of the abutment teeth. The patient would not accept any major surgical procedures. After removing the failed bridge and extracting the roots, alveoloplasty was performed for an aesthetic implant restoration with prosthetic soft tissue. Four implants were placed immediately, and a fixed provisional restoration was delivered on the same day. (**b**) Initial radiograph: insufficient bone and soft tissue to support an ideal implant restoration. (**c**) Aesthetic problems with her smile. (**d**) Clinical photograph of the definitive implant restoration with pink porcelain. The restoration is screw-retained. (**e**) Radiographic view. The implants at 5 years. (**f**) Patient smile with prosthesis in place

1. Cases with a severe bone loss:
   - Due to trauma or congenital defects
   - From previous major implant failure (difficult to recover by surgery)
2. Full-arch implant cases (or similar treatment concept)
   - Based on the patient's requirement and/or due to its necessity
3. Need to avoid surgical trauma (less invasive surgery is required)
   - Systemic illness
   - Based on the patient's requirement

If we choose to provide a superstructure with prosthetic soft tissue, we should be aware of the position of the transition line between natural and artificial gingiva, especially for the high lip line patients. To avoid aesthetic failures in these cases, it is very important to know the relationship between the smile line (lip line) and the gingival line and to configure them in the proper positions when the restoration is made. If the "Superstructure–natural Gum junction line" is exposed when patients smile, this will be an aesthetic failure. To prevent this, sufficient alveoloplasty must be performed.

3.9 Summary

Implant site preparation is critical for enhancing the prognosis of implant restoration and achieving a predictable aesthetic, functional, hygienic result in the aesthetic zone. This treatment option should be made available to patients in order to improve negative situations using hard and soft tissue augmentation or resective procedure to make an ideal implant site. It is also important to understand the concept, method, materials, and procedure, especially the timing of treatment, so that we can provide proper treatment approach for each patient to achieve a long-term aesthetic implant success.

References

1. Grunder U. Stability of the mucosal topography around single-tooth implants and adjacent teeth: 1-year results. Int J Periodontics Restorative Dent. 2000;20(1):11–7.
2. Kan JY, Rungcharassaeng K, Umezu K, Kois JC. Dimensions of peri-implant mucosa: an evaluation of maxillary anterior single implants in humans. J Periodontol. 2003;74(4):557–62.
3. Saadoun AP, Touati B. Soft tissue recession around implants: is it still unavoidable?--Part I. Pract Proced Aesthet Dent. 2007;19(1):55–62. quiz 64.
4. Touati B. Biologically driven prosthetic options in implant dentistry. Pract Proced Aesthet Dent. 2004;16(7):517–20.
5. Pontoriero R, Celenza F Jr, Ricci G, Carnevale G. Rapid extrusion with fiber reaction: a combined orthidontic-periodontic treatment modality. Int J Periodontics Restorative Dent. 1987;7(5):30–43.
6. López SG, Gaya MVO, Capilla MV. Esthetic restoration with orthodontic traction and single-tooth implant: case report. Int J Periodontics Restorative Dent. 2005;25:239–45.
7. Mantzikos T, Shamus I. Case report: forced eruption and implant site development. Angle Orthod. 1998;68:179–86.
8. Mantzikos T, Shamus I. Forced eruption and implant site development: soft tissue response. Am J Orthod Dentfacical Orthop. 1997;112:596–606.
9. Kwon EY, Lee JY, Choi J. Effect of slow forced eruption on the vertical levels of the interproximal bone and papilla and the width of the alveolar ridge. Korean J Orthod. 2016;46(6):379–85.
10. Maeda S, Sasaki T. Modality and risk management for orthodontic extrusion procedures in interdisciplinary treatment for generating proper bone and tissue contours for the planned implant: a case report. Int J Implant Dent. 2015;1(1):26.
11. Chochlidakis KM, Geminiani A, Papaspyridakos P, Singh N, Ercoli C, Chen CJ. Buccal bone thickness around single dental implants in the maxillary esthetic zone. Quintessence Int. 2016;48(4):295–308. [Epub ahead of print].
12. Cosyn J, Eghbali A, Hanselaer L, De Rouck T, Wyn I, Sabzevar MM, Cleymaet R, De Bruyn H. Four modalities of single implant treatment in the anterior maxilla: a clinical, radiographic, and aesthetic evaluation. Clin Implant Dent Relat Res. 2013;15(4):517–30.

13. Kan JY, Rungcharassaeng K, Lozada J. Immediate placement and provisionalization of maxillary anterior single implants: 1-year prospective study. Int J Oral Maxillofac Implants. 2003;18(1):31–9.
14. Wöhrle PS. Single-tooth replacement in the aesthetic zone with immediate provisionalization: fourteen consecutive case reports. Pract Periodontics Aesthet Dent. 1998;10(9):1107–14.
15. Razavi T, Palmer RM, Davies J, Wilson R, Palmer PJ. Accuracy of measuring the cortical bone thickness adjacent to dental implants using cone beam computed tomography. Clin Oral Implants Res. 2010;21(7):718–25.
16. Lee CT, Chiu TS, Chuang SK, Tarnow D, Stoupel J. Alterations of the bone dimension following immediate implant placement into extraction socket: systematic review and meta-analysis. J Clin Periodontol. 2014;41(9):914–26.
17. Lee EA, Gonzalez-Martin O, Fiorellini J. Lingualized flapless implant placement into fresh extraction sockets preserves buccal alveolar bone: a cone beam computed tomography study. Int J Periodontics Restorative Dent. 2014;34(1):61–8.
18. Morimoto T, Tsukiyama Y, Morimoto K, Koyano K. Facial bone alterations on maxillary anterior single implants for immediate placement and provisionalization following tooth extraction: a superimposed cone beam computed tomography study. Clin Oral Implants Res. 2015;26(12):1383–9.
19. Roe P, Kan JY, Rungcharassaeng K, Caruso JM, Zimmerman G, Mesquida J. Horizontal and vertical dimensional changes of peri-implant facial bone following immediate placement and provisionalization of maxillary anterior single implants: a 1-year cone beam computed tomography study. Int J Oral Maxillofac Implants. 2012;27(2):393–400.
20. Cooper LF, Reside GJ, Raes F, Garriga JS, Tarrida LG, Wiltfang J, Kern M, De Bruyn H. Immediate provisionalization of dental implants placed in healed alveolar ridges and extraction sockets: a 5-year prospective evaluation. Int J Oral Maxillofac Implants. 2014;29(3):709–17.
21. Kan JY, Rungcharassaeng K, Lozada JL, Zimmerman G. Facial gingival tissue stability following immediate placement and provisionalization of maxillary anterior single implants: a 2- to 8-year follow-up. Int J Oral Maxillofac Implants. 2011;26(1):179–87.
22. Malchiodi L, Cucchi A, Ghensi P, Nocini PF. Evaluation of the esthetic results of 64 nonfunctional immediately loaded postextraction implants in the maxilla: correlation between interproximal alveolar crest and soft tissues at 3 years of follow-up. Clin Implant Dent Relat Res. 2013;15(1):130–42.
23. Araújo MG, Sukekava F, Wennström JL, Lindhe J. Ridge alterations following implant placement in fresh extraction sockets: an experimental study in the dog. J Clin Periodontol. 2005;32(6):645–52.
24. Botticelli D, Berglundh T, Lindhe J. Hard-tissue alterations following immediate implant placement in extraction sites. J Clin Periodontol. 2004;31(10):820–8.
25. Carlsson GE, Bergman B, Hedegård B. Changes in contour of the maxillary alveolar process under immediate dentures. A longitudinal clinical and x-ray cephalometric study covering 5 years. Acta Odontol Scand. 1967;25(1):45–75.
26. Chen ST, Darby IB, Reynolds EC. A prospective clinical study of non-submerged immediate implants: clinical outcomes and esthetic results. Clin Oral Implants Res. 2007;18(5):552–62.
27. Degidi M, Daprile G, Nardi D, Piattelli A. Immediate provisionalization of implants placed in fresh extraction sockets using a definitive abutment: the chamber concept. Int J Periodontics Restorative Dent. 2013;33(5):559–65.
28. Demircan S, Demircan E. Dental cone beam computed tomography analyses of the anterior maxillary bone thickness for immediate implant placement. Implant Dent. 2015;24(6):664–8.
29. Sanz M, Cecchinato D, Ferrus J, Pjetursson EB, Lang NP, Lindhe J. A prospective, randomized-controlled clinical trial to evaluate bone preservation using implants with different geometry placed into extraction sockets in the maxilla. Clin Oral Implants Res. 2010;21(1):13–21.
30. Vera C, De Kok IJ, Reinhold D, Limpiphipatanakorn P, Yap AK, Tyndall D, Cooper LF. Evaluation of buccal alveolar bone dimension of maxillary anterior and premolar teeth: a cone beam computed tomography investigation. Int J Oral Maxillofac Implants. 2012;27(6):1514–9.

31. Arora H, Ivanovski S. Correlation between pre-operative buccal bone thickness and soft tissue changes around immediately placed and restored implants in the maxillary anterior region: a 2-year prospective study. Clin Oral Implants Res. 2016;29:1188–94. [Epub ahead of print].
32. Ferrus J, Cecchinato D, Pjetursson EB, Lang NP, Sanz M, Lindhe J. Factors influencing ridge alterations following immediate implant placement into extraction sockets. Clin Oral Implants Res. 2010;21(1):22–9.
33. Tarnow DP, Chu SJ. Human histologic verification of osseointegration of an immediate implant placed into a fresh extraction socket with excessive gap distance without primary flap closure, graft, or membrane: a case report. Int J Periodontics Restorative Dent. 2011;31(5):515–21.
34. Grunder U, Gracis S, Capelli M. Influence of the 3-D bone-to-implant relationship on esthetics. Int J Periodontics Restorative Dent. 2005;25(2):113–9.
35. Spray JR, Black CG, Morris HF, Ochi S. The influence of bone thickness on facial marginal bone response: stage 1 placement through stage 2 uncovering. Ann Periodontol. 2000;5(1):119–28.
36. Zhang W, Skrypczak A, Weltman R. Anterior maxilla alveolar ridge dimension and morphology measurement by cone beam computerized tomography (CBCT) for immediate implant treatment planning. BMC Oral Health. 2015;15:65.
37. Kan JY, Roe P, Rungcharassaeng K, Patel RD, Waki T, Lozada JL, Zimmerman G. Classification of sagittal root position in relation to the anterior maxillary osseous housing for immediate implant placement: a cone beam computed tomography study. Int J Oral Maxillofac Implants. 2011;26(4):873–6.
38. Chung SH, Park YS, Chung SH, Shon WJ. Determination of implant position for immediate implant placement in maxillary central incisors using palatal soft tissue landmarks. Int J Oral Maxillofac Implants. 2014;29(3):627–33.
39. Chappuis V, Bornstein MM, Buser D, Belser U. Influence of implant neck design on facial bone crest dimensions in the esthetic zone analyzed by cone beam CT: a comparative study with a 5-to-9-year follow-up. Clin Oral Implants Res. 2016;27(9):1055–64.
40. Rosa AC, da Rosa JC, Dias Pereira LA, Francischone CE, Sotto-Maior BS. Guidelines for selecting the implant diameter during immediate implant placement of a fresh extraction socket: a case series. Int J Periodontics Restorative Dent. 2016;36(3):401–7.
41. Jensen OT. Dental extraction, immediate placement of dental implants, and immediate function. Oral Maxillofac Surg Clin North Am. 2015;27(2):273–82.
42. Koh RU, Rudek I, Wang HL. Immediate implant placement: positives and negatives. Implant Dent. 2010;19(2):98–108.
43. Kois JC. Predictable single-tooth peri-implant esthetics: five diagnostic keys. Compend Contin Educ Dent. 2004;25(11):895–6. 898, 900 passim; quiz 906–7.
44. Kan JY, Morimoto T, Rungcharassaeng K, Roe P, Smith DH. Gingival biotype assessment in the esthetic zone: visual versus direct measurement. Int J Periodontics Restorative Dent. 2010;30(3):237–43.
45. Lemes HD, Sartori IA, Cardoso LC, Ponzoni D. Behaviour of the buccal crestal bone levels after immediate placement of implants subjected to immediate loading. Int J Oral Maxillofac Surg. 2015;44(3):389–94.
46. Olsson M, Lindhe J, Marinello CP. On the relationship between crown form and clinical features of the gingiva in adolescents. J Clin Periodontol. 1993;20(8):570–7.
47. Seibert J, Lindhe J. Esthetics and periodontal therapy. In: Lindhe J, editor. Textbook of clinical periodontology. 2nd ed. Copenhagen: Munksgaard; 1989. p. 477–514.
48. Weisgold A. Gmtoun of the full crown restoration. Alpha Omegan. 1977;10:77–89.
49. Schropp L, Wenzel A. Timing of single implant placement and long-term observation of marginal bone levels. Eur J Oral Implantol. 2016;9(Suppl 1):107–22.
50. Berberi AN, Sabbagh JM, Aboushelib MN, Noujeim ZF, Salameh ZA. A 5-year comparison of marginal bone level following immediate loading of single-tooth implants placed in healed alveolar ridges and extraction sockets in the maxilla. Front Physiol. 2014;5:29.
51. De Rouck T, Collys K, Wyn I, Cosyn J. Instant provisionalization of immediate single-tooth implants is essential to optimize esthetic treatment outcome. Clin Oral Implants Res. 2009;20(6):566–70.

52. Gamborena I, Blatz MB. Evolution, contemporary protocols for anterior single-tooth implants. IL: Quintessence Publishing; 2015. p. 163–322.
53. Schoenbaum TR, Chang YY, Klokkevold PR, Snowden JS. Abutment emergence modification for immediate implant provisional restorations. J Esthet Restor Dent. 2013;25(2):103–7.
54. Su H, Gonzalez-Martin O, Weisgold A, Lee E. Considerations of implant abutment and crown contour: critical contour and subcritical contour. Int J Periodontics Restorative Dent. 2010;30(4):335–43.
55. Urban IA, Klokkevold PR, Takei HH. Abutment-supported papilla: a combined surgical and prosthetic approach to papilla reformation. Int J Periodontics Restorative Dent. 2016;36(5):665–71.
56. Tarnow DP, Chu SJ, Salama MA, Stappert CF, Salama H, Garber DA, Sarnachiaro GO, Sarnachiaro E, Gotta SL, Saito H. Flapless postextraction socket implant placement in the esthetic zone: part 1. The effect of bone grafting and/or provisional restoration on facial-palatal ridge dimensional change-a retrospective cohort study. Int J Periodontics Restorative Dent. 2014;34(3):323–31.
57. Chu SJ, Salama MA, Garber DA, Salama H, Sarnachiaro GO, Sarnachiaro E, Gotta SL, Reynolds MA, Saito H, Tarnow DP. Flapless postextraction socket implant placement, part 2: the effects of bone grafting and provisional restoration on peri-implant soft tissue height and thickness- a retrospective study. Int J Periodontics Restorative Dent. 2015;35(6):803–9.
58. Vignoletti F, Sanz M. Immediate implants at fresh extraction sockets: from myth to reality. Periodontol. 2014;66(1):132–52.
59. Langer B, Langer L. Subepithelial connective tissue graft technique for root coverage. J Periodontol. 1985;56(12):715–20.
60. Ross SB, Pette GA, Parker WB, Hardigan P. Gingival margin changes in maxillary anterior sites after single immediate implant placement and provisionalization: a 5-year retrospective study of 47 patients. Int J Oral Maxillofac Implants. 2014;29(1):127–34.
61. Rungcharassaeng K, Kan JY, Yoshino S, Morimoto T, Zimmerman G. Immediate implant placement and provisionalization with and without a connective tissue graft: an analysis of facial gingival tissue thickness. Int J Periodontics Restorative Dent. 2012;32(6):657–63.
62. Horváth A, Mardas N, Mezzomo LA, Needleman IG, Donos N. Alveolar ridge preservation. A systematic review. Clin Oral Investig. 2013;17(2):341–63.
63. MacBeth N, Trullenque-Eriksson A, Donos N, Mardas N. Hard and soft tissue changes following alveolar ridge preservation: a systematic review. Clin Oral Implants Res. 2016;26:982–1004. [Epub ahead of print] Review.
64. Mardas N, Trullenque-Eriksson A, MacBeth N, Petrie A, Donos N. Does ridge preservation following tooth extraction improve implant treatment outcomes: a systematic review: group 4: therapeutic concepts & methods. Clin Oral Implants Res. 2015;26(Suppl 11):180–201.
65. Sottosanti JS. Aesthetic extractions with calcium sulfate and the principles of guided tissue regeneration. Pract Periodontics Aesthet Dent. 1993;5(5):61–9. quiz 69.
66. Iasella JM, Greenwell H, Miller RL, Hill M, Drisko C, Bohra AA, Scheetz JP. Ridge preservation with freeze-dried bone allograft and a collagen membrane compared to extraction alone for implant site development: a clinical and histologic study in humans. J Periodontol. 2003;74(7):990–9.
67. Lekovic V, Kenney EB, Weinlaender M, Han T, Klokkevold P, Nedic M, Orsini M. A bone regenerative approach to alveolar ridge maintenance following tooth extraction. Report of 10 cases. J Periodontol. 1997;68(6):563–70.
68. Saadoun AP, Le Gall MG, Touati B. Current trends in implantology: part II--treatment planning, aesthetic considerations, and tissue regeneration. Pract Proced Aesthet Dent. 2004;16(10):707–14. quiz 716.
69. Al-Sabbagh M. Implants in the Esthetic Zone. Dent Clin. 2006;50(3):391–407.
70. Schoenbaum TR, Chang YY. Dentist-technician collaboration in the digital age: enhancing outcomes through photography, teamwork, and technology. J Calif Dent Assoc. 2011;39(8):559–67.
71. Zadeh HH. Implant site development: clinical realities of today and the prospects of tissue engineering. J Calif Dent Assoc. 2004;32(12):1011–20.

72. Maló P, de Araújo Nobre M, Lopes A, Francischone C, Rigolizzo M. "All-on-4" immediate-function concept for completely edentulous maxillae: a clinical report on the medium (3 years) and long-term (5 years) outcomes. Clin Implant Dent Relat Res. 2012;14(Suppl 1):e139–50.
73. Maló P, de Araújo Nobre M, Lopes A, Ferro A, Gravito I. All-on-4® treatment concept for the rehabilitation of the completely edentulous mandible: a 7-year clinical and 5-year radiographic retrospective case series with risk assessment for implant failure and marginal bone level. Clin Implant Dent Relat Res. 2015;17(Suppl 2):e531–41.

Guided Bone Regeneration (GBR) for Implants in the Aesthetic Zone

4

Joan Pi-Anfruns and Bach Le

Abstract

Guided bone regeneration follows the principles of guided tissue regeneration, where an occlusive membrane is utilized to provide a barrier and allow bone regeneration to occur at a specific oral defect. Particulate bone substitutes are utilized to provide a scaffold and direct bone formation, which will occur by subsequent remodeling of the graft material. The success of the grafting procedure is directly dependent on a number of factors, including the host's ability to heal, the proper execution of the procedure, and the materials utilized. Adequate postoperative management, including administration of antibiotics and regular follow-ups, will minimize the incidence of complications. With a success rate above 90%, guided bone regeneration procedures have become a predictable approach to regenerate deficient sites for the dental implant patient.

4.1 Historical Background of GBR

Bone grafting is an essential component of the surgeon's armamentarium for successful treatment outcomes in implant dentistry. Deficiencies of the maxillary and mandibular arches may occur as a result of dental extractions and as residual defects following surgical treatment of pathology, congenital alveolar defects, and trauma.

J. Pi-Anfruns (✉)
Division of Diagnostic and Surgical Sciences, Division of Regenerative and Constitutive Sciences, Dental Implant Center, UCLA School of Dentistry, Los Angeles, CA, USA
e-mail: jpianfruns@dentistry.ucla.edu

B. Le
Department of Oral and Maxillofacial Surgery, Herman Ostrow School of Dentistry at USC, Los Angeles, CA, USA

Private Practice, Whittier, CA, USA

Todd R. Schoenbaum (ed.), *Implants in the Aesthetic Zone*,
https://doi.org/10.1007/978-3-319-72601-4_4

Subsequently, regenerative procedures in the form of bone grafts are often performed to solve these problems. Guided bone regeneration (GBR) is a technique by which barrier membranes are utilized in combination with particulate bone substitutes to direct the formation of new bone. The principles of GBR are based on the concept of guided tissue regeneration (GTR), where unwanted epithelial cells are prevented from entering the site of bone regeneration. Melcher [1] first described the concept of GTR in 1976, showing that the repair potential of periodontal tissues depended on the cell type allowed to repopulate an exposed root surface, defining the nature of the attachment. These findings were later confirmed by Nyman and co-workers [2], confirming that new connective tissue attachment could form on a previously periodontally involved root surface, provided cells that originated from the periodontal ligament were enabled to repopulate the root surface during healing. In 1988, Dahlin and co-workers [3] applied the same principles of GTR for the healing of bone defects, demonstrating that when fibroblasts and other connective tissue cells were prevented from entering a bone defect, bone regeneration was possible by repopulation of cells of osteogenic potential. Subsequent to this development, the term guided bone regeneration was born.

4.2 Rationale and Biological Principles of GBR

The effects of bone remodeling following tooth extraction may prevent dental implant placement and compromise functional and aesthetic outcomes. Guided bone regeneration in association with dental implant procedures can be utilized to augment deficient alveolar ridges, cover implant fenestrations and dehiscences, allow immediate implant placement in residual osseous defects and post-extraction sites, and treat peri-implant disease [4]. These defects can be localized to a single tooth or extend to multiple teeth. Horizontal defects around implants will lead to thread exposure, dehiscence, or fenestration, most commonly on the buccal surface. Vertical defects around implants will lead to placement of shorter implants than desired, long clinical crowns, increased functional demands, and unaesthetic results.

As with native bone repair, grafted bone heals in three major phases: inflammation, proliferation, and remodeling. Guided bone regeneration is based on the concept of using a resorbable or non-resorbable barrier membrane to stabilize the blood clot and create a space into which bone cells can grow without interference of the faster proliferating soft tissue cells [3].

4.3 Preoperative Evaluation for the Aesthetic Zone

The proper placement and successful restoration of a dental implant is directly dependent on a three-dimensional evaluation of the alveolar bone morphology and soft tissue contours. This prosthetically driven approach as described in Chap. 1 is dictated by the aesthetic and functional demands of the restoration and soft tissue. The preoperative evaluation can be divided into three phases: laboratory, clinical, and radiographic.

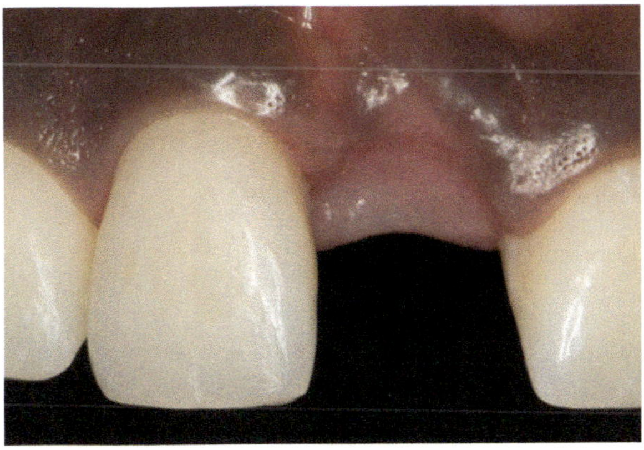

Fig. 4.1 Evaluation of edentulous site #9. Thick biotype present with adequate zone of keratinized mucosa will make successful outcomes more predictable

The laboratory evaluation involves obtaining study models and generating a pre-prosthetic wax-up. This wax-up should include both the deficient ridge and teeth to be restored. From this wax-up, a radiographic guide is fabricated.

The clinical evaluation should include an assessment of the thickness (biotype) and width of soft tissue, gingival display at maximum smile, smile line, lip support, and position of the adjacent teeth. Thick biotype and abundant keratinized tissue is preferred for optimal aesthetic outcomes (Fig. 4.1).

In situations where the soft tissue is not adequate (<2 mm width or thin biotype), soft tissue grafting procedures to improve the quality and quantity are recommended prior to guided bone regeneration procedures.

The radiographic evaluation is done in three dimensions utilizing a CBCT with the radiographic guide as described in Chap. 2. The advancements in cone-beam computerized tomography (CBCT) allow clinicians to plan and execute procedures with high levels of accuracy, precision, and predictability, improving outcomes in highly demanding situations as in the aesthetic zone.

4.4 Flap Design and Soft Tissue Considerations

The success of guided bone regeneration procedures is greatly dependent on a thorough assessment and careful management of the soft tissue of the recipient site. An adequate zone of keratinized gingiva (KG) is key to providing stability to the wound edges. A minimum width of 2 mm of KG is required at each wound edge. Moreover, the biotype of the surrounding soft tissue will also influence the success of the procedure. Flaps that are less than 1.2 mm thick are more susceptible to wound dehiscence [5], the most commonly encountered complication, which will compromise the success of GBR.

Primary wound closure, tension-free adaptation of the wound edges, and undisturbed healing are key to successful regeneration of the deficient site. Therefore, a proper flap design should be planned. In anticipation of the augmentation procedure, the flap should have enough freedom or mobility to allow tension-free closure. The crestal incision should extend at least to one adjacent tooth to each side. The

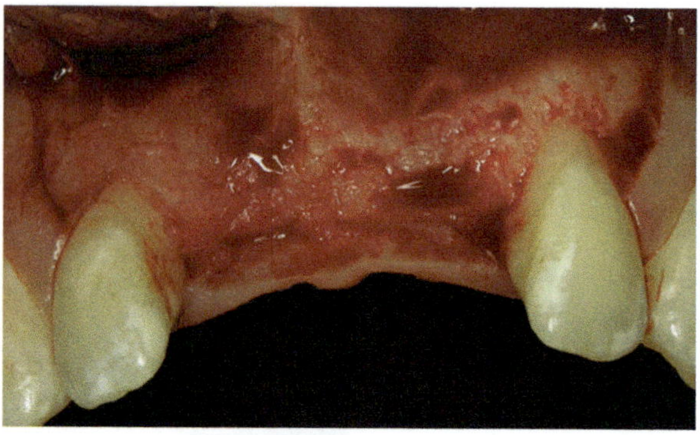

Fig. 4.2 Flap design for GBR. Extension of the flap to one adjacent tooth. The placement of vertical releasing incisions at the distobuccal line angles and wide-based trapezoid-designed flap are crucial to successful GBR

vertical releasing incisions should be placed away from the aesthetic zone whenever possible and at the distobuccal line angles of the adjacent teeth. In aesthetic areas, papilla-sparring incisions should be used to prevent papilla loss around the adjacent teeth. The flap should be trapezoid-shaped with a wide base to ensure adequate blood supply (Fig. 4.2).

4.5 Preparation of the Recipient Site

Preparation of the recipient site is another key factor in successful GBR procedures. During guided bone regeneration, vascular channels (several small perforations of the cortical bone at the recipient site) are recommended. The biological rationale for this is to access the bone marrow space, increasing blood supply and facilitating the migration of cells and nutrients into the defect site [6–8]. In an animal study utilizing a GBR model, Lee and co-workers showed that perforations of the recipient bed improved neo-angiogenesis in bone grafts and increased osteoneogenesis, especially in the early healing phase. Moreover, the vascular channels will in turn increase the number of osteoclastic tunnels or cutting cones [9, 10]. These cutting cones are essential in bone remodeling because they are immediately followed by capillaries and osteoblasts, which lay down the osteoid to fill the cutting cone.

These vascular channels can be rounded perforations of 1–2 mm in diameter or longitudinal channels and can be created using a wide range of instruments. Bone scrapers, fissure burs, and ultrasonic cutting devices have all been utilized for this purpose. Regardless of the instrument used or shape of the perforation, the depth of the channels must penetrate into the marrow space, allowing for blood flow into the grafted site (Fig. 4.3).

When creating the vascular channels, care should be taken not to damage the adjacent teeth, nerves, vessels, or flap itself during preparation.

4.6 Graft Materials and Selection

An ideal bone graft material possesses the three characteristics of bone formation: osteogenesis, osteoinduction, and osteoconduction. Osteogenesis refers to the

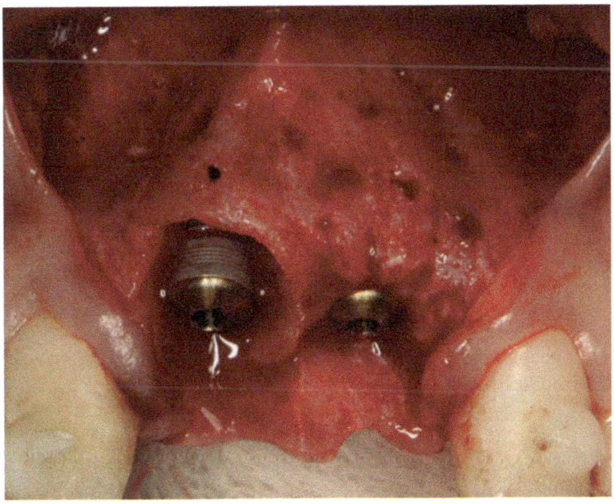

Fig. 4.3 Vascular channels created with a #1 round bur to provide additional blood supply to the grafted site. Note the active bleeding from within the medullary space. With simultaneous implant placement, vascular channels should be created prior to implant placement to avoid damage to the implant surface

B.G. ~ 4 months healing

natural process of bone formation. Osteoinduction is the process by which osteogenesis is induced, and it implies the recruitment of immature cells and the stimulation of these cells to develop into preosteoblasts. Osteoconduction refers to the provision of a scaffold which bone can grow into.

As with normal bone repair, bone grafts heal in three major phases: inflammation, proliferation, and remodeling [11–15]. The inflammatory phase begins immediately following the injury and will continue for about 5 days. Inflammation is caused by blood vessel injury and triggers hemostasis. During this phase, the action of the platelets and vasoconstriction will allow a blood clot to form, initiating the healing process. At this stage, neutrophils and macrophages debride the wound site, reducing the bacterial load. The proliferation phase of graft healing will last about 3 weeks and result in the production of a disorganized osteoid or new bone woven by the bone graft cells. In the remodeling phase that follows, the immature bone is resorbed and replaced by organized lamellar bone. The entire process may take months, depending on the patient and the characteristics of the bone graft material used for regeneration.

Bone grafts can be classified according to the source from which they were obtained. Autogenous grafts are composed of bone harvested from the patient being treated, allografts are taken from another individual of the same species (cadaver), xenografts are from a different species than the recipient (animal), and alloplastic grafts are composed of synthetic materials (Table 4.1).

Bone graft substitutes vary in origin, composition, structure, particle size, and resorption time. A single bone graft material can be selected, or a combination of materials can be used to maximize specific properties of each material [16, 17]. Ideally, the resorption rate of any bone graft substitute should be similar to that of new bone formation. Resorption rates will be influenced by certain properties of the material such as crystallinity, particle size, surface area, and porosity but also by local factors like pH, presence of cells, water content, and the overall healing capacity of the patient [18]. Autogenous bone has a higher and more unpredictable resorption rate than other materials and is not recommended for use alone in GBR procedures [19]. Xenografts, on the

Don't use autogenous — mix w/ xenograft

Table 4.1 Resorption rates of various particulate graft materials from fastest (green) to slowest (red)

AUTOGENOUS	same individual
ALLOGRAFT	different individual
ALLOPLAST	synthetic materials
XENOGRAFTS	different species

No one material is ideal for all clinical scenarios, and the material should be selected based on the desired resorption rate

other hand, have shown to retain their overall volume stability for as long as 11 years [19, 20], though this may not be desirable in all clinical situations.

The presence of pores in bone graft substitutes is essential for new bone formation because they allow migration and proliferation of cells, thus promoting angiogenesis. In addition, a porous surface improves mechanical interlocking between the bone graft substitute and the surrounding natural bone, providing greater mechanical stability at this critical interface [21]. The micro- and macroporosity of the graft particle will influence the bioresorbability of the material. The recommended pore size range for a bone substitute is 100–400 μm [22]. It has been shown that a higher porosity leads to faster osteogenesis, likely due to a larger surface area [23]. The structure of the pores is another key factor that determines the effectiveness of the biomaterial. The pores may either be part of a network (interconnected) or contained. Interconnected pores have been shown to be advantageous because a continuous porous structure facilitates the ingrowth of new bone [24].

The selection of a bone graft material depends on several factors. The rate of resorption of the graft material and the shape and size of the defect are important factors to consider when deciding what type of graft material is best suited. As mentioned, autogenous bone alone should not be used for GBR because of its very fast resorption rate. It does, however, provide viable nutrients when used in combination with other graft materials. Xenografts, on the other hand, have no viable cells but will provide the longest volumetric stability over time. Therefore, these materials can be combined to provide the best environment for new bone formation based on their combined ability to provide and recruit the necessary cells and to protect the augmentation volume over time. In regard to the shape and size of the defect, a circumferential or four-wall defect is more favorable than a two- or one-wall defect, and a single tooth defect is more favorable than several adjacent missing teeth.

4.7 Barrier Membranes

The biologic principle of GBR relies on the use of a mechanical barrier to protect the blood clot, isolate the bony defect, prevent penetration of connective tissue, and allow bone precursor cells to populate the defect. Barrier membranes can be

Table 4.2 Advantages and disadvantages of resorbable and non-resorbable membranes for use in GBR

RESORBABLE MEMBRANES		NON-RESORBABLE MEMBRANES	
Advantages	**Disadvantages**	**Advantages**	**Disadvantages**
• eliminates need for removal surgery • lower cost • lower complication rates	• unpredictable degree of resorption • unfavorable mechanical properties • not indicated for large grafts	• space maintaining • occlusive yet allow cell migration	• require removal • higher cost • higher complication rates

Note that individual patient needs and clinician preferences will strongly influence material selection

resorbable or non-resorbable, and their selection should vary depending on the nature of the defect to be regenerated. For instance, in cases were a localized horizontal deficiency requires a minor GBR procedure, a resorbable membrane can be utilized. If the defect is vertical or a combined vertical-horizontal defect, then a non-resorbable reinforced membrane is recommended to provide additional support and prevent collapse. Barrier membranes should be trimmed and rounded to remove any sharp edges in order to prevent perforation of the soft tissues. This is especially important with non-resorbable membranes and titanium mesh (Table 4.2).

4.7.1 Resorbable Membranes

Resorbable membranes currently used in GBR are made of natural or synthetic polymers. The most common used are collagen and aliphatic polyesters (polyglycolide or polylactide). Collagen membranes are most commonly manufactured from type I collagen of bovine or equine origin. These membranes can be treated chemically or by radiation to strengthen the bonds of the collagen fibers, extending their resorption times. This process is known as *cross-linking*. Some collagen membranes can be side-specific, where a specific side is intended to face the bone or soft tissue. These are usually indicated by the manufacturer, and one should ensure the proper application of these membranes. Resorbable synthetic membranes, as those made of polylactide or polyglycolide, have extended resorption times and resorb via hydrolytic degradation. Their handling and clinical manageability are more complex, making them less user-friendly and therefore less popular than the above.

4.7.2 Non-resorbable Membranes

Currently available non-resorbable membranes consist of titanium mesh and polytetrafluoroethylene (PTFE). First introduced in 1969 by Boyne et al. [25], titanium mesh has excellent mechanical properties for the stabilization of bone grafts, but its rigidity, stiffness, and sharp edges lead to significantly higher incidences of exposure. Similarly, its higher macroporosity makes it more challenging to remove, as the soft tissue integrates with the pores and becomes embedded to the mesh.

High-density PTFE (d-PTFE) membranes have been well documented since their introduction in 1993 [26, 27]. With a submicron pore size of 0.2 μm, bacterial

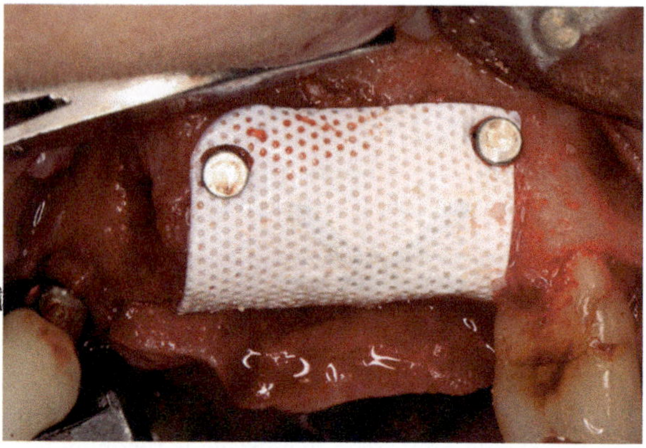

Fig. 4.4 Non-resorbable, titanium-reinforced d-PTFE membrane secured with two fixation pins for horizontal and vertical GBR in the anterior maxilla prior to implant placement

infiltration into the bone augmentation site is eliminated, protecting the underlying graft material. Another advantage of this type of membrane is that soft tissue does not attach to the surface, making it easy to remove by pulling on the membrane.

4.7.3 Fixation

Fixation of the membrane will be required in certain clinical situations where additional support is needed to stabilize the graft. In small, self-contained defects where a resorbable membrane is utilized, stabilization may not be required (one- or two-teeth defect). In contrast, larger defects where a non-resorbable membrane is need for support, fixation of the membrane is required in order to prevent it from moving during healing. Stability of the graft material is crucial to successful GBR. Fixation can be achieved with tacks, pins, or screws. Tacks and pins have similar designs and therefore behave similarly. Some incorporate a retentive element that can provide additional retention, ideal in cases where a non-resorbable membrane is required. Fixation screws, on the other hand, are generally reserved for titanium mesh and can be harder to remove as they may become partially buried by newly formed bone (Fig. 4.4).

Membranes utilized in GBR, regardless of their composition, must fulfill the following five features in order to achieve successful bone regeneration [28]:

4.8 Biocompatibility

Barrier membranes should not be harmful to the surrounding living tissues or the patient.

4.9 Create and Maintain a Space for Bony Ingrowth

Maintenance of a suitable space for regeneration is a key factor to successful GBR. Membrane thickness, composition, and stiffness will determine the support provided to the site. If the membrane selected is not able to maintain the desired space, it may affect the outcome of the grafting procedure. Flexible membranes such as those made of resorbable collagen may need the support of fixation pins or tenting screws to provide adequate space for successful regeneration.

4.10 Occlusivity

Periosteum – supplies nutrients for bone formation

The occlusivity of the membrane is determined by its porosity and the ability to avoid fibrous tissue formation within the site. On the other hand, membrane pores facilitate the diffusion of critical fluids, oxygen, and nutrients from the periosteum, which are vital for bone formation. Large pores will allow the penetration of faster-moving cells (epithelial cells or gingival fibroblasts) and provide an easier pathway for bacterial contamination. If the pores are too small, on the other hand, it may inhibit nutrient exchange to the site. Currently available membranes for GBR contain pores that allow nutrient exchange while excluding soft tissue cells.

4.11 Tissue Integration

Tissue integration is key in stabilizing the healing wound process. The barrier membrane must be able to adapt to the borders of the neighboring bone. A membrane that is too stiff is not able to adapt to the contours of the recipient site. Poorly adapted membranes cannot fully prevent migration of soft tissues into the graft site and are more likely to perforate through the flaps during healing.

4.12 Clinical Manageability

Barrier membranes need to be manageable during the surgical procedure. If a membrane is too stiff, it may not be easily contoured, and its sharp edges are more likely to lead to perforation of the soft tissue. On the other hand, softer membranes are more difficult to handle once hydrated.

4.13 Suturing Principles for GBR

Adequate approximation and closure of the wound edges is fundamental to successful GBR procedures and requires the use of sutures. Sutures should be biocompatible, retain adequate strength during the critical period of healing, and induce minimal tissue reactions [29]. Sutures are made from resorbable or non-resorbable materials and may be fabricated by either mono- or multifilament fibers [30]. Studies have shown that multifilament, braided sutures (i.e., silk) are more likely to be contaminated by bacteria than monofilament sutures [31, 32], which induces increased inflammation.

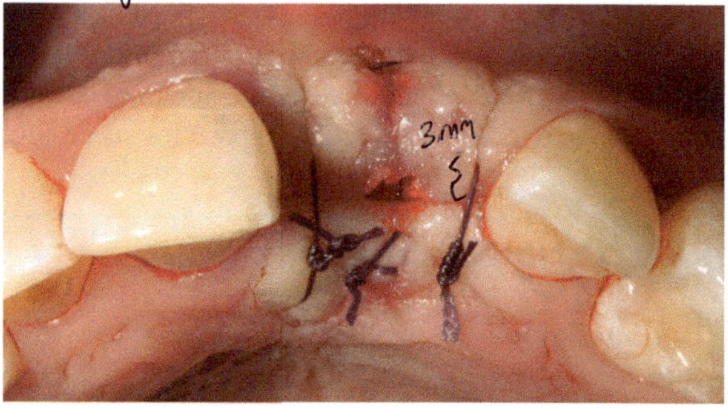

Fig. 4.5 Closure of flap following GBR for horizontal augmentation provided by one horizontal mattress suture in the center of the wound and two single interrupted sutures at the wound edges

Another important aspect of suturing is tension control. High tensions exerted by sutures and applied to the wound edges may lead to tearing of the soft tissue margins [33]. These soft tissue dehiscences may prolong the healing time [34], cause additional resorption of the underlying bone [35], jeopardize the healing results [36], create irregular soft tissue contours, and result in an overall reduction of the final graft volume.

Vascularity of the wound edges is another key factor for successful wound closure. Sutures that are placed too tight and in high quantities will compromise the microperfusion and restrict blood supply. Reduced blood supply to the wound edges will compromise the success of GBR treatment.

Closure of the flaps in GBR should be achieved first with horizontal mattress sutures to create two contact surfaces of at least 3 mm thick, followed by alternating single interrupted sutures [37] (Fig 4.5).

4.14 Postoperative Care

Following guided bone regeneration procedures, as with any bone grafting procedure, oral antibiotics and pain medication should be prescribed to prevent infection and manage postoperative pain.

Postoperative edema, hematoma, and bleeding are common with GBR, and patients should be advised accordingly. Patients should avoid using a toothbrush directly around the wound for at least 1 week to prevent wound dehiscence. Rinses with a bacteriostatic/bactericidal agent are recommended to minimize bacterial accumulation on sutures.

A non-chewing diet should be recommended, and the use of a removable prosthesis over the grafted site is strongly discouraged. Unless otherwise indicated, follow-ups should occur at 1–2 weeks after surgery to monitor wound healing. Sutures should not be removed before 1 week, and it is recommended to maintain them for 2 weeks whenever possible.

4.15 Complications and Management

Wound dehiscence and membrane exposure is the most commonly reported complication in GBR procedures [38], followed by infection [39]. In order to prevent wound dehiscence, several factors may be considered:

4.15.1 Preoperative Factors

Some systemic diseases like diabetes mellitus and chronic corticosteroid therapy will jeopardize healing. Social habits like smoking, excess alcohol consumption, and recreational drug use can also interfere in the wound healing process. Patients in this group should be instructed on proper oral hygiene habits prior to surgery to minimize plaque accumulation and bacterial contamination.

4.15.2 Intraoperative Factors

As with any other surgical procedure, adequate flap design and clean and sharp incisions should be considered. Adequate muscle and flap release should allow sufficient flap elongation to achieve tension-free closure. Moreover, soft tissues should be handled gently to prevent tearing. As discussed, adequate barrier fixation and mattress sutures will prevent displacement of the membrane and further prevent wound dehiscence.

4.15.3 Postoperative Factors

Instruction of proper oral hygiene habits will minimize plaque accumulation and bacterial contamination during the postoperative period. Antibiotic and anti-inflammatory medication can reduce the chances of infection and reduce wound tension. Removable prosthesis that applies pressure to the site should be avoided to minimize movement of the membrane and graft.

References

1. Melcher AH. On the repair potential of periodontal tissues. J Periodontol. 1976;47(5):256–60.
2. Nyman S, et al. New attachment following surgical treatment of human periodontal disease. J Clin Periodontol. 1982;9(4):290–6.
3. Dahlin C, et al. Healing of bone defects by guided tissue regeneration. Plast Reconstr Surg. 1988;81(5):672–6.

4. Simion M, Trisi P, Piattelli A. Vertical ridge augmentation using a membrane technique associated with osseointegrated implants. Int J Periodontics Restorative Dent. 1994;14(6):496–511.
5. Burkhardt R, Lang NP. Role of flap tension in primary wound closure of mucoperiosteal flaps: a prospective cohort study. Clin Oral Implants Res. 2010;21:50–4.
6. Lee SH, Lim P, Yoon HJ. The influence of cortical perforation on guided bone regeneration using synthetic bone substitutes: a study of rabbit cranial defects. Int J Oral Maxillofac Implants. 2014;29:464–71.
7. Nishimura I, Shimizu Y, Ooya K. Effects of cortical bone perforation on experimental guided bone regeneration. Clin Oral Implants Res. 2004;15:293–300.
8. Hämmerle CH, Schmid J, Lang NP, Olah AJ. Temporal dynamics of healing in rabbit cranial defects using guided bone regeneration. J Oral Maxillofac Surg. 1995;53:167–74.
9. Cha JK, Kim CS, Choi SH, Cho KS, Chai JK, Jung UW. The influence of perforating the autogenous block bone and the recipient bed in dogs. Part II: histologic analysis. Clin Oral Implants Res. 2012;23:987–92.
10. Shapiro F. Cortical bone repair. The relationship of the lacunar-canalicular system and intercellular gap junctions to the repair process. J Bone Joint Surg Am. 1988;70:1067–81.
11. Siddiqui NA, Owen JM. Clinical advances in bone regeneration. Curr Stem Cell Res Ther. 2013;8:192.
12. Roberts TT, Rosenbaum AJ. Bone grafts, bone substitutes and orthobiologics: the bridge between basic science and clinical advancements in fracture healing. Organogenesis. 2012;8:114.
13. Einhorn TA. The cell and molecular biology of fracture healing. Clin Orthop Relat Res. 1998;355:S7.
14. Aghaloo T, Felsenfeld AL. Principles of repair and grafting of bone and cartilage. In: Bagheri SC, Horswell BB, Khan HA, editors. Current therapy in oral and maxillofacial surgery. Philadelphia: Saunders; 2012.
15. Ulma R, Aghaloo T, Freymiller E. Wound healing. In: Fonseca RJ, Barber HD, Powers MP, Frost DE, editors. Oral and maxillofacial trauma. 4th ed. St. Louis: Elsevier; 2013. p. 9.
16. Urban IA, Nagursky H, Lozada JL, Nagy K. Horizontal ridge augmentation with a collagen membrane and a combination of particulated autogenous bone and anorganic bovine bone-derived mineral: a prospective case series in 25 patients. Int J Periodontics Restorative Dent. 2013;33:299.
17. Rickert D, Sauerbier S, Nagursky H, Menne D, Vissink A, Raghoebar GM. Maxillary sinus floor elevation with bovine bone mineral combined with either autogenous bone or autogenous stem cells: a prospective randomized clinical trial. Clin Oral Implants Res. 2011;22:251.
18. LeGeros RZ. Properties of osteoconductive biomaterials: calcium phosphates. Clin Orthop Relat Res. 2002;395:81–98.
19. Mordenfeld A, Hallman M, Johansson CB, Albrektsson T. Histological and histomorphometrical analyses of biopsies harvested 11 years after maxillary sinus floor augmentation with deproteinized bovine and autogenous bone. Clin Oral Implants Res. 2010;21(9):961–70.
20. Lundgren S, Cricchio G, Hallman M, Jungner M, Rasmusson L, Sennerby L. Sinus floor elevation procedures to enable implant placement and integration: techniques, biological aspects and clinical outcomes. Periodontol. 2017;73(1):103–20.
21. Karageorgiou V, Kaplan D. Porosity of 3D biomaterial scaffolds and osteogenesis. Biomaterials. 2005;26:5474–91.
22. Hannink G, Arts JJC. Bioresorbability, porosity and mechanical strength of bone substitutes: what is optimal for bone regeneration? Injury. 2011;42:S22–5.
23. Hing KA. Bioceramic bone graft substitutes: influence of porosity and chemistry. Int J Appl Ceram Technol. 2005;2:184–99.
24. Blokhuis TJ, Termaat MF, den Boer FC, Patka P, Bakker FC, Haarman HJ. Properties of calcium phosphate ceramics in relation to their in vivo behavior. J Trauma. 2000;48:179–86.
25. Boyne PJ, Cole MD, Stringer D, Shafqat JP. A technique for osseous restoration of deficient edentulous maxillary ridges. J Oral Maxillofac Surg. 1985;43:87–91.

26. Bartee BK. Evaluation of new polytetrafluoroethylene-guided tissue regeneration membrane in healing extraction sites. Compendium. 1998;19:1256–8. 1260, 1262–4.
27. Bartee BK. The use of high-density polytetrafluoroethylene membrane to treat osseous defects clinical reports. Implant Dent. 1995;4:21–6.
28. Scantlebury TV. 1982–1992: a decade of technology development for guided tissue regeneration. J Periodontol. 1993;64:1129–37.
29. Leknes KN, Røynstrand IT, Selvig KA. Human gingival tissue reactions to silk and expanded polytetrafluoroethylene sutures. J Periodontol. 2005;76(1):34–42.
30. Edlich RF, Panek PH, Rodeheaver GT, Turnbull VG, Kurtz LD, Edgerton MT. Physical and chemical configuration of sutures in the development of surgical infection. Ann Surg. 1973;177:679–88.
31. Lilly GE. Reaction of oral tissues to suture materials. Oral Surg Oral Med Oral Pathol. 1968;26:128–33.
32. Lilly GE, Armstrong JH, Salem JE, Cutcher JL. Reaction of oral tissues to suture materials. Oral Surg Oral Med Oral Pathol. 1968;26:592–9.
33. Burkhardt R, Preiss A, Joss A, Lang NP. Influence of suture tension to the tearing characteristics of the soft tissues: an in vitro experiment. Clin Oral Implants Res. 2008,19:314–9.
34. Selvig KA, Kersten B, Chamberlain A, Wikesjö UME, Nilveus R. Regenerative surgery of intrabony periodontal defects using e-PTFE barrier membranes. Scanning electron microscopic evaluation of retrieved membranes versus clinical healing. J Periodontol. 1992;63:974–8.
35. Wilderman M, Wentz F, Orban B. Histogenesis of repair after mucogingival surgery. J Periodontol. 1960;31:283–99.
36. Nowzari H, Slots J. Microorganism in polytetrafluoroethylene barrier membranes for guided tissue regeneration. J Clin Periodontol. 1994;21:203–10.
37. Tinti C, Parma-Benfenati S. Vertical ridge augmentation: surgical protocol and retrospective evaluation of 48 consecutively inserted implants. Int J Periodontics Restorative Dent. 1998;18(5):434–43.
38. Hitti R, Kerns D. Guided bone regeneration in the oral cavity: a review. Open Pathol J. 2011;5:33–45.
39. Pi-Anfruns J. Complications in implant dentistry. Alpha Omegan. 2014;107(1):8–12.

Soft Tissue Management for Implants in the Aesthetic Zone

5

Perry R. Klokkevold

Abstract

While implant success depends on a multitude of factors, soft tissue management is critical to the aesthetic success of anterior implant tooth replacement in the partially edentulous patient. The peri-implant soft tissue appearance should emulate and match natural periodontal aesthetics. Ideally, peri-implant soft tissues blend imperceptibly with and mimic the surrounding periodontal soft tissues of the natural dentition. Achieving that goal requires an understanding of periodontal and peri-implant anatomy and an appreciation for factors that influence soft tissue contours around teeth and dental implant restorations. In addition to mastering surgical objectives and techniques, clinicians must be able to evaluate and accurately diagnose the existing periodontal condition.

5.1 Introduction

Soft tissue management is critical to the aesthetic success of anterior tooth replacement with implants in the partially edentulous patient. The peri-implant soft tissue appearance should emulate and match the natural periodontal aesthetics. In the ideal aesthetic outcome, peri-implant soft tissues will blend imperceptibly with and mimic the surrounding periodontal soft tissues of the natural dentition. Achieving that goal requires an understanding of periodontal and peri-implant anatomy and an appreciation for factors that influence soft tissue contours around teeth and dental

P. R. Klokkevold
Section of Periodontics, University of California, Los Angeles, CA, USA
e-mail: pklokkevold@dentistry.ucla.edu

Todd R. Schoenbaum (ed.), *Implants in the Aesthetic Zone*,
https://doi.org/10.1007/978-3-319-72601-4_5

implant restorations. And, in the case of deficient contours, it may require soft tissue augmentation procedures to reconstruct or enhance missing structure and volume.

This chapter describes soft tissue aesthetics, soft tissue management, and surgical strategies to enhance the aesthetic predictability for implants in the partially edentulous patient.

5.2 Ideal Soft Tissue Aesthetics

What is ideal periodontal (soft tissue) aesthetics? Certainly, the criteria for soft tissue aesthetics will vary from one individual to another. Each individual is unique. Upon smiling, the amount of gingival display will range from very little or no visible soft tissues to an excessive amount of soft tissue exposure, sometimes referred to as a "gummy smile," and everything in between (Fig. 5.1). The amount of gingival display for a given individual will differ and will likely influence the degree of his/her concern with soft tissue aesthetics. However, regardless of gingival display, individual personal preference and aesthetic demands may vary from frank indifference to an obsessive attention to detail and a need for perfection, even when soft tissues are not visible in their normal smile.

While some individuals will have little concern about aesthetics, most will be at least moderately concerned. It is important to assess each individual's aesthetic desires and to determine whether their expectations are realistic relative to the limits of their presenting circumstances. If not, and especially if the patient has truly unrealistic expectations, it is imperative to clearly discuss treatment options along with anticipated outcomes and to reach an understanding about the goals and limitations of treatment prior to initiating therapy.

In general, the ideal periodontal soft tissue aesthetics will consist of healthy, coral pink soft tissues that circumscribe the crowns and fill the interproximal spaces. The papillae will be peaked up to the contact point, and, with the exception of the midline papilla, they will be balanced and symmetrical with the corresponding contralateral papilla and tightly adapted to the tooth surfaces. The gingival margins follow the cementoenamel junction forming a smooth arch around each crown with a zenith that is slightly distal to or coincident with the midline of each tooth. The zenith or peak of the gingival margin typically aligns with the long axis of the tooth

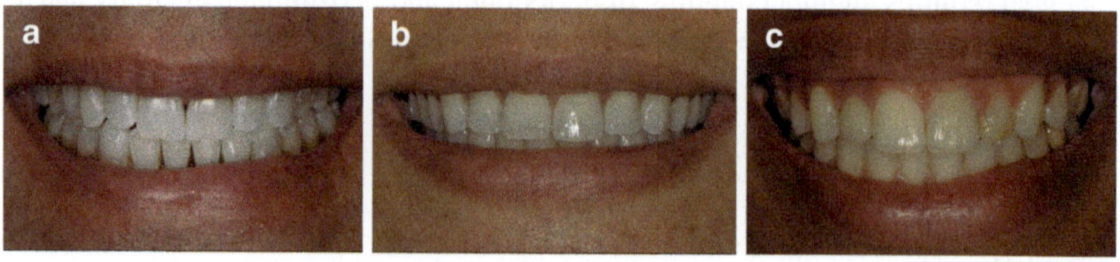

Fig. 5.1 (**a**) Patient with low smile line. There is limited or no gingival display upon smiling. (**b**) Patient with average smile line. There is a partial gingival display upon smiling. (**c**) Patient with high smile line. There is significant gingival display upon smiling

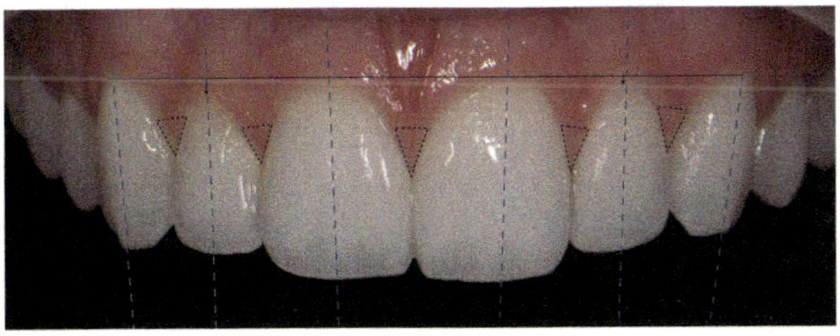

Fig. 5.2 Ideal periodontal aesthetics in a natural dentition without restoration or missing teeth. Soft tissue contours are bilaterally symmetrical. Interproximal spaces are filled with papilla peaked up to the contact point. The gingival margin is influenced by the axial inclination of each tooth; it follows the cementoenamel junction with zenith located coincident or slightly distal to the midline as depicted with a dotted line through the long axis of the tooth

and will be influenced by the position and prominence of the tooth within the alveolus. The gingival margin height of smaller teeth, such as the lateral incisors, will often be 1–2 mm lower (more coronal) than the gingival margins of the adjacent, larger teeth. The gingival margins of the centrals and canines will be fairly equivalent in height. Healthy periodontal tissues are firm, knife edged, and closely adherent to the tooth surfaces. As an example, Fig. 5.2 shows aesthetically ideal, healthy periodontal soft tissues surrounding a natural dentition without restorations or missing teeth.

5.3 Soft Tissue Deficits with Dental Implants

The dimensions of periodontal tissues are greater with natural teeth present than when missing or replaced with dental implants. Tooth loss whether caused by disease or trauma often results in loss of hard and soft tissue volume. Aesthetic tooth replacement with dental implants is most challenging when there is a lack of tissue volume to support and surround the implant restoration. State-of-the-art advances in dental materials, digital technologies, laboratory techniques, and artistic skills have made it possible to fabricate very realistic prosthetic tooth restorations that are indistinguishable from natural teeth. Consequently, it is the lack of tissue volume that presents the most significant challenge for the successful aesthetic replacement of missing teeth with implants, especially in anterior partially edentulous patients.

First and foremost, there must be an adequate volume of the bone in the area to support implant(s) in the proper prosthetically driven position. See Chap. 2 for details of diagnostic imaging, implant planning, and implant simulation and Chaps. 3, 4, 7 for details of bone augmentation/preservation procedures for situations when bone reconstruction is indicated. Adequate bone volume and proper implant position are essential elements that must be present prior to considering the nuances of achieving soft tissue aesthetics. Assuming an adequate bone volume and appropriate implant position, soft tissue deficits may still present a challenge for aesthetic tooth replacement. Common peri-implant soft tissue problems include recession (Fig. 5.3) and deficient papillae (Fig. 5.4).

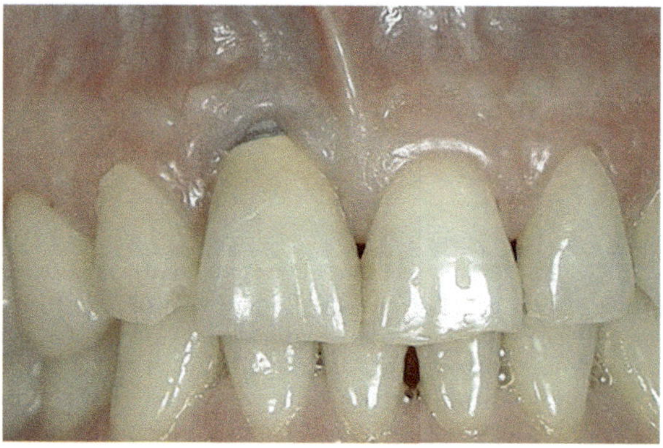

Fig. 5.3 Gingival recession on labial surface of single tooth implant replacing the right central incisor (#8). A wide diameter implant was placed immediately at the time of extraction with intact socket walls, including the buccal plate of the bone. It was restored about 5 months later after integration. Gingival margins were relatively even at delivery of final restoration and remained stable for some time but subsequently receded over the next 18–24 months due to buccal plate remodeling

Adequate bone
Anterior maxilla
- place implants 2mm palatal to center of original tooth position
- center (M-D)
- 3-4 mm apical to desired gingival margin

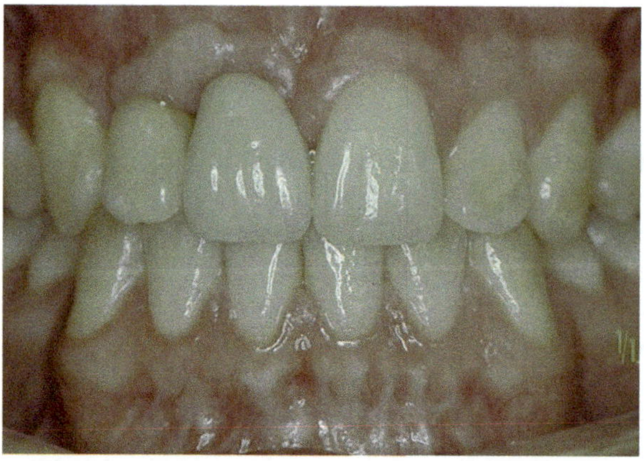

Fig. 5.4 The papilla between adjacent implants #7 and #8 is noticeably deficient as compared to the contralateral papilla between natural teeth #9 and #10. The soft tissue between two implants is primarily supported by the alveolar crest of the bone. There are no inserting connective tissue fibers (around implants) to aid in the supracrestal support of soft tissues (*Restorative treatment by Dr. John Beumer, UCLA*)

Proper implant position is critical to achieving and maintaining optimal soft tissue aesthetics. In general, implants placed in the anterior maxilla should be positioned slightly (~2 mm) palatal to the center of the original (ideal) tooth position. This compensates for the existing or anticipated horizontal alveolar bone remodeling/resorption of the buccal plate and facilitates the maintenance of the bone on the labial surface of the implant. Unless the buccal-lingual alveolar ridge dimension is substantial, the use of wide diameter implants should be avoided in the anterior maxilla for the same reason (i.e., preservation and maintenance of buccal bone).

Standard, or sometimes narrow, diameter implants should be placed in the center (mesial-distal) of the tooth position and approximately 3–4 mm apical to the desired gingival margin to allow proper emergence of the restoration from the tissue. Again, this assumes there is an adequate volume and location of the bone to support the implant or there is a plan to reconstruct it. Perhaps the most critical aspect of implant position relative to soft tissue management is the labial inclination. The position and angulation of existing maxillary anterior alveolar bone will often require that implants are placed with a labial inclination and a long axis that projects through the facial aspect of a planned restoration. Fortunately, there is a moderately wide range of labial-palatal angulations that can be managed prosthetically with angled or custom abutments, from a vertical direction that emerges through the cingulum to a facial direction that emerges through the cervical area of the labial aspect. However, if the long axis of the implant emerges through or apical to the desired gingival margin, there will almost certainly be excessive soft tissue recession resulting in a long clinical crown, regardless of prosthetic maneuvering with angled abutments and customization. Placing implants with a facial inclination that projects apical to the desired gingival margin must be avoided.

The other important soft tissue management principle is preservation of the interproximal papilla. It is well known that loss of bone and periodontal attachment leads to gingival recession and loss of interdental papilla height. It has also been well established that surgical manipulation of soft tissues, especially the interdental papilla, will result in retraction and loss of soft tissue height—aka "black triangles" in the proximal space. The presence of periodontitis with attachment loss and bone loss makes this latter concern much more likely and significant. For this reason, surgical treatment of periodontal disease is avoided in the anterior maxilla; nonsurgical therapy is preferred over surgical therapy to prevent or minimize loss of interdental soft tissue height. Even in the absence of periodontitis, surgical flap reflection of papillae can result in black triangles. Surgical manipulation of interproximal soft tissues should be minimized or avoided.

5.4 Periodontal Anatomy

Soft tissue contours in the natural dentition are supported coronal to the alveolar bone crest by the normal periodontal attachment apparatus. The supracrestal periodontal anatomy consists of the gingival sulcus, the long junctional epithelial attachment, and the connective tissue attachment. The outer oral surface of the gingiva consists of several layers of keratinized squamous epithelium extending from the mucogingival junction up to the free gingival margin. In periodontal health, the gingival sulcus is lined with just a few cell layers of nonkeratinized squamous epithelium. Apical to the gingival sulcus, a thin, single layer of epithelium forms an intimately adapted, relatively weak "adhesion" attachment, via hemi-desmosomes, to the crown and/or root surface. Apical to the long junctional epithelial attachment, the tissue is firmly attached to the tooth with perpendicular connective tissue (Sharpey's) fibers that insert into the cementum. As part of the normal periodontal attachment apparatus, a multidirectional network of dense collagen fibers intertwine and connect soft tissues to the teeth and bone. This periodontal attachment stabilizes teeth and creates a soft tissue matrix that is relatively immobile. Teeth are non-shedding, mineralized tissues that emerge into the oral cavity through the periodontium. The periodontal attachment apparatus is a unique structure in the body that is responsible for creating and maintaining a seal or barrier around the teeth, which are constantly exposed to the oral microbial flora. Healthy, non-inflamed periodontal tissues are resistant to gentle periodontal probe penetration and tissue retraction away from teeth. When periodontal health is maintained, long-term soft tissue attachment and stability are predictable.

The biologic dimensions of the periodontal attachment apparatus and gingival sulcus have been described histologically by Gargiulo and co-workers [1]. While there is a range of biologic width dimensions around teeth that vary from one individual to another, from one tooth to another, and from one tooth surface to another, the average dimension of the facial soft tissues is estimated to be about 3 mm, and the average interproximal "papilla" dimension has been shown to be about 4.5 mm [1–3]. The critical "papilla" height dimension, measured from the interproximal crest of the bone to the contact point between crowns of natural teeth, is approximately 5 mm [4]. Interproximal vertical dimensions >5 mm (bone crest to contact) are less likely to be completely filled by papilla in the natural dentition. An important distinction of the healthy periodontal attachment apparatus, as compared to the peri-implant soft tissues, is that teeth have a supracrestal zone (~1 mm) of connective tissue attachment with inserting fibers that provides a structural scaffold to support periodontal tissues coronal to the level of the bone, even when alveolar bone is very thin or missing. For example, it is common in the anterior maxilla to have a stable, intact periodontal connective tissue attachment without periodontal probing pocket depth over a root surface with a bony dehiscence. An inserting connective tissue attachment zone does not exist around implants. Consequently, the only "seal" around implants is achieved by the relatively weak adhesion of long junctional epithelium. The thickness and density of circumferential collagen fibers in the surrounding soft tissues can help to stabilize the peri-implant seal, but there are no inserting fibers. Unsupported tissues that surround implants, especially thin mucosa, will easily retract away from the implant/restoration.

5.5 Factors that Influence Soft Tissue Aesthetics

Periodontal soft tissue aesthetics are influenced by many factors including tooth shape, tooth position, proximity of adjacent teeth, periodontal biotype, supporting bone, and periodontal health. All of these factors will also influence peri-implant soft tissue aesthetics. The primary difference being that implants do not have inserting connective tissue fibers and therefore rely almost entirely on the bone and adjacent teeth to provide structural support for soft tissues. Additionally, the implant diameter is typically narrower than the tooth it is replacing. Consequently, peri-implant tissues must be full and maintain greater volume in order to have a similar appearance as the natural periodontium.

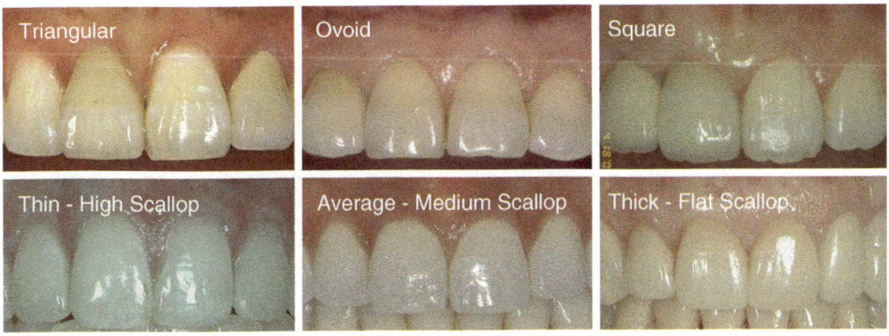

Fig. 5.5 (**a**) Triangular-shaped teeth typically present with highly scalloped gingiva and tall interproximal papilla height. (**b**) Ovoid-shaped teeth will present with an average gingival scallop and an average interproximal papilla height. (**c**) Square-shaped teeth tend to present with a shallow gingival scallop and short interproximal papilla height

5.5.1 Tooth Shape, Position, and Proximity

Tooth shape influences the interproximal space and the resultant interdental papilla height. The overall gingival architecture varies from relatively flat, short papillae between square-shaped teeth to highly scalloped, tall papillae between triangular-shaped teeth (Fig. 5.5). Tall, thin papillae are particularly vulnerable to loss when manipulated and/or when teeth are lost.

Tooth position influences the soft tissue contours. Gingival margins of teeth that are prominent (labial) in the arch will tend to be thinner, positioned more apical, and will be more susceptible to recession. Similarly, gingival margins in patient with a thin biotype will tend to be more susceptible to recession, whereas teeth that are more palatal in position will tend to have thicker labial tissue, and the gingival margins will be less susceptible to recession. Likewise, gingival margins in a patient with a thick biotype will be more resistant to recession of the gingival margin.

The normal approximation and contact between adjacent maxillary anterior teeth form a pyramidal-shaped space that is occupied by interdental papilla. The base of the pyramid is supported by the interproximal crestal bone and bordered by the cervical contours of adjacent teeth with the papilla peak rising coronal up to the contact point. Again, the interproximal tissues, adjacent to teeth, are supported coronal to the bone crest by connective tissue fibers inserting into the cementum on the root surfaces. If adjacent teeth are crowded, in close approximation or possibly overlapping one another, the interproximal space may be diminished or absent causing the papilla to be blocked out. Conversely, when adjacent teeth are separated by >2.4 mm, the papilla will be less likely to fill the interproximal space [5]. In a study evaluating the effect of interproximal distance on papilla presence, the authors reported that the interproximal papilla was always deficient when the interproximal distance between roots was >4.0 mm [6]. When there is a diastema, the interproximal soft tissues will be flat (Fig. 5.6). This phenomenon

Teeth separated by diastema >2.4 mm, absent papilla
Roots distance >4.00 mm

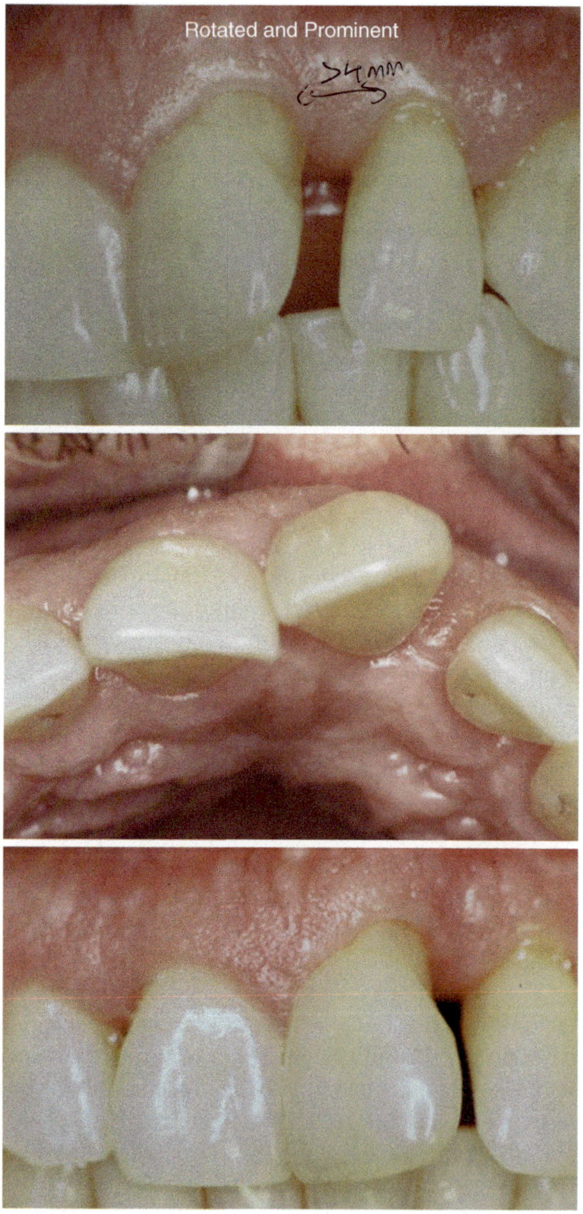

Fig. 5.6 Adjacent teeth that are not in close proximity fail to form the typical pyramid-shaped interproximal space. Consequently, interdental tissues remain flat without a peaked papilla. This case demonstrates the effect of a diastema space on the interproximal tissues. The tissue is flat when the interdental space is >4 mm with diastema

tooth #9 - more labial and therefore tissues more apical and prone to recession

will also be observed when a tooth is missing without a properly contoured prosthetic tooth replacement to support the papilla (Fig. 5.7). On the other hand, when teeth are replaced with a properly contoured provisional restoration (i.e., pontic), the interproximal papilla can be maintained (Fig. 5.8).

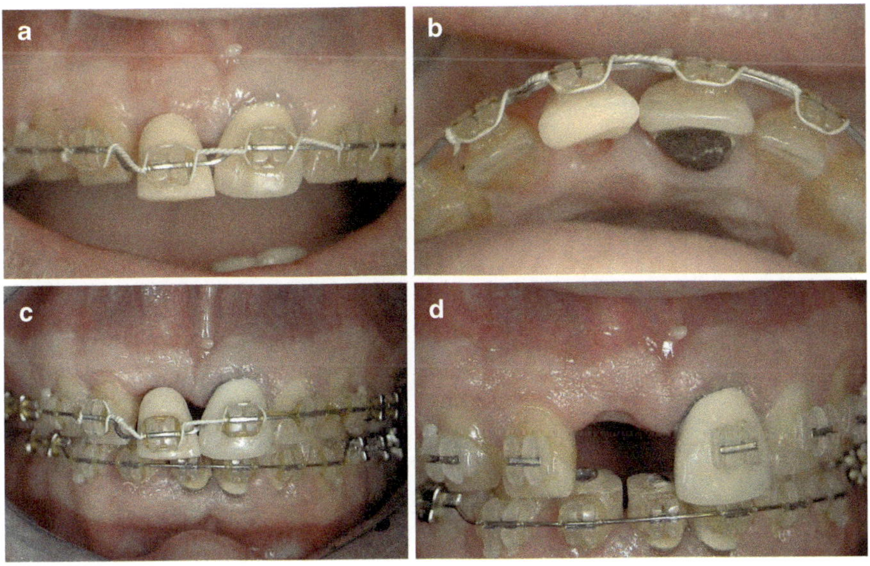

Fig. 5.7 Without a properly contoured provisional restoration to support soft tissues, the interproximal papilla height will flatten during the healing period following tooth extraction. (**a**, **b**) A relatively flat veneer is attached with a bracket to the orthodontic arch wire to serve as a temporary tooth replacement following extraction of the right maxillary central incisor. (**c**, **d**) Following about 6 months of healing, the gingival architecture is flattened with loss of papilla height adjacent to the neighboring teeth. Note the lack of prosthetic contours at the interproximal gingival level

5.5.2 Periodontal Biotype/Bone Support

Periodontal biotype is an important assessment to make when planning implant placement to replace missing anterior teeth. Maintaining soft tissue aesthetics in individuals with a thick biotype is fairly predictable. However, maintenance of soft tissue aesthetics in an individual with a thin biotype is very challenging. Soft tissue management in patients with thin biotype is critical.

Gingival morphology follows the shape of the underlying bone. It is difficult to build aesthetically acceptable gingiva in areas with deficient supporting bone. Bone augmentation is essential when there is moderate to severe loss of tissue height, especially when implants will be used to replace missing teeth. Soft tissue augmentation can be used to replace greater volumes in an edentulous (pontic) space than in areas occupied by implant restorations, especially adjacent implants (Fig. 5.9) [7].

When considering the surgical placement of implants, clinicians must consider the approach (conventional two-stage approach versus a one-stage approach) and the timing of implant placement (immediate versus delayed or staged placement). For sites that require bone augmentation, the approach may be to bone graft the ridge first and place the implant(s) after healing, or the simultaneous implant placement and bone graft at the same time. All of these approaches can provide a

- augment edentulous areas w/ soft tissue before placing implants

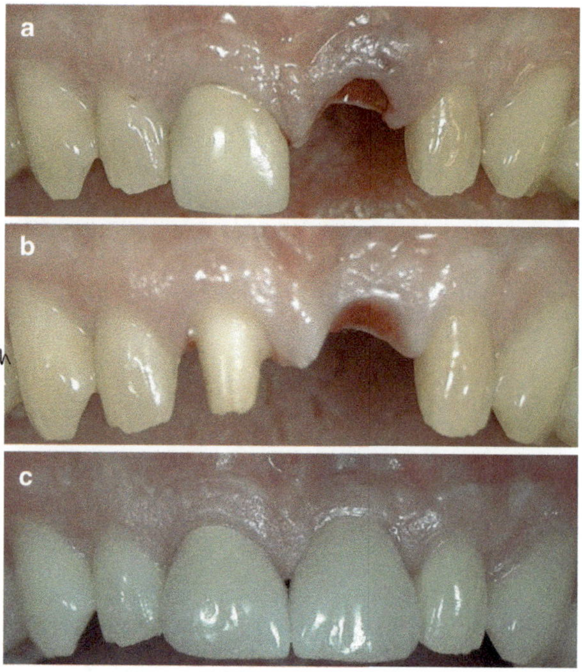

- ovate pontic can maintain interproximal papilla for 6 months post-extraction

Fig. 5.8 This case shows how the use of a properly contoured provisional restoration (cantilevered ovate pontic) can maintain the interproximal papilla from extraction to 6 months post-extraction healing. (**a**) Maxillary left central incisor #9 extracted without hard or soft tissue grafting. Note the contours of the interproximal tissues around extraction socket. (**b**) The site was allowed to heal with an ovate pontic used to support interproximal tissues. Subsequently, an implant was placed with a full-thickness flap using a papilla preservation design. The provisional restoration (cantilevered pontic) was used throughout the posttreatment healing periods. (**c**) Final restoration with maintained gingival architecture at 5-year follow-up

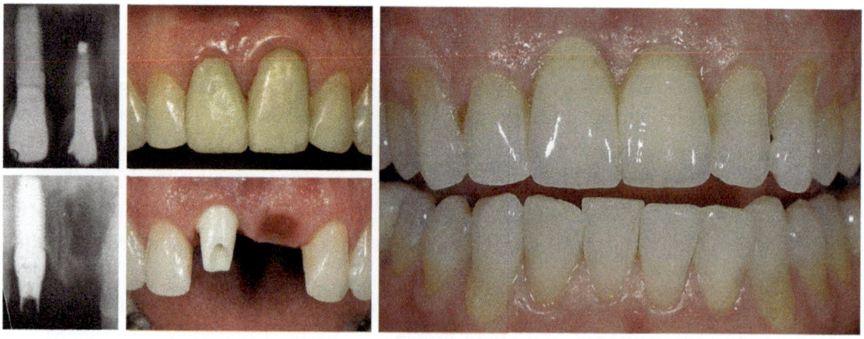

Fig. 5.9 Greater soft tissue volume can be created in edentulous ridge "pontic space" than can be achieved between two adjacent implants. This case shows extraction of a failed endodontically treated tooth, which is adjacent to an existing restored implant. Radiograph following extraction showing complete buccal-palatal loss of the bone. Following complete degranulation, the extraction socket was grafted with particulate bone allograft and a soft tissue graft harvested from the palate. The result is an edentulous site with substantial tissue thickness that can be shaped to create the appearance of full interproximal papilla. The site was provisionalized with an ovate pontic that was cantilevered from the adjacent implant (*Restorative treatment by Dr. Edward McLaren, UCLA*)

successful outcome if patient selection is appropriate and techniques are performed properly [8–11]. Again, bone support is essential to achieving and maintaining soft tissue aesthetics.

Wound healing following any surgical intervention will often result in retraction and recession of soft tissue contours observed as gingival margin recession and loss of interdental papilla height. For this reason, whenever possible, soft tissue anatomy should be preserved, and surgical manipulation should be minimized. Papillae are particularly vulnerable to changes with surgical manipulation. Surgical procedures, such as papilla preservation techniques, should be used to effectively maintain interproximal tissue height [12–14].

When evaluating soft tissue aesthetics, it is important to recognize that soft tissues are supported by the bone and remaining teeth. Without careful management, loss of bone and lack of teeth will result in soft tissue deficiency. When a tooth is lost, the normal process of extraction socket wound healing results in loss of tissue dimensions. The alveolar socket walls remodel leading to shrinkage of alveolar dimensions [15]. This is especially true for the horizontal dimension [16, 17]. The buccal plate is particularly susceptible loss of dimension as part of the normal remodeling process. Regardless of extraction socket bone graft/preservation techniques, the alveolar dimensions are diminished after tooth extraction. A recent systematic review estimated that the mean horizontal dimension is reduced by 3.8 mm and the mean vertical dimension is reduced by 1.2 mm within 6 months after extraction [18]. Although the soft tissue dimensions remain fairly consistent before and after extraction socket remodeling, they are supported by the underlying bone and therefore tend to be reduced by a similar dimension following tooth loss. The loss of dimension is greater when the labial bone is very thin or nonexistent, especially when socket preservation is not performed. Post-extraction management of hard and soft tissues is critical.

In the absence of teeth, soft tissue contours are only supported by and follow the contours of the underlying bone. Likewise, when missing teeth are replaced with dental implants, the soft tissues are primarily supported by and follow the contours of the bone. Since there are no inserting connective tissue fibers attached to implants or the restorative components, peri-implant soft tissues rely on supporting the bone and adjacent teeth. This is why it is virtually impossible to create a full natural papilla height between implants (see Fig. 5.4). Furthermore, it is important to support soft tissues with provisional restorations such as an ovate pontic during transitional periods of healing prior to implant placement/restoration.

Soft tissue thickness ranges from 1 to 3 mm. Thus, soft tissue height supported only by underlying bone and implants will generally be limited to 3 mm or less. The average interproximal papilla height between implants is approximately 3.4 mm, compared to approximately 4.5 mm between natural teeth [19].

5.5.3 Periodontal Health/Disease

Although it is an obvious statement, it cannot be emphasized enough to state that periodontal health is essential for the achievement and maintenance of soft tissue aesthetics. Gingivitis and periodontitis are bacterial-driven inflammatory diseases that cause swelling and edema of soft tissues adjacent to contaminated tooth surfaces. Periodontitis, by definition, involves attachment loss and bone loss as well. Since teeth (and implants too for that matter) are non-shedding, hard structures, a bacterial biofilm builds on the surfaces especially within the sulcus/pocket in the absence of proper oral hygiene. Left undisturbed, the biofilm evolves into a pathogenic microflora, which perpetuates a chronic inflammatory response in the tissues. At the early stages, prior to significant attachment and bone loss, edematous tissues cover root surfaces and fill interproximal spaces and may give patients a false sense of "normal" soft tissue contours. However, inflamed tissues are not adherent to tooth surfaces, tend to bleed easily, and are not stable. They are edematous, easily retract away from the tooth, and are highly susceptible to recession. Perhaps most critical to this concern is the fact that when inflammation is resolved and/or when inflamed tissues are surgically manipulated, they will shrink dramatically resulting in recession and open interproximal spaces; without a proper assessment, the result may be unexpected poor soft tissue aesthetics. Periodontal health must be established prior to treatment in order to anticipate and achieve predictable results.

5.5.4 Aesthetic Prognostic Factors

The patient's chief complaint, aesthetic expectations, tooth positions, gingival form, osseous crest position, periodontal biotype, tooth shape, and ridge deficiency all play an important role in deriving an accurate aesthetic treatment plan for the patient. Therefore, developing the necessary skill and knowledge to examine and recognize problems of these components is essential to clinical success.

A diagnostic wax-up of the proposed prosthetic restoration as well as a 3D diagnostic scan and implant simulation can be very insightful for visualizing the final outcome and will shed light on the tissue deficiencies. This assessment will facilitate decision-making and development of the surgical treatment plan.

The most favorable prognostic factors include labial bone that is ≤3 mm from the desired gingival margin, intact interdental bone height, tooth position that is coronal and palatal, thick periodontal biotype, and a flat gingival architecture [2, 20]. The least favorable prognostic factors include loss or lack of labial bone >3 mm from desired gingival margin and deficient interdental bone height, tooth position that is apical and facial, thin periodontal biotype, and a highly scalloped gingival architecture (Fig. 5.10) [2, 20]. Greater gingival recession occurs around implants with labial bone loss [21].

5.6 Techniques for Soft Tissue Augmentation

Many of the techniques for soft tissue augmentation around dental implants have been adopted from periodontal soft tissue augmentation procedures. Techniques include free gingival grafts (FGGs), pedicle grafts, subepithelial connective tissue grafts (SCTGs), and various non-autogenous materials. Flap management may

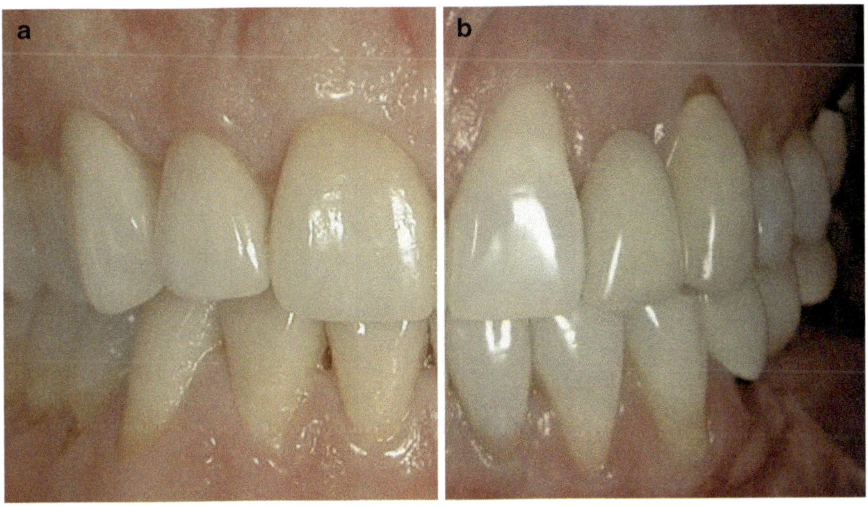

Fig. 5.10 It is essential to evaluate each patient for his/her presenting circumstances to determine risk factors and treatment prognosis. (**a**) Best aesthetic prognosis includes thick periodontal biotype, bone ≤3 mm from gingival margin, high interproximal bone height, relatively flat gingival architecture, tooth position that is coronal and palatal, and square-shaped teeth. (**b**) Least favorable aesthetic prognosis includes thin periodontal biotype, bone >3 mm from gingival margin, reduced interproximal bone height, highly scalloped gingival architecture with tall papillae, tooth position that is apical and labial, and triangular-shaped teeth

include coronally advanced flap (CAF), split-thickness flap, or variations of a pouch procedure. Papilla preservation procedures are essential especially if there is attachment and/or bone loss. Biologics such as enamel matrix derivative (EMD) and growth factors can be used to enhance healing of soft tissue grafts [22, 23]. More recently, the use of autologous blood products such as leukocyte- and platelet-rich fibrin (L-PRF) has been advocated as an adjunct to soft tissue grafting [24].

Free gingival grafts utilize keratinized surface tissue, including the epithelial layer, harvested from the palate that is transplanted and secured to a prepared recipient site. The epithelial surface is left exposed (i.e., it is not covered by a flap). The advantage of FGGs is the predictable increase in tissue thickness and zone of keratinized tissue at the recipient site. The aesthetic disadvantage is that FGGs tend to be distinct and visibly noticeable due to the difference in color from adjacent tissues. FGGs maintain the color of the donor tissue, which may not be aesthetic.

Subepithelial connective tissue grafts (SCTGs) are aesthetically advantageous because they blend, imperceptibly, with adjacent tissues. SCTGs increase tissue thickness, especially when placed under the recipient flap. Although SCTGs can be used as a free graft without overlying flap coverage, this method can be less successful in achieving increased tissue thickness. Thus, SCTGs should be placed under a flap or into a pouch. Many variations of the flap design have been used to improve blood supply for SCTGs including full-thickness flap, split-thickness flap, lateral pedicle flap, double-papilla flap, and pouch techniques to achieve root coverage and to enhance soft tissue thickness around teeth. Figure 5.11 shows an example of a

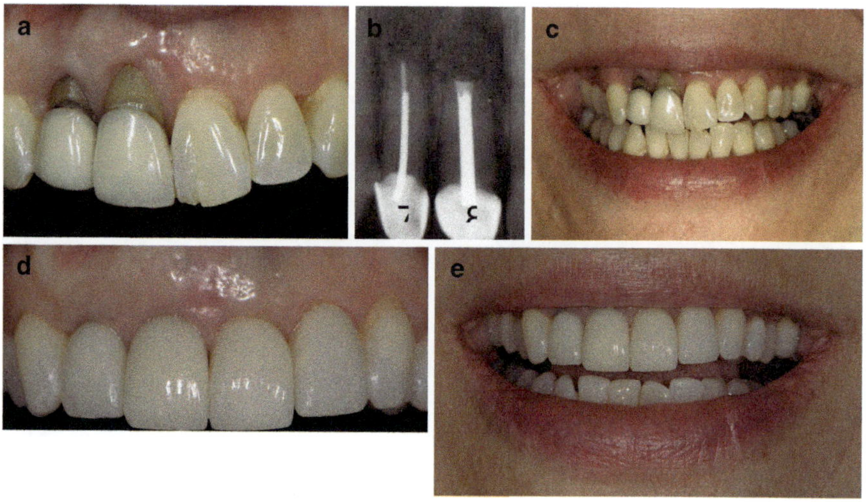

Fig. 5.11 (**a**, **c**) Severe gingival recession on the labial surface of the maxillary right lateral and central incisor caused by inadvertent surgical manipulation of tissues during apical surgery. (**b**) Radiograph of the maxillary right lateral and central incisor showing evidence of endodontics and apical surgery. (**d**, **e**) The recession was treated with a subepithelial connective tissue graft using a pouch procedure. The advantages of this technique include preservation of papillae (no incisions) and good blending of grafted soft tissues with adjacent gingival tissues. Note the tooth contours and rotations were corrected with new crown and veneer restorations (*Restorative treatment by Dr. Todd Schoenbaum, UCLA*)

root coverage procedure using a pouch technique. Many of these techniques as well as some unique variations have been adapted for use around implants [25].

Several studies have shown that there is rapid labial and vertical bone loss after extractions [15, 26, 27], and immediate implant placement does not stop the resorption process [28–30]. Furthermore, it has been demonstrated that soft and hard tissues grafted in augmentation procedures to enhance aesthetics undergo extensive shrinkage within 3–6 months [31, 32]. Thus, soft tissue augmentation is thought to be advantageous [33]. Interestingly, in contrast to this tenant, a recent systematic review and meta-analysis of soft tissue changes following immediate implant placement with or without simultaneous augmentation found that CT grafts offered no advantage [34].

5.7 Immediate Implant Placement for Predictability and Aesthetics

Immediate implant placement in a one-stage approach, with a healing abutment or provisional restoration that is attached to the implant, provides more predictable preservation of the interproximal peri-implant gingival tissue with less treatment time [10, 35]. This approach to implant placement is minimally invasive and, when used for appropriate cases, is perhaps the best approach to achieving soft tissue aesthetics with implant tooth replacement.

A potential disadvantage of immediate implant placement is that it may result in progressive recession of the gingival labial margin over the implant restoration [36, 37]. Therefore, a prudent strategy is to simultaneously enhance the quality and quantity of labial soft tissue [38]. One of the most effective ways to minimize collapse of the implanted socket and improve the labial gingival biotype is to simultaneously fill the labial socket void with particulate bone and augment the labial gingival tissue with soft tissue [15, 26, 27, 33].

An effective augmentation technique used with flapless immediate implant placement in a one-stage approach is the bone and crescent-shaped free gingival grafting technique originally described by Han and Jeong [25]. In this technique, the space between the inner surface of the labial bony wall and the labial surface of the implant is filled with slow-resorbing bone allograft or xenograft to help preserve the horizontal dimension of the ridge. A crescent-shaped soft tissue graft is harvested from the palate and transplanted into the labial recipient site coronal to the particulate bone graft. It is important for graft survival that the outer surface of the crescent graft fits snug with the bleeding lamina propria of the labial gingiva. Proper suturing ensures good proximity and prevents the graft from being displaced coronally out of the recipient site. See Cases 2 and 3 described below.

The advantage of this approach to soft tissue augmentation is simplicity and minimal surgical morbidity. In addition to providing a sealed protection for the bone graft, it augments the labial soft tissue. Preparation of the recipient site involves no incisions and no soft tissue flap reflection. Only the inner aspect of the gingival sulcus is de-epithelialized. The surrounding soft tissues remain intact, maintaining all existing connective tissue fibers and blood supply. The palatal donor site wound is small (~3 × 4 × 3 mm) and epithelializes quickly with minimal discomfort. Multiple grafts can be harvested simultaneously to treat multiple immediate implants. This simple gingival augmentation technique frequently improves an unfavorable initial gingival margin.

5.8 Applications/Case Presentations

When treatment planning an anterior case, it is important to determine what aspects of the soft and hard tissues need to be preserved for a predictable aesthetic result. For example, if the initial vertical position of the interdental papillae is aesthetically acceptable, it is prudent to preserve them rather risk loss with surgical elevation. Determining the tissues to be preserved will aid in the decision-making and selection of an appropriate surgical approach.

5.9 Case 1 (Deficient Bone Volume)

Some cases that lack sufficient bone volume for proper implant placement require a staged approach. Figure 5.12 shows the case of a 59-year-old healthy female who presents with a maxillary left central incisor (#9) that was deemed hopeless due to

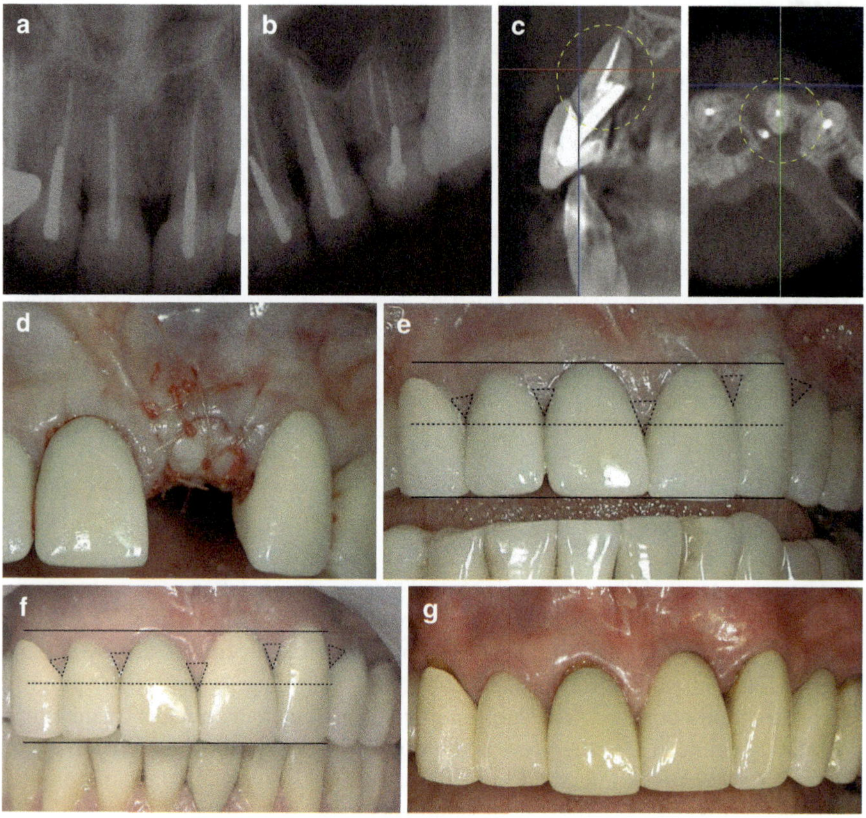

Fig. 5.12 This patient required extraction of the maxillary left central incisor due to post-perforation, deep probing pocket depth, and bone loss localized to the palatal surface. (**a**, **b**) Preoperative periapical radiographs showing multiple teeth with endodontics, posts, and crowns. (**c**) Preoperative CBCT cross-sectional image of maxillary left central incisor #9. Due to the lack of the bone on the facial and palatal surfaces, this site is not a candidate for immediate implant placement. (**d**) Using a staged approach, a simple extraction without incisions or soft tissue reflection was completed. The site was carefully and meticulously degranulated and grafted with particulate bone allograft, which was covered by a resorbable barrier and sealed with a free gingival graft harvested from the palate. The site was immediately provisionalized with a removable partial denture utilizing an ovate pontic. Subsequently, after 6-month healing, a narrow diameter implant was placed. (**e**) Preoperative clinical photograph of maxillary anterior teeth. There is a lack of symmetry due to a missing left lateral incisor. The prognosis is challenging due to a thin periodontal biotype and multiple crowns, which can hinder optimal biofilm control. (**f**) Postoperative clinical photograph of the maxillary anterior teeth after delivery of final restoration. There is good maintenance of soft tissue contours including levels of marginal gingiva and interproximal papillae. (**g**) The 8-year follow-up shows some labial gingival recession affecting both the natural teeth and the implant. Interproximal papilla heights are maintained *(Restorative treatment by Dr. Ben Wu, UCLA)*

a palatal post-perforation. There were deep palatal probing pocket depth and severe localized bone loss on the palatal surface. Clinical examination revealed a thin periodontal biotype with normal interproximal probing depth (≤3 mm) for all teeth. All maxillary teeth were endodontically treated and restored with posts and full-coverage crowns. Except for localized periodontitis on the palatal aspect of tooth #9, there was periodontal health.

Three-dimensional CBCT imaging and implant simulation revealed a lack of bone volume with no bone on the facial surface and no bone on the palatal surface of the maxillary left central incisor. Thus, immediate implant placement was not a viable option. The treatment plan required extraction and bone augmentation. The critical decision was to extract the tooth and graft the alveolar ridge (socket) without incisions and without soft tissue flap reflection. Surgical manipulation of soft tissue in this case would cause significant retraction that would be difficult to reconstruct. The site was meticulously degranulated and grafted with mineralized, freeze-dried bone allograft, covered with a biodegradable collagen membrane and a free gingival graft (used as a biological barrier covering the extraction socket orifice). The tooth was provisionally replaced with a removable prosthesis using an ovate pontic design shaped to support the interproximal papilla.

Six months later, a narrow diameter implant was placed in the proper position. A subepithelial connective tissue graft was place over the ridge at the time of implant placement to enhance the soft tissue thickness. Following another 4 months, the implant was exposed and restored with a single crown. The final restoration and surrounding soft tissues are aesthetic with contours that are similar to the pretreatment appearance. Long-term (8 years) follow-up reveals gingival margin recession across all maxillary anterior teeth, both natural and implant, yet the interproximal papillae height was maintained. This latter finding is consistent with reports in the literature that indicate individuals with a thin periodontal biotype are more susceptible to gingival recession over 2–8 years, while interproximal papillae are maintained [39].

5.10 Case 2 (Severe Localized Periodontal Bone Loss)

Careful evaluation of the existing periodontal parameters will aid in the proper diagnosis and lead to appropriate treatment plan. Figure 5.13 shows the case of a 36-year-old healthy female who presents with severe localized bone loss affecting the maxillary lateral incisors. Clinical examination revealed normal attachment and bone levels around adjacent teeth (centrals and canines). The periodontal biotype was average to thin. There is slight gingival recession and drifting of the right lateral incisor with a slight diastema. Three-dimensional CBCT imaging and implant simulation revealed adequate bone volume for proper implant position and

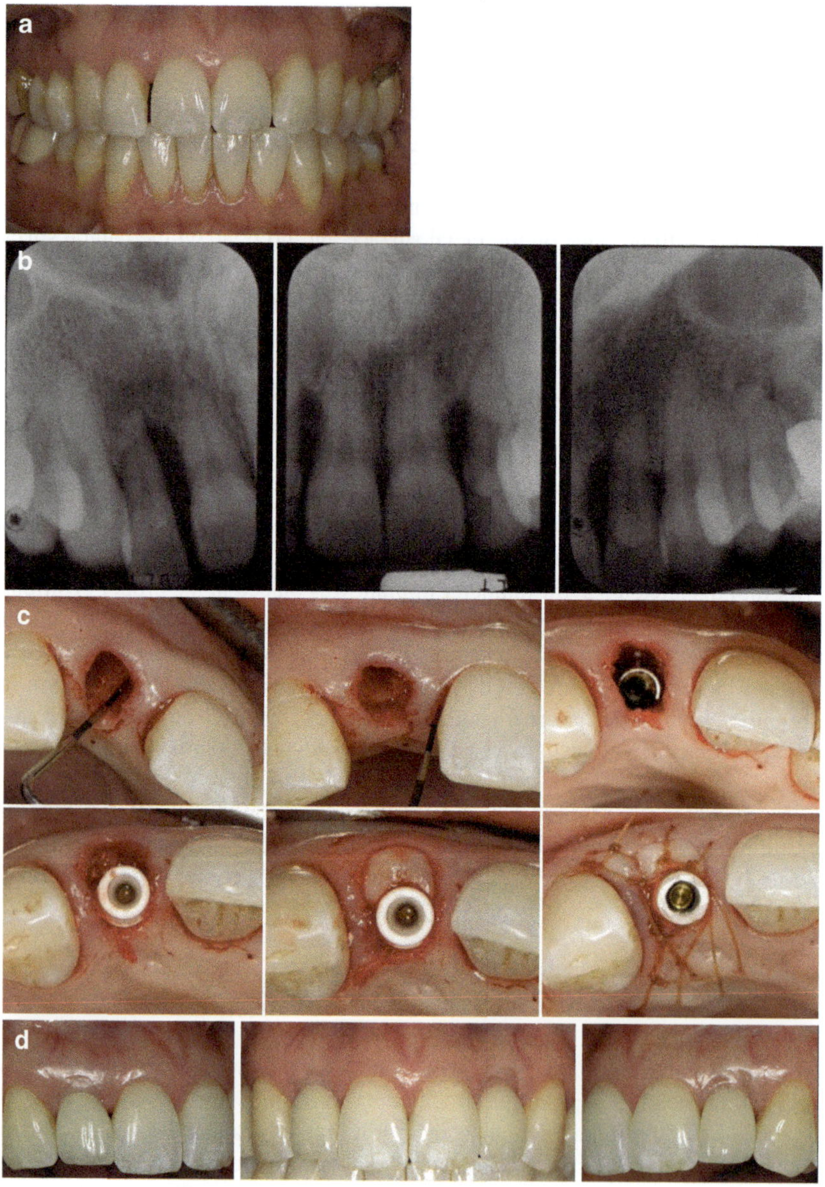

Fig. 5.13 Localized aggressive periodontitis case with severe localized bone loss affecting the maxillary lateral incisors, #7 and 10. (**a**) Preoperative clinical photo. Notice that both maxillary lateral incisors are beginning to migrate toward the facial. There is a diastema between the right maxillary lateral and central incisor with flattened interproximal tissue. (**b**) Preoperative periapical radiographs of maxillary anteriors showing severe localized bone loss around the lateral incisors. (**c**) Sequential series of clinical photos demonstrating the treatment steps including extraction, assessment of bone levels and tissue attachment, implant placement in palatal position, bone grafting labial extraction socket, placement of provisional abutment, placement of crescent-shaped gingival graft, and suturing of the graft. (**d**) Clinical photograph of case 4 years after delivery of final restorations. (**e**) Periapical radiographs demonstrating good bone levels and osseointegration of implants 4 years after treatment (*Courtesy of Dr. Thomas Han and Dr. Dan Nelson*)

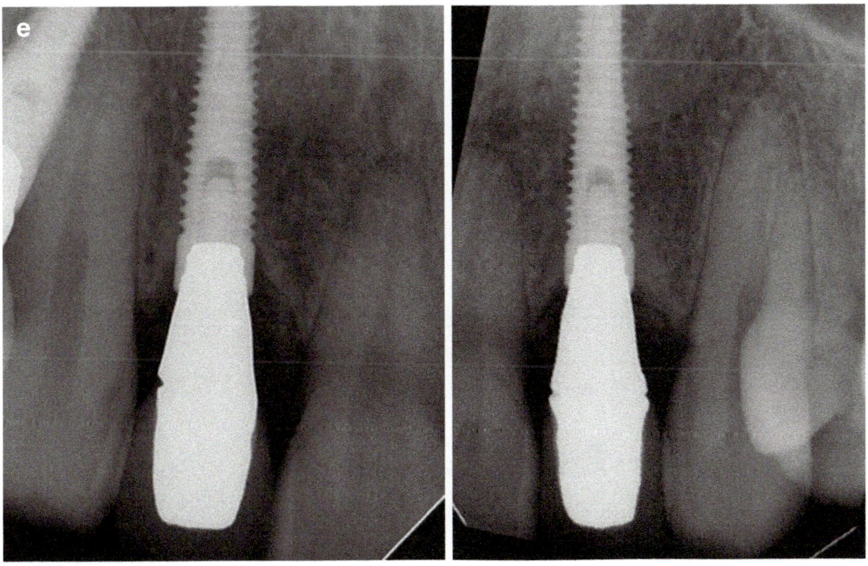

Fig. 5.13 (continued)

placement. Based on clinical and radiographic examination, it was deemed possible to replace the lateral incisors with immediate implant placement and immediate provisional restorations.

Importantly, this procedure was performed without incisions and without soft tissue flap reflection. The labial aspect of the extraction socket was grafted with mineralized, freeze-dried bone allograft. Crescent-shaped soft tissue grafts were harvested from the palate and secured over the bone graft in the labial socket to enhance the soft tissue biotype. The implants were immediately provisionalized with temporary crowns to support the interproximal soft tissues. Long-term (4 years) follow-up reveals excellent soft tissue aesthetics with good bone support and implant stability.

5.11 Case 3 (Moderate Localized Bone Loss Associated with Endodontic Lesion)

Figure 5.14 shows the case of a 38-year-old healthy female who presents with moderate localized bone loss associated with a failing endodontically treated maxillary left central incisor. The adjacent lateral incisor is also endodontically treated and restored with a full-coverage crown. Clinical examination revealed normal attachment and bone levels around adjacent teeth. The periodontal biotype was average. There was deep periodontal probing on the mesial of tooth #9 and fistula on the facial gingiva. The tooth was deemed hopeless. Three-dimensional CBCT imaging

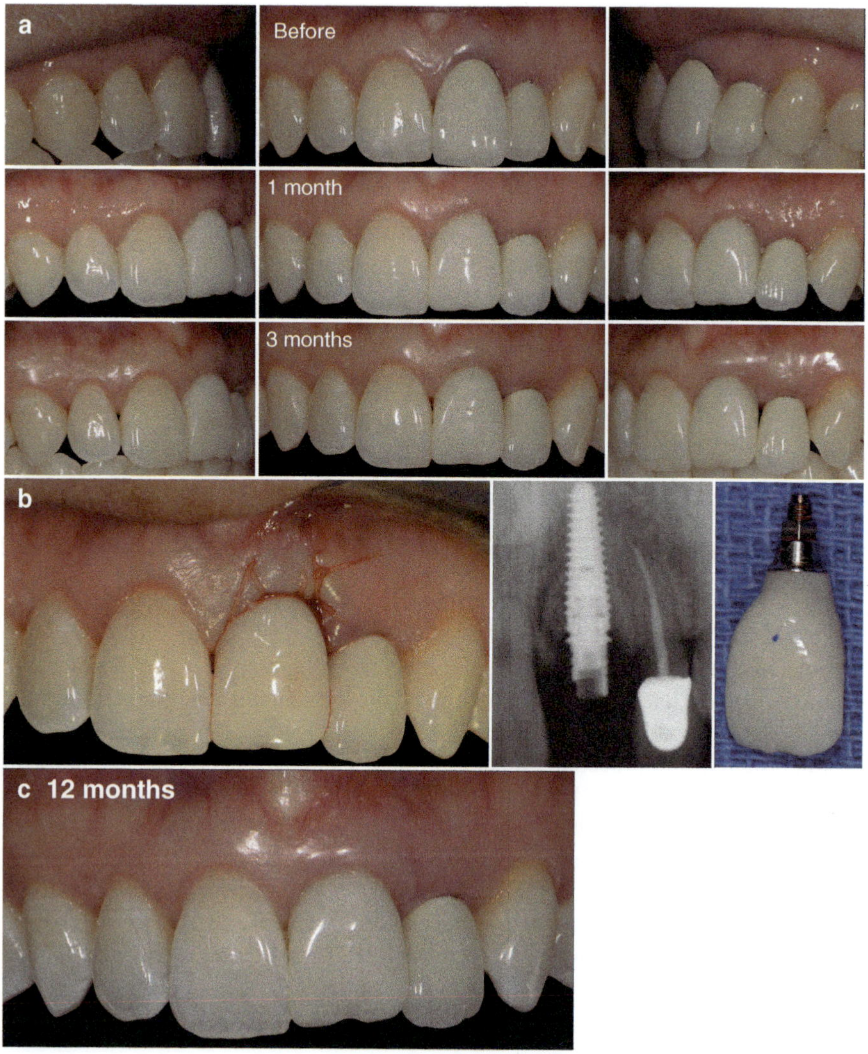

Fig. 5.14 Case presentation of an immediate implant placement with immediate (prefabricated) provisional restoration to replace an endodontically failing maxillary left central incisor, #9. (**a**) Clinical photographs of maxillary anterior teeth before treatment, 1 month after treatment, and 3 months after treatment. (**b**) Clinical photograph and periapical radiograph immediately after extraction, implant placement, bone graft, crescent-shaped gingival graft, and provisionalization. (**c**) Clinical photograph of maxillary anterior teeth 12 months after treatment. The immediately placed provisional restoration remains in place. Gingival tissues are preserved at the preoperative levels

and implant simulation revealed adequate bone volume for proper implant position and placement. Based on clinical and radiographic examination, it was deemed possible to replace the central incisor with an immediate implant and immediate prefabricated provisional restoration.

The tooth was extracted, socket was meticulously degranulated, and an implant was placed using a computer-generated surgical guide. There were no incisions and no soft tissue flap reflection. The labial aspect of the socket was grafted with mineralized, freeze-dried bone allograft. The prefabricated provisional restoration was delivered. Contacts and occlusion were carefully checked and adjusted to prevent interference. A crescent-shaped soft tissue graft was harvested from the palate and secured over the bone graft to enhance the labial soft tissue thickness. Follow-up evaluation reveals excellent soft tissue aesthetics.

5.12 Case 4 (Severe Labial Bone Loss with Moderate Gingival Recession)

Figure 5.15 shows the case of a 55-year-old healthy male who presents with severe localized bone loss associated with a traumatized, endodontically failing maxillary left central incisor. The tooth became progressively more mobile and began extruding and drifting to the facial. Clinical examination revealed normal attachment and bone levels around adjacent teeth. The periodontal biotype was thick. Three-dimensional CBCT imaging and implant simulation revealed adequate bone volume for proper implant position and placement. Based on clinical and radiographic examination, it was deemed possible to replace the central incisor with an immediate implant and immediate prefabricated provisional restoration.

The tooth was extracted. A full-thickness flap was prepared with papilla-sparing incisions. The socket was meticulously degranulated. An implant was placed using a computer-generated surgical guide. The prefabricated provisional restoration was delivered. Contacts and occlusion were carefully checked and adjusted to prevent interference. As anticipated from the implant simulation, there was a bony dehiscence on the labial aspect of the implant. It was grafted with mineralized, freeze-dried bone allograft. The particulate bone graft material was covered, and the soft tissue thickness was augmented with several layers of L-PRF barrier membrane. The flap was coronally repositioned and sutured at the desired gingival margin position. Follow-up evaluation (1 year) reveals excellent soft tissue aesthetics.

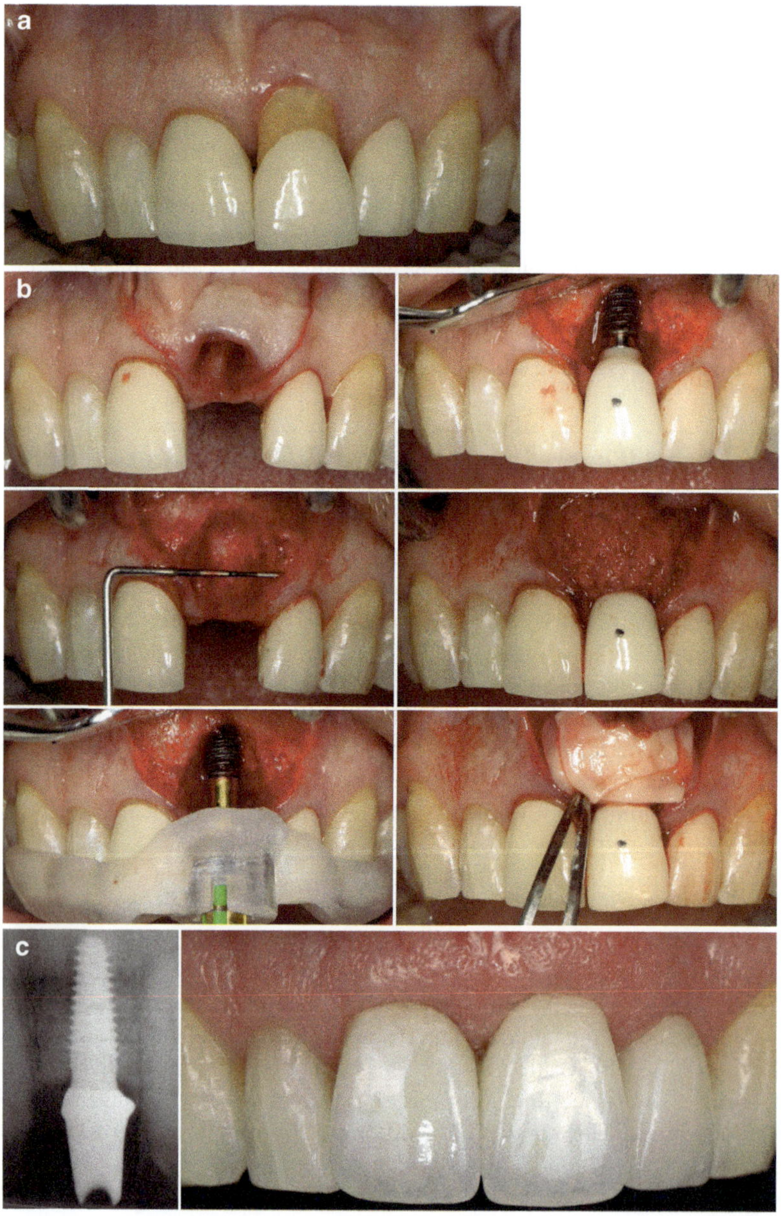

Fig. 5.15 Case presentation of an immediate implant placement with immediate (prefabricated) provisional restoration to replace an endodontically failing maxillary left central incisor, #9. (**a**) Preoperative clinical photo of maxillary anterior teeth. Notice the maxillary left central incisor area has drifted coronal and facial. There is a diastema between the right maxillary lateral and central incisor with flattened interproximal tissue. (**b**) Preoperative sequential series of clinical photos demonstrating the treatment steps including extraction, flap reflection, implant placement in palatal position utilizing a computer-generated surgical guide, bone grafting labial dehiscence defect with particulate bone allograft, placement of prefabricated provisional restoration, and placement of several layers of L-PRF membrane. (**c**) Clinical photograph 1 year later after delivery of final restorations, including crown #8, implant crown #9, and veneer #10 (*Courtesy of Dr. Thomas Han and Dr. Todd Schoenbaum*)

Conclusions

Aesthetic failures frequently begin with an inadequate examination of the existing soft and hard tissues, which leads to an incorrect diagnosis and ultimately to an inappropriate treatment plan. The wrong treatment plan combined with selection of inappropriate surgical approaches or techniques can result in poor aesthetic outcomes.

The clinical science in dentistry has evolved to where placement of dental implants and restoring them requires sufficient knowledge in several disciplines of dentistry. In addition to mastering surgical objectives and techniques, clinicians must be able to evaluate and accurately diagnose the existing periodontal condition. Furthermore, proper restorative management of soft tissues is critical to achieving and maintaining aesthetics. Hence, there are multiple aspects of diagnosis that are essential for the development of an appropriate treatment plan necessary for a successful outcome in aesthetic implant dentistry.

The soft tissue management and minimally invasive surgical approach to aesthetics presented in this chapter are based on sound biological principles and offer a predictable way to preserve and enhance aesthetics of anterior partially edentulous cases.

References

1. Gargiulo AW, Wentz FM, Orban B. Dimensions and relations of the dentogingival junction in humans. J Periodontol. 1961;32:261–7.
2. Kan JY, Rungcharassaeng K, Umezu K, Kois JC. Dimensions of peri-implant mucosa: an evaluation of maxillary anterior single implants in humans. J Periodontol. 2003;74:557–62.
3. Vacek JS, Gher ME, Assad DA, Richardson AC, Giambarresi LI. The dimensions of the human dentogingival junction. Int J Periodontics Restorative Dent. 1994;14:154–65.
4. Tarnow DP, Magner AW, Fletcher P. The effect of the distance from the contact point to the crest of bone on the presence or absence of the interproximal dental papilla. J Periodontol. 1992;63:995–6.
5. Martegani P, Silvestri M, Mascarello F, Scipioni T, Ghezzi C, Rota C, Cattaneo V. Morphometric study of the interproximal unit in the esthetic region to correlate anatomic variables affecting the aspect of soft tissue embrasure space. J Periodontol. 2007;78:2260–5.
6. Cho HS, Jang HS, Kim DK, Park JC, Kim HJ, Choi SH, Kim CK, Kim BO. The effects of interproximal distance between roots on the existence of interdental papillae according to the distance from the contact point to the alveolar crest. J Periodontol. 2006;77:1651–7.
7. Schoenbaum TR, Klokkevold PR, Chang YY. Immediate implant-supported provisional restoration with a root-form pontic for the replacement of two adjacent anterior maxillary teeth: a clinical report. J Prosthet Dent. 2013;109:277–82.
8. Buser D, Bornstein MM, Weber HP, Grutter L, Schmid B, Belser UC. Early implant placement with simultaneous guided bone regeneration following single-tooth extraction in the esthetic zone: a cross-sectional, retrospective study in 45 subjects with a 2- to 4-year follow-up. J Periodontol. 2008;79:1773–81.
9. Chen ST, Darby IB, Reynolds EC, Clement JG. Immediate implant placement postextraction without flap elevation. J Periodontol. 2009;80:163–72.
10. Kan JY, Rungcharassaeng K, Lozada J. Immediate placement and provisionalization of maxillary anterior single implants: 1-year prospective study. Int J Oral Maxillofac Implants. 2003;18:31–9.
11. Klokkevold PR, Han TJ, Camargo PM. Aesthetic management of extractions for implant site development: delayed versus staged implant placement. Pract Periodontics Aesthet Dent. 1999;11:603–10. quiz 612.

12. Azzi R, Takei HH, Etienne D, Carranza FA. Root coverage and papilla reconstruction using autogenous osseous and connective tissue grafts. Int J Periodontics Restorative Dent. 2001;21:141–7.
13. Han TJ, Takei HH. Progress in gingival papilla reconstruction. Periodontol. 1996;11:65–8.
14. Takei HH, Han TJ, Carranza FA Jr, Kenney EB, Lekovic V. Flap technique for periodontal bone implants. Papilla preservation technique. J Periodontol. 1985;56:204–10.
15. Lekovic V, Kenney EB, Weinlaender M, Han T, Klokkevold P, Nedic M, Orsini M. A bone regenerative approach to alveolar ridge maintenance following tooth extraction. Report of 10 cases. J Periodontol. 1997;68:563–70.
16. Araujo MG, Lindhe J. Dimensional ridge alterations following tooth extraction. An experimental study in the dog. J Clin Periodontol. 2005;32:212–8.
17. Araujo MG, Wennstrom JL, Lindhe J. Modeling of the buccal and lingual bone walls of fresh extraction sites following implant installation. Clin Oral Implants Res. 2006;17:606–14.
18. Hammerle CH, Araujo MG, Simion M, Osteology Consensus G. Evidence-based knowledge on the biology and treatment of extraction sockets. Clin Oral Implants Res. 2012;23(Suppl 5):80–2.
19. Tarnow D, Elian N, Fletcher P, Froum S, Magner A, Cho SC, Salama M, Salama H, Garber DA. Vertical distance from the crest of bone to the height of the interproximal papilla between adjacent implants. J Periodontol. 2003;74:1785–8.
20. Kois JC. Predictable single-tooth peri-implant esthetics: five diagnostic keys. Compend Contin Educ Dent. 2004;25:895–6. 898, 900 passim; quiz 906–897.
21. Benic GI, Mokti M, Chen CJ, Weber HP, Hammerle CH, Gallucci GO. Dimensions of buccal bone and mucosa at immediately placed implants after 7 years: a clinical and cone beam computed tomography study. Clin Oral Implants Res. 2012;23:560–6.
22. Miron RJ, Dard M, Weinreb M. Enamel matrix derivative, inflammation and soft tissue wound healing. J Periodontal Res. 2015;50:555–69.
23. Rasperini G, Roccuzzo M, Francetti L, Acunzo R, Consonni D, Silvestri M. Subepithelial connective tissue graft for treatment of gingival recessions with and without enamel matrix derivative: a multicenter, randomized controlled clinical trial. Int J Periodontics Restorative Dent. 2011;31:133–9.
24. Hehn J, Schwenk T, Striegel M, Schlee M. The effect of PRF (platelet-rich fibrin) inserted with a split-flap technique on soft tissue thickening and initial marginal bone loss around implants: results of a randomized, controlled clinical trial. Int J Implant Dent. 2016;2:13.
25. Han TJ, Jeong CW. Bone and crescent shaped free gingival grafting for anterior immediate implant placement: technique and case report. J Implant Adv Clin Dent. 2009;1:23–33.
26. Araujo MG, Sukekava F, Wennstrom JL, Lindhe J. Ridge alterations following implant placement in fresh extraction sockets: an experimental study in the dog. J Clin Periodontol. 2005;32:645–52.
27. Nevins M, Camelo M, De Paoli S, Friedland B, Schenk RK, Parma-Benfenati S, Simion M, Tinti C, Wagenberg B. A study of the fate of the buccal wall of extraction sockets of teeth with prominent roots. Int J Periodontics Restorative Dent. 2006;26:19–29.
28. Chiapasco M, Consolo U, Bianchi A, Ronchi P. Alveolar distraction osteogenesis for the correction of vertically deficient edentulous ridges: a multicenter prospective study on humans. Int J Oral Maxillofac Implants. 2004;19:399–407.
29. Covani U, Cornelini R, Barone A. Bucco-lingual bone remodeling around implants placed into immediate extraction sockets: a case series. J Periodontol. 2003;74:268–73.
30. Schropp L, Kostopoulos L, Wenzel A. Bone healing following immediate versus delayed placement of titanium implants into extraction sockets: a prospective clinical study. Int J Oral Maxillofac Implants. 2003;18:189–99.
31. Allen EP, Gainza CS, Farthing GG, Newbold DA. Improved technique for localized ridge augmentation. A report of 21 cases. J Periodontol. 1985;56:195–9.
32. Seibert JS. Treatment of moderate localized alveolar ridge defects. Preventive and reconstructive concepts in therapy. Dent Clin N Am. 1993;37:265–80.

33. Kan JY, Rungcharassaeng K, Lozada JL. Bilaminar subepithelial connective tissue grafts for immediate implant placement and provisionalization in the esthetic zone. J Calif Dent Assoc. 2005;33:865–71.
34. Khzam N, Arora H, Kim P, Fisher A, Mattheos N, Ivanovski S. Systematic review of soft tissue alterations and esthetic outcomes following immediate implant placement and restoration of single implants in the anterior maxilla. J Periodontol. 2015;86:1321–30.
35. Kan JY, Rungcharassaeng K. Site development for anterior single implant esthetics: the dentulous site. Compend Contin Educ Dent. 2001;22:221–6. 228, 230-221; quiz 232.
36. Bengazi F, Wennstrom JL, Lekholm U. Recession of the soft tissue margin at oral implants. A 2-year longitudinal prospective study. Clin Oral Implants Res. 1996;7:303–10.
37. Grunder U. Stability of the mucosal topography around single-tooth implants and adjacent teeth: 1-year results. Int J Periodontics Restorative Dent. 2000;20:11–7.
38. Nozawa T, Enomoto H, Tsurumaki S, Ito K. Biologic height-width ratio of the buccal supra-implant mucosa. Eur J Esthet Dent. 2006;1:208–14.
39. Kan JY, Rungcharassaeng K, Lozada JL, Zimmerman G. Facial gingival tissue stability following immediate placement and provisionalization of maxillary anterior single implants: a 2- to 8-year follow-up. Int J Oral Maxillofac Implants. 2011;26:179–87.

Growth Factors for Site Preparation: Current Science, Indications, and Practice

6

Tara Aghaloo and Rachel Lim

Abstract

Implant restoration of the dentition poses many challenges in cases of limited bony foundation. Many patients suffer from loss of teeth and supporting bony structures through mechanisms including trauma, congenital abnormalities, or resorption secondary to tooth loss. In addition to classic alveolar ridge augmentation techniques and materials, growth factors are being studied to improve patient outcomes, especially in cases of larger, more challenging defects, in previously failed graft sites, and in stringent aesthetic cases. In this chapter, we will discuss three growth factors which are most commonly studied and US Food and Drug Administration approved: bone morphogenetic protein-2 (BMP-2), platelet-derived growth factor (PDGF), and platelet-rich protein/platelet-rich fibrin (PRP/PRF). Currently, growth factors are utilized in a wide variety of clinical situations, including guided bone regeneration, peri-implant defects, sinus augmentation, and socket augmentation. Furthermore, we will explore the future of growth factor usage, with new factors in various stages of investigation, combinations of materials, and viable cell therapy. Though much work has been done in the last few decades to reveal the clinical relevance of growth factors, much more research, both basic and clinical, must be performed to improve current technologies, develop predictable protocols, and evaluate long-term results.

T. Aghaloo (✉)
Section of Oral and Maxillofacial Surgery, UCLA School of Dentistry, Los Angeles, CA, USA
e-mail: taghaloo@dentistry.ucla.edu

R. Lim
Department of Oral and Maxillofacial Surgery, University of Washington, Seattle, WA, USA

Todd R. Schoenbaum (ed.), *Implants in the Aesthetic Zone*,
https://doi.org/10.1007/978-3-319-72601-4_6

6.1 Introduction

Many patients suffer from significant loss of the periodontium and surrounding bony structures through mechanisms including periodontal disease, trauma, congenital abnormalities, tumors, or resorption secondary to tooth loss. In these situations, achieving a stable site for reconstruction through implant placement can pose clinical challenges and may require augmentation to optimize the supporting structures [1]. Furthermore, aesthetic zone sites require more stringent planning, with factors such as gingival biotype and space limitations significantly affecting the final result, and in which proper placement of the implant is paramount to an ideal outcome [2]. In smaller bony defects, successful treatment with guided bone regeneration (GBR; see Chap. 4) using autografts, allografts, or xenografts has been well documented [3]. However, larger or more challenging defects in previously failed graft sites or implant sites in medically compromised patients will require more complex therapy to achieve a successful outcome. In such cases, traditional techniques and materials may not achieve sufficient bone regeneration, compromising the prosthetic rehabilitation and final outcome.

One of the main techniques that have been implemented since its development in the 1980s is guided bone regeneration, which has resulted in predictable regeneration of contained defects through usage of grafting materials and/or barrier membranes [1, 3]. In cases requiring significant bone regeneration, secondary techniques have been employed concurrently with GBR to overcome limitations of scaffold material and to recruit the desired cell types for regeneration. Over the past decade, molecular mediators, such as growth factors, have been extensively studied for their potential to combat challenging clinical scenarios by accelerating the healing process and aid in regeneration of the missing maxillofacial tissues [4]. Growth factors naturally occur in the body and are capable of stimulating growth, proliferation, and differentiation of cells. Growth factors regulate many of the key cellular events that are required for tissue repair and regeneration. The clinical application of these biologic agents aims to provide faster healing, implant osseointegration, and expedited establishment of functionality. Currently, growth factors are utilized in a wide variety of clinical situations including intrabony defects, barrier membranes for GBR, peri-implant defects, sinus augmentation, and socket augmentation. In this chapter, we will focus on US Food and Drug Administration (FDA)-approved growth factors: bone morphogenetic protein (BMP-2), platelet-derived growth factor (PDGF), and platelet-rich plasma (PRP)/platelet-rich fibrin (PRF).

Bone forms through three distinct mechanisms, and bone grafting materials are classified based on their ability to activate these mechanisms. Osteo*conductive* materials possess the ability to passively act as a scaffold and allow substitution of new bone. Osteoconduction requires good surrounding bone that can be resorbed and replaced with new native bone from the host. Although osteoconductive materials are readily available and inexpensive, large and complex bone defects or medically compromised patients with poor healing potential generally cannot regenerate bone from only scaffold grafting material. Osteo*inductive* materials can actively recruit undifferentiated mesenchymal stem cells to the graft site and stimulate osteoblastic differentiation. Bringing these cells to the site and driving bone formation is a huge advantage of inductive materials. However, most off the shelf bone grafts do not contain these properties. Osteo*genic* materials transplant live bone cells which can actively form new bone at the recipient site [5]. Osteogenesis is the most powerful of the three mechanisms, but only autogenous bone possesses these properties. Unfortunately, not all patients are candidates for autogenous bone harvesting since it often requires a second surgical site, increased morbidity, and longer surgical time. When determining the appropriate growth factor for a specific patient, evaluating the bone or soft tissue enhancing properties of the material is important. Since no graft material can possess all the ideal properties—biocompatibility, biodegradability, promotion of vascularity, mechanical properties similar to bone, selectivity for osteogenic cell adherence and survival, ease of manipulation, availability, and low cost—growth factors may improve or enhance our currently utilized materials.

6.2 Bone Morphogenetic Protein-2 (BMP-2)

Bone morphogenetic proteins (BMPs) are secreted glycoproteins that belong to the transforming growth factor-beta (TGF-β) superfamily. These glycoproteins are classified as morphogens, with roles in dictating tissue patterning in embryonic development, and are potent regulators of bone and cartilage formation and repair. Many studies have demonstrated that BMP's can induce mesenchymal stem cell differentiation into bone and cartilage, making them promising molecules for tissue engineering and bone therapy [6]. In 1965, Urist first discovered BMP as a substance in the extracellular bone matrix which was capable of inducing ectopic osteogenesis when implanted in extraskeletal rabbit muscle pouches [7]. Since the classification of BMP's in the late 1980s, more than 20 members have been identified, though not all are osteogenic [8, 9]. Specifically, BMP-2 is most commonly utilized for its osteoinductive properties, which allows it to actively promote chemotaxis to the graft site and stimulate osteoblastic differentiation and bone formation [10, 11]. BMP-2 has been extensively studied and increasingly applied in orthopedic surgery to improve the results of bone therapy. In 2002, recombinant human BMP-2 and BMP-7 (rhBMP-2 and rhBMP-7) were approved by the FDA for orthopedic applications including (1) promoting fusion of lower spine vertebrae, (2) acute tibia fractures, and (3) tibia nonunion [12]. As patients become more medically compromised or when conventional grafting techniques fail, growth factors have been utilized for new applications such as posttraumatic osteonecrosis of the femoral head [13].

In oral and maxillofacial reconstruction, BMP-2 has demonstrated ability to control bone formation, contour, and density through endochondral formation [1]. Randomized clinical trials demonstrate predictable bone formation in localized alveolar bone defects associated with tooth extraction and sinus augmentation when placed on an absorbable collagen sponge (ACS) [14–16]. These successes led to FDA approval for these dental indications in 2007 (Infuse, Medtronic, Nashville, TN). Since its approval, clinicians and researchers continue to expand the off-label uses of rhBMP-2/ACS to include onlay grafting, lateral ridge augmentation, extensive maxillofacial reconstruction, and mandibular continuity defects (Fig. 6.1) [4, 17–25]. These more complicated defects generally require a more compressive resistant scaffold (such as titanium mesh) [26, 27].

rhBMP-2/ACS is often combined with a xenograft or allograft for alveolar ridge or sinus augmentation, resulting in further off-label utilization (Fig. 6.1) [27–32]. In addition, improved soft tissue compression resistance can be obtained by combining rhBMP-2/ACS with additional graft materials or titanium mesh. Specifically, combination with osteoconductive materials may decrease the BMP-2 dose needed to regenerate bone defects. Clinically FDA-approved supraphysiologic BMP-2 doses have been associated with many side effects including major swelling, inflammation, seromas, wound breakdown, heterotopic bone formation, cystic bone cavities, immunogenicity, BMP antibody formation, osteolysis through osteoclast activation, and bone cyst formation [33–39]. Currently, BMP-2 use for oral and maxillofacial defects has not been optimized due to high costs, nonideal carriers, and suboptimal bone formation, resulting in limited clinical use. However, in patients with

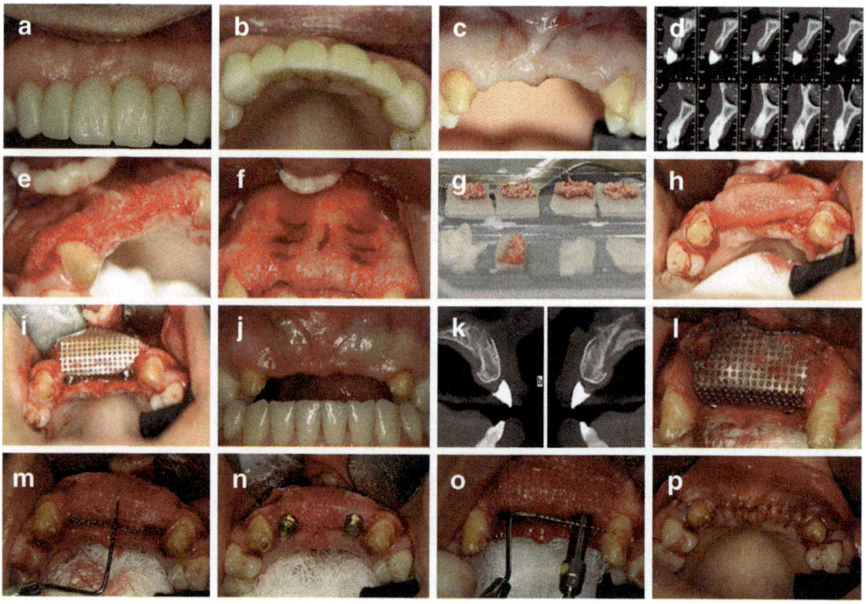

Fig. 6.1 rhBMP-2 for anterior maxillary ridge augmentation. (**a**) Buccal and (**b**) occlusal view of resorbed alveolar ridge with temporary fixed partial denture. (**c**) Clinical and (**d**) radiographic (*CBCT* cone-beam CT scan) preoperative alveolar ridge. (**e**) After flap reflection, (**f**) cortical bone decortication is performed to release undifferentiated mesenchymal stem cells from the trabecular bone that can respond to the rhBMP-2. (**g**) rhBMP-2/ACS is combined with autograft and alloplast grafting materials and covered with a (**h**) BMP-2 sponge before (**i**) titanium mesh is applied to resist soft tissue compression. (**j**) Wound healing after 7 months and (**k**) CBCT scan before implant placement. (**l**) Titanium mesh is seen at the time of implant placement for removal and reveals (**m**) an increased volume of bone for (**n**) implant placement. (**o**) Adequate ridge dimensions are seen, and (**p**) soft tissue coverage is performed without difficulty

Table 6.1 Advantages and disadvantages of rhBMP-2

rhBMP-2	
Advantages	Disadvantages
Osteoinductive	Cost
Angiogenesis	Swelling
No donor site	Few studies
Reliable RCT studies	Short-term studies
Low infection risk	Wound dehiscence
FDA approval	No compression resistance

previously failed bone grafts, severely medically compromised patients, or when other graft materials are contraindicated, BMP-2 is a promising alternative [40, 41]. Advantages and disadvantages of rhBMP-2 must be considered when making decisions about utilizing specific growth factors (Table 6.1).

6.3 Platelet-Derived Growth Factor (PDGF)

Platelet-derived growth factor (PDGF) is one of the most extensively studied growth factors in implantology due to its potential for both soft tissue and hard tissue repair. In the late 1980s, Lynch discovered PDGF's capability for periodontal regeneration in an animal study of beagle dogs with periodontitis-affected teeth [42]. Preliminary results suggested that application of PDGF and insulin-like growth factor (IGF-1) had potential to enhance regeneration of the bone and cementum. PDGF originates from platelets during clotting and is released in response to soft or hard tissue injury. PDGF promotes chemotaxis, angiogenesis, and platelet activation [43–46]. Interestingly, in vitro and in vivo studies have shown that PDGF can attract gingival and periodontal ligament fibroblasts, cementoblasts, and osteoblasts. In dentistry, rhPDGF-BB (Gem 21S, Osteohealth, Shirley, NY) is US FDA approved to treat intrabony defects and gingival recession defects in combination with a beta-tricalcium phosphate carrier. It has been shown to improve clinical attachment levels, osseous fill, and reduce gingival recession [1, 47, 48]. Similar to BMP-2, PDGF off-label use is extremely common, especially in implant dentistry. PDGF has shown some success when combined with xenografts, allografts, and alloplasts in socket grafting, sinus augmentation, and alveolar ridge augmentation [49–57].

PDGF is also a major mitogenic factor produced by connective tissue cells (such as fibroblasts and smooth muscle cells) to play roles in embryogenesis and wound healing. In addition to chemotactic effects, PDGF induces macrophages to produce and secrete growth factors for various phases of healing. Studies show that PDGF is able to stimulate production of relevant matrix molecules such as fibronectin, collagen, and hyaluronic acid [58, 59]. PDGF is related to production and secretion of collagenase by fibroblasts, which suggests a role in soft tissue remodeling. Furthermore, PDGF is shown to have effects on the vascular system, with receptors expressed on capillary endothelial cells. It is implicated in regulation of vascular tone by constriction of blood vessels, as well as cardiac angiogenesis [60]. In wound healing, platelets release PDGF in response to injury and cause a decrease in

Table 6.2 Advantages and disadvantages of rhPDGF-BB

rhPDGF-BB	
Advantages	Disadvantages
Osteoconductive	Not osteoinductive
Angiogenesis	Only FDA for periodontal defects
Promotes soft tissue healing	Lack of controlled studies
Cost	Minimal data

platelet aggregation. Its vascular properties validate its use, which led to FDA approval for many years to treat chronic foot ulcers in diabetic patients [61]. PDGF aids in both hard and soft tissue healing, but it does not have osteoinductive properties. In addition, overactivity of PDGF is implicated with pathologic growth stimulation in tumorigenesis, as well as benign conditions of atherosclerosis and fibrotic conditions [45]. Similar to BMP-2, rhPDGF has specific advantages and disadvantages that should be considered before choosing this material for clinical use (Table 6.2).

6.4 Platelet-Rich Plasma (PRP)/Platelet-Rich Fibrin (PRF)

In 1998, Marx proposed a method to concentrate autologous platelet factors through treatment and of centrifugation of whole blood. Platelets release α-granules which contain numerous proteins necessary for healing and assist in processes of chemotaxis, mitogenesis, angiogenesis, collagen synthesis, and bone matrix formation [62]. This preparation is applied directly to wound and surgical sites to promote bone and soft tissue regeneration and repair [63–65]. A significant increase in platelets with PRP preparation may be associated with increased growth factor concentration and thus improved healing. Specifically, PDGF, transforming growth factor-ß (TGF-ß), vascular endothelial growth factor (VEGF), and IGF-1 have been shown to be increased in PRP preparations [65–67].

Some studies demonstrate favorable bone formation when PRP is added to conventional bone grafts, while others show conflicting results. Variations in growth factor concentration and platelet activity are seen with different patient gender, age, and PRP preparation methods [68–74]. Even though results are inconsistent, PRP has been successfully utilized to graft extraction sockets, augment the maxillary sinus, enhance alveolar ridges, and improve soft tissue thickness [70, 75–78]. In clinical practice, clinicians are consistently searching for less invasive and more cost-effective methods to enhance outcomes. PRP has fallen out of favor in recent years because it required expensive, bulky centrifuges that needed large volumes of blood and complicated anticoagulant preparations. Additionally, clinical results were highly inconsistent and outcomes unpredictable [79].

An increasingly popular development in the use of growth factors requires less autologous blood and comes at a lower cost [80, 81]. Platelet-rich fibrin (PRF)

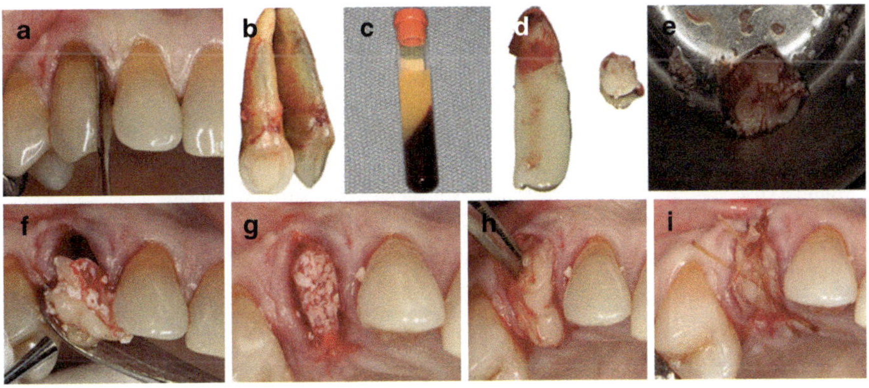

Fig. 6.2 Socket augmentation with PRF. (**a**, **b**) Extraction is performed with minimal trauma. (**c**) PRF is prepared in a 10 mL tube to form a (**d**) membrane and a plug that is combined with the (**e**) bone substitute material. (**f**, **g**) The socket is grafted, and the (**h**) PRF membrane is placed over the graft and sutured (**i**)

requires only 8–10 mL of autologous blood (compared to 60 mL needed for PRP), no anti-coagulants, and a small desktop centrifuge. The platelets are concentrated in the buffy coat and contain key growth factors including PDGF, transforming growth factor-beta (TGF-β), vascular endothelial growth factor (VEGF), insulin-like growth factor (IGF), thrombospondin, fibronectin, vitronectin, and interleukin-1 (IL-1), IL-6, and IL-4 [62, 82, 83]. Similar to PRP, favorable studies can be found that demonstrate a trend toward improved soft tissue and bone healing in extraction sockets, though not statistically significant (Fig. 6.2) [84]. Mostly case series are available for other augmentation procedures such as sinus augmentation, where bone gain was seen, implants survived, and vital bone was biopsied [85]. Another study utilized autogenous block bone grafts covered by a PRF membrane resulting in less bone resorption after healing [86]. Although these studies show favorable results, they are preliminary and few in number. Other studies show conflicting results where PRF did not significantly enhance bone regeneration or soft tissue healing [84, 87].

As PRF becomes increasingly utilized for a variety of clinical indications, it is imperative that well-designed and well-controlled studies be performed to validate the preliminary results. In addition, manufacturing processes for autologous platelet concentrates are highly variable, and there are many systems and preparations available on the market for soft and hard tissue application. L-PRF contains leukocytes that may enhance immune function or increase growth factor production. A-PRF may enhance growth factor presence through recruitment of macrophages and granulocytes in the clot. Both need much more investigation to determine if any significant clinical effects exist [88–91]. As the field becomes more complicated, it often makes interpreting and generalizing the results of available studies difficult and requires more stringent review of these clinical studies (Table 6.3).

Table 6.3 Advantages and disadvantages of PRF

PRF	
Advantages	Disadvantages
Small amount blood	Additional training
Multiple growth factors	Clinically significant growth factor concentrations
Many techniques: sticky bone/membrane	Varied preparations and protocols
Minimal cost	Not occlusive or barrier membrane
Possible less surgical time, less graft material	Inconclusive studies soft tissue/bone healing
Autologous source	
Decreased swelling/hematoma	

6.5 Future of Growth Factors in Implant Dentistry

Although only BMP-2, PDGF, and platelet concentrates are FDA approved for clinical use in patients for dental use, there are other growth factors which are in various stages of investigation. Some of these factors have shown great promise for bone and/or soft tissue healing and will likely undergo clinical studies in the near future. In addition, cellular-based products are also available that have very few case reports in oral surgical applications. These are important areas where proper research must be done to determine their indications, success rates, limitations, and protocols for use in implant dentistry.

6.5.1 Fibroblast Growth Factor (FGF)

One of the most important factors of ensuring implant success is the creation of a well-formed soft tissue seal. The microbial insults are strongly associated with the destructive inflammation of peri-implantitis, leading to implant failure due to resorption of bone and soft tissue [92]. Accordingly, research is being done to improve this soft tissue seal through manipulating the bone-implant and bone-gingiva contact. One method is through utilization of fibroblast growth factor (FGF), deposited via nanotubule carrier or collagen sponge. The FGF family consists of proteins which aid in the proliferation, migration, and differentiation of periodontal ligament (PDL) cells, as well as the production of extracellular matrix (ECM) [93]. Specifically, FGF-2 is being studied for its ability to increase bone deposition in areas of peri-implant defects as well as intrabony defects [1]. In a study on critical-sized defects in rat calvarial bone, Kigami et al. found that usage of FGF-2 on absorbable collagen sponge increased formation of blood vessels and concentration of osteoblast and osteoclast cells; however, the increase in angiogenesis was the most prominent finding. Their work recommended studies using scaffolds that could deliver FGF-2 more continuously than absorbable collagen sponge, which by 4 weeks, only showed 64% cumulative release of FGF-2 [94].

In a study by Nagayasu-Tanaka et al., FGF-2 on hydroxypropyl cellulose carrier was used on customized titanium implants, which were created to have low contact with the existing bone in beagle dogs. They evaluated bone-implant interface at 4, 8, and 12 weeks and found that FGF-2 significantly promoted bone formation at 4 weeks and increased the ISQ value by about ten compared to control. However, the increase in ISQ value peaked at 4 weeks and remained fairly constant even at 12 weeks for both the FGF-2-impregnated implants and control, suggesting that FGF-2 accelerates bone formation but does not alter it over a longer timeframe. Notably, FGF-2 was most remarkable in improving bone formation in areas delayed by gaps between implant and bone [95]. Several studies demonstrated that the use of FGF increased the amount of bone-to-implant contact, for improved osseointegration. In 2001, McCracken et al. found that addition of FGF in an activated fibrinogen matrix on titanium-aluminum-vanadium implants significantly increased the amount of bone-to-implant contact ($p < 0.05$) compared to controls. This study also demonstrated a greater percentage volume of bone deposition adjacent to the implants, which supported the hypothesis that FGF could increase bone formation around implants in a rat model [96].

6.5.2 Nell-1

NELL-1 is a potent pro-osteogenic protein, first discovered in locations of excessive bone growth in calvarial sutures of patients with craniosynostosis [97]. To date, NELL-1 has demonstrated induction of the bone in several preclinical models including increased bone deposition in osteoporotic mice, distraction osteogenesis, and increased rates of spinal fusion in various animal models. In 2006, Cowan et al. studied NELL-1 in the craniofacial complex through administration on distracted intermaxillary sutures in mice, demonstrating that NELL-1 induced bone formation at rates similar to BMP-2 and accelerated chondrocyte hypertrophy and endochondral bone formation [98]. The ability of NELL-1 to induce bone formation in the palatal suture demonstrates potential for usage in palatal defect healing. According to a study by Cowan et al., NELL-1 has potential to synergistically enhance osteogenic differentiation of mesenchymal stem cells when used with BMP-2. This study confirmed the osteochondral specificity of NELL-1 signaling, and potential for enhanced therapeutic BMP-2 bone regeneration [99, 100]. NELL-1 is currently being studied for clinical applications including vertebral compression fractures, osteoporosis, as well as potential to promote development of cartilage. While there is currently no existing literature on the application of NELL-1 in patients or to implant dentistry, the characterization of NELL-1 as an osteogenic protein posits NELL-1 as an important factor for consideration in future studies.

6.6 Allografts with Viable Cells

Alternative methods of enhancing bone regeneration include usage of mesenchymal stem cells with bone allograft material. Autograft bone, harvested most commonly from the patient's iliac crest, is the gold standard for bone augmentation because it is histocompatible and non-immunogenic. Furthermore, autograft bone provides the three pillars of bone growth: osteoconductive scaffold, osteoinductive factors, and osteogenic cells [101]. However, the process of harvesting autogenous bone presents many clinical downfalls, such as donor site morbidity, increased surgical time, risk of infection, and limited availability [102].

A new approach being investigated is the use of bone allograft combined with bone marrow mesenchymal stem cells (BMSCs) to maintain osteoconductivity, osteoinductivity, and osteogenicity. Since their discovery in 1966, mesenchymal stem cells (MSCs) have been characterized with ability for self-renewal as well as multipotential to differentiate into bone, cartilage, fat, nerve, muscle, and tendon, depending on external cues in the local environment [103]. For MSC's to be directed to a particular lineage of differentiation, they require appropriate density, spatial organization, and local factors [104]. Furthermore, MSCs are part of the bony repair callus and differentiates into bone or cartilage based on stability. Vasculature and angiogenesis are additional requirements for osteogenic differentiation. Current growth factor systems rely on the body's inherent local cells, including MSC's and osteoprogenitor cells, to help regenerate bone.

Several new products are now on the market that combine various formulations of endogenous bone forming cells with osteoinductive growth factors (Trinity® Evolution™, Osteocel® Plus, and Osiris BIO^{4}™). Trinity® Evolution™ (TE) is a cryopreserved allograft consisting of viable cancellous bone matrix and demineralized cortical bone matrix, with mesenchymal stem cells, osteoprogenitors, and osteoinductive proteins, and osteoconductive matrix [105]. In 2016, a prospective clinical study was performed, which observed the usage of TE in anterior cervical discectomy and fusion. Degree of fusion was assessed based on radiographic appearance, function, and residual pain, performed with a series of clinical tests by examiners. This study reported fusion rates of 94% with TE, similar to previously reported fusion rates of autografts in similar conditions. Overall, the study concluded that TE had a high rate of single-level cervical fusion with no serious adverse events. Though inconclusive, current data of bone allografts with MSCs are favorable and offer an alternative to autografts, allografts, and growth factors. Clinical trials are currently being conducted, with usage of MSCs with allograft in transforaminal lumbar body fusion, anterior cervical discectomy and fusion, and foot and ankle fusion [101, 106, 107]. Favorable results of allograft and MSC usage include new bone formation at site of implantation, with satisfactory clinical and radiographic success in situations of stable internal or external skeletal fixation. In implant dentistry, although generally favorable, few case series are available to support the use of MSC/allograft technology [108].

Conclusions

What is the future of growth factors in implant dentistry? This is a question that is posed by patients, clinicians, researchers, and industry. Much work has been done in the last few decades, but in many situations, the clinical relevance, predictability, and protocols have not been fully understood. It is unclear whether all patients will require or benefit from growth factors to assist with wound healing

Table 6.4 Growth factor uses

Growth factor uses
All patients
Compromised wounds
Complex hard/soft tissue defects
Previously failed surgeries
Medically compromised patients

and augmentation or if they are only relevant in medically compromised patients and those with previously failed procedures (Table 6.4). What is clear is that the field is looking for materials and methods to enhance bone and soft tissue healing, allowing treatment of more complex patients and wounds. Growth factors, and possibly stem cells, are a plausible answer to current limitations. However, much more research, both basic and clinical, needs to be done to improve current technologies, develop predictable protocols, and evaluate long-term results.

References

1. Suarez-Lopez Del Amo F, et al. Biologic agents for periodontal regeneration and implant site development. Biomed Res Int. 2015;2015:957518.
2. Higginbottom FL. Implants as an option in the esthetic zone. J Oral Maxillofac Surg. 2005;63(9 Suppl 2):33–44.
3. Aghaloo TL, Moy PK. Which hard tissue augmentation techniques are the most successful in furnishing bony support for implant placement? Int J Oral Maxillofac Implants. 2007;22(Suppl):49–70.
4. Schliephake H. Clinical efficacy of growth factors to enhance tissue repair in oral and maxillofacial reconstruction: a systematic review. Clin Implant Dent Relat Res. 2015;17(2):247–73.
5. Miyazaki M, et al. An update on bone substitutes for spinal fusion. Eur Spine J. 2009;18(6):783–99.
6. Reddi AH. Morphogenesis and tissue engineering of bone and cartilage: inductive signals, stem cells, and biomimetic biomaterials. Tissue Eng. 2000;6(4):351–9.
7. Urist MR. Bone: formation by autoinduction. Science. 1965;150(3698):893–9.
8. Lavery K, et al. BMP-2/4 and BMP-6/7 differentially utilize cell surface receptors to induce osteoblastic differentiation of human bone marrow-derived mesenchymal stem cells. J Biol Chem. 2008;283(30):20948–58.
9. Poon B, et al. Bone morphogenetic protein-2 and bone therapy: successes and pitfalls. J Pharm Pharmacol. 2016;68(2):139–47.
10. Wozney JM. Overview of bone morphogenetic proteins. Spine (Phila Pa 1976). 2002;27(16 Suppl 1):S2–8.
11. Yamaguchi A, Komori T, Suda T. Regulation of osteoblast differentiation mediated by bone morphogenetic proteins, hedgehogs, and Cbfa1. Endocr Rev. 2000;21(4):393–411.
12. Valdes MA, et al. Recombinant bone morphogenic protein-2 in orthopaedic surgery: a review. Arch Orthop Trauma Surg. 2009;129(12):1651–7.
13. Carreira AC, et al. Bone morphogenetic proteins: structure, biological function and therapeutic applications. Arch Biochem Biophys. 2014;561:64–73.
14. Boyne PJ, et al. De novo bone induction by recombinant human bone morphogenetic protein-2 (rhBMP-2) in maxillary sinus floor augmentation. J Oral Maxillofac Surg. 2005;63(12):1693–707.
15. Triplett RG, et al. Pivotal, randomized, parallel evaluation of recombinant human bone morphogenetic protein-2/absorbable collagen sponge and autogenous bone graft for maxillary sinus floor augmentation. J Oral Maxillofac Surg. 2009;67(9):1947–60.

16. Fiorellini JP, et al. Randomized study evaluating recombinant human bone morphogenetic protein-2 for extraction socket augmentation. J Periodontol. 2005;76(4):605–13.
17. Carter TG, et al. Off-label use of recombinant human bone morphogenetic protein-2 (rhBMP-2) for reconstruction of mandibular bone defects in humans. J Oral Maxillofac Surg. 2008;66(7):1417–25.
18. Herford AS, Boyne PJ. Reconstruction of mandibular continuity defects with bone morphogenetic protein-2 (rhBMP-2). J Oral Maxillofac Surg. 2008;66(4):616–24.
19. Herford AS. rhBMP-2 as an option for reconstructing mandibular continuity defects. J Oral Maxillofac Surg. 2009;67(12):2679–84.
20. Fallucco MA, Carstens MH. Primary reconstruction of alveolar clefts using recombinant human bone morphogenic protein-2: clinical and radiographic outcomes. J Craniofac Surg. 2009;20(Suppl 2):1759–64.
21. Chin M, et al. Repair of alveolar clefts with recombinant human bone morphogenetic protein (rhBMP-2) in patients with clefts. J Craniofac Surg. 2005;16(5):778–89.
22. Herford AS, et al. Bone morphogenetic protein-induced repair of the premaxillary cleft. J Oral Maxillofac Surg. 2007;65(11):2136–41.
23. Canan LW Jr, et al. Human bone morphogenetic protein-2 use for maxillary reconstruction in cleft lip and palate patients. J Craniofac Surg. 2012;23(6):1627–33.
24. Cicciu M, et al. Recombinant human bone morphogenetic protein type 2 application for a possible treatment of bisphosphonates-related osteonecrosis of the jaw. J Craniofac Surg. 2012;23(3):784–8.
25. Alonso N, et al. Evaluation of maxillary alveolar reconstruction using a resorbable collagen sponge with recombinant human bone morphogenetic protein-2 in cleft lip and palate patients. Tissue Eng Part C Methods. 2010;16(5):1183–9.
26. Edmunds RK, et al. Maxillary anterior ridge augmentation with recombinant human bone morphogenetic protein 2. Int J Periodontics Restorative Dent. 2014;34(4):551–7.
27. Misch CM, et al. Vertical bone augmentation using recombinant bone morphogenetic protein, mineralized bone allograft, and titanium mesh: a retrospective cone beam computed tomography study. Int J Oral Maxillofac Implants. 2015;30(1):202–7.
28. Tarnow DP, et al. Maxillary sinus augmentation using recombinant bone morphogenetic protein-2/acellular collagen sponge in combination with a mineralized bone replacement graft: a report of three cases. Int J Periodontics Restorative Dent. 2010;30(2):139–49.
29. Jung RE, et al. A randomized-controlled clinical trial evaluating clinical and radiological outcomes after 3 and 5 years of dental implants placed in bone regenerated by means of GBR techniques with or without the addition of BMP-2. Clin Oral Implants Res. 2009;20(7):660–6.
30. Jensen OT, et al. BMP-2/ACS/allograft for combined maxillary alveolar split/sinus floor grafting with and without simultaneous dental implant placement: report of 21 implants placed into 7 alveolar split sites followed for up to 3 years. Int J Oral Maxillofac Implants. 2014;29(1):e81–94.
31. Butura CC, Galindo DF. Implant placement in alveolar composite defects regenerated with rhBMP-2, anorganic bovine bone, and titanium mesh: a report of eight reconstructed sites. Int J Oral Maxillofac Implants. 2014;29(1):e139–46.
32. Bowler D, Dym H. Bone morphogenic protein: application in implant dentistry. Dent Clin North Am. 2015;59(2):493–503.
33. Chan DS, et al. Wound complications associated with bone morphogenetic protein-2 in orthopaedic trauma surgery. J Orthop Trauma. 2014;28(10):599–604.
34. Garrett MP, et al. Formation of painful seroma and edema after the use of recombinant human bone morphogenetic protein-2 in posterolateral lumbar spine fusions. Neurosurgery. 2010;66(6):1044–9. discussion 1049.
35. Hustedt JW, Blizzard DJ. The controversy surrounding bone morphogenetic proteins in the spine: a review of current research. Yale J Biol Med. 2014;87(4):549–61.
36. James AW, et al. A review of the clinical side effects of bone morphogenetic protein-2. Tissue Eng Part B Rev. 2016;22(4):284–97.

37. Lebl DR. Bone morphogenetic protein in complex cervical spine surgery: a safe biologic adjunct? World J Orthop. 2013;4(2):53–7.
38. Neovius E, et al. Alveolar bone healing accompanied by severe swelling in cleft children treated with bone morphogenetic protein-2 delivered by hydrogel. J Plast Reconstr Aesthet Surg. 2013;66(1):37–42.
39. Woo EJ. Adverse events reported after the use of recombinant human bone morphogenetic protein 2. J Oral Maxillofac Surg. 2012;70(4):765–7.
40. Zetola A, et al. Recombinant human bone morphogenetic protein-2 (rhBMP-2) in the treatment of mandibular sequelae after tumor resection. Oral Maxillofac Surg. 2011;15(3):169–74.
41. Herford AS, Miller M, Signorino F. Maxillofacial defects and the use of growth factors. Oral Maxillofac Surg Clin North Am. 2017;29(1):75–88.
42. Lynch SE, et al. A combination of platelet-derived and insulin-like growth factors enhances periodontal regeneration. J Clin Periodontol. 1989;16(8):545–8.
43. Canalis E, McCarthy T, Centrella M. Growth factors and the regulation of bone remodeling. J Clin Invest. 1988;81(2):277–81.
44. Hauschka PV, et al. Growth factors in bone matrix. Isolation of multiple types by affinity chromatography on heparin-Sepharose. J Biol Chem. 1986;261(27):12665–74.
45. Heldin CH, Westermark B. Mechanism of action and in vivo role of platelet-derived growth factor. Physiol Rev. 1999;79(4):1283–316.
46. Grotendorst GR, et al. Stimulation of granulation tissue formation by platelet-derived growth factor in normal and diabetic rats. J Clin Invest. 1985;76(6):2323–9.
47. Howell TH, et al. A phase I/II clinical trial to evaluate a combination of recombinant human platelet-derived growth factor-BB and recombinant human insulin-like growth factor-I in patients with periodontal disease. J Periodontol. 1997;68(12):1186–93.
48. Nevins M, et al. Platelet-derived growth factor stimulates bone fill and rate of attachment level gain: results of a large multicenter randomized controlled trial. J Periodontol. 2005;76(12):2205–15.
49. Nevins ML, Reynolds MA. Tissue engineering with recombinant human platelet-derived growth factor BB for implant site development. Compend Contin Educ Dent. 2011;32(2):18–20-7. quiz 28, 40.
50. Nevins ML, et al. Recombinant human platelet-derived growth factor BB for reconstruction of human large extraction site defects. Int J Periodontics Restorative Dent. 2014;34(2):157–63.
51. Froum SJ, et al. A histomorphometric comparison of Bio-Oss alone versus Bio-Oss and platelet-derived growth factor for sinus augmentation: a postsurgical assessment. Int J Periodontics Restorative Dent. 2013;33(3):269–79.
52. Simion M, Rocchietta I, Dellavia C. Three-dimensional ridge augmentation with xenograft and recombinant human platelet-derived growth factor-BB in humans: report of two cases. Int J Periodontics Restorative Dent. 2007;27(2):109–15.
53. De Angelis N, De Lorenzi M, Benedicenti S. Surgical combined approach for alveolar ridge augmentation with titanium mesh and rhPDGF-BB: a 3-year clinical case series. Int J Periodontics Restorative Dent. 2015;35(2):231–7.
54. Chiang T, et al. Reconstruction of the narrow ridge using combined ridge split and guided bone regeneration with rhPDGF-BB growth factor-enhanced allograft. Int J Periodontics Restorative Dent. 2014;34(1):123–30.
55. Wallace SC, Snyder MB, Prasad H. Postextraction ridge preservation and augmentation with mineralized allograft with or without recombinant human platelet-derived growth factor BB (rhPDGF-BB): a consecutive case series. Int J Periodontics Restorative Dent. 2013;33(5):599–609.
56. Funato A, et al. A novel combined surgical approach to vertical alveolar ridge augmentation with titanium mesh, resorbable membrane, and rhPDGF-BB: a retrospective consecutive case series. Int J Periodontics Restorative Dent. 2013;33(4):437–45.
57. Urban IA, et al. Horizontal guided bone regeneration in the posterior maxilla using recombinant human platelet-derived growth factor: a case report. Int J Periodontics Restorative Dent. 2013;33(4):421–5.

58. Steed DL. Clinical evaluation of recombinant human platelet-derived growth factor for the treatment of lower extremity ulcers. Plast Reconstr Surg. 2006;117(7 Suppl):143S–9S. discussion 150S-151S.
59. Antoniades HN. Human platelet-derived growth factor (PDGF): purification of PDGF-I and PDGF-II and separation of their reduced subunits. Proc Natl Acad Sci U S A. 1981;78(12):7314–7.
60. Andrae J, Gallini R, Betsholtz C. Role of platelet-derived growth factors in physiology and medicine. Genes Dev. 2008;22(10):1276–312.
61. Steed DL. Clinical evaluation of recombinant human platelet-derived growth factor for the treatment of lower extremity diabetic ulcers. Diabetic Ulcer Study Group. J Vasc Surg. 1995;21(1):71–8. discussion 79-81.
62. Dohan DM, et al. Platelet-rich fibrin (PRF): a second-generation platelet concentrate. Part II: platelet-related biologic features. Oral Surg Oral Med Oral Pathol Oral Radiol Endod. 2006;101(3):e45–50.
63. Bielecki T, Gazdzik TS, Szczepanski T. Re: "The effects of local platelet rich plasma delivery on diabetic fracture healing". What do we use: platelet-rich plasma or platelet-rich gel? Bone. 2006;39(6):1388. author reply 1389.
64. Kaigler D, et al. Platelet-derived growth factor applications in periodontal and peri-implant bone regeneration. Expert Opin Biol Ther. 2011;11(3):375–85.
65. Marx RE, et al. Platelet-rich plasma: growth factor enhancement for bone grafts. Oral Surg Oral Med Oral Pathol Oral Radiol Endod. 1998;85(6):638–46.
66. Weibrich G, et al. Growth factor levels in platelet-rich plasma and correlations with donor age, sex, and platelet count. J Craniomaxillofac Surg. 2002;30(2):97–102.
67. Dugrillon A, et al. Autologous concentrated platelet-rich plasma (cPRP) for local application in bone regeneration. Int J Oral Maxillofac Surg. 2002;31(6):615–9.
68. Khairy NM, et al. Effect of platelet rich plasma on bone regeneration in maxillary sinus augmentation (randomized clinical trial). Int J Oral Maxillofac Surg. 2013;42(2):249–55.
69. Kutkut A, et al. Extraction socket preservation graft before implant placement with calcium sulfate hemihydrate and platelet-rich plasma: a clinical and histomorphometric study in humans. J Periodontol. 2012;83(4):401–9.
70. Geurs N, et al. Using growth factors in human extraction sockets: a histologic and histomorphometric evaluation of short-term healing. Int J Oral Maxillofac Implants. 2014;29(2):485–96.
71. Roffi A, et al. Does PRP enhance bone integration with grafts, graft substitutes, or implants? A systematic review. BMC Musculoskelet Disord. 2013;14:330.
72. Eskan MA, et al. Platelet-rich plasma-assisted guided bone regeneration for ridge augmentation: a randomized, controlled clinical trial. J Periodontol. 2014;85(5):661–8.
73. Torres J, et al. Effect of platelet-rich plasma on sinus lifting: a randomized-controlled clinical trial. J Clin Periodontol. 2009;36(8):677–87.
74. Tonelli P, et al. Counting of platelet derived growth factor and transforming growth factor-beta in platelet-rich-plasma used in jaw bone regeneration. Minerva Stomatol. 2005;54(1-2):23–34.
75. Antonello Gde M, et al. Evaluation of the effects of the use of platelet-rich plasma (PRP) on alveolar bone repair following extraction of impacted third molars: prospective study. J Craniomaxillofac Surg. 2013;41(4):e70–5.
76. Kassolis JD, Reynolds MA. Evaluation of the adjunctive benefits of platelet-rich plasma in subantral sinus augmentation. J Craniofac Surg. 2005;16(2):280–7.
77. Raghoebar GM, et al. Does platelet-rich plasma promote remodeling of autologous bone grafts used for augmentation of the maxillary sinus floor? Clin Oral Implants Res. 2005;16(3):349–56.
78. Torres J, et al. Platelet-rich plasma may prevent titanium-mesh exposure in alveolar ridge augmentation with anorganic bovine bone. J Clin Periodontol. 2010;37(10):943–51.
79. Moy P, et al. Hard and soft tissue augmentation. In: Moy P, Pozzi A, Beumer J, editors. Fundmentals of implant dentistry. Chicago: Quintessence; 2016. p. 205–58.

80. Dohan DM, et al. Platelet-rich fibrin (PRF): a second-generation platelet concentrate. Part I: technological concepts and evolution. Oral Surg Oral Med Oral Pathol Oral Radiol Endod. 2006;101(3):e37–44.
81. Davis VL, et al. Platelet-rich preparations to improve healing. Part I: workable options for every size practice. J Oral Implantol. 2014;40(4):500–10.
82. Khorshidi H, et al. Comparison of the mechanical properties of early leukocyte- and platelet-rich fibrin versus PRGF/Endoret membranes. Int J Dent. 2016;2016:1849207.
83. Schar MO, et al. Platelet-rich concentrates differentially release growth factors and induce cell migration in vitro. Clin Orthop Relat Res. 2015;473(5):1635–43.
84. Suttapreyasri S, Leepong N. Influence of platelet-rich fibrin on alveolar ridge preservation. J Craniofac Surg. 2013;24(4):1088–94.
85. Mazor Z, et al. Sinus floor augmentation with simultaneous implant placement using Choukroun's platelet-rich fibrin as the sole grafting material: a radiologic and histologic study at 6 months. J Periodontol. 2009;80(12):2056–64.
86. Moussa M, El-Dahab OA, El Nahass H. Anterior maxilla augmentation using palatal bone block with platelet-rich fibrin: a controlled trial. Int J Oral Maxillofac Implants. 2016;31(3):708–15.
87. Yoon JS, Lee SH, Yoon HJ. The influence of platelet-rich fibrin on angiogenesis in guided bone regeneration using xenogenic bone substitutes: a study of rabbit cranial defects. J Craniomaxillofac Surg. 2014;42(7):1071–7.
88. Cieslik-Bielecka A, et al. L-PRP/L-PRF in esthetic plastic surgery, regenerative medicine of the skin and chronic wounds. Curr Pharm Biotechnol. 2012;13(7):1266–77.
89. Ghanaati S, et al. Advanced platelet-rich fibrin: a new concept for cell-based tissue engineering by means of inflammatory cells. J Oral Implantol. 2014;40(6):679–89.
90. Simonpieri A, et al. Simultaneous sinus-lift and implantation using microthreaded implants and leukocyte- and platelet-rich fibrin as sole grafting material: a six-year experience. Implant Dent. 2011;20(1):2–12.
91. Dohan Ehrenfest DM, et al. Do the fibrin architecture and leukocyte content influence the growth factor release of platelet concentrates? An evidence-based answer comparing a pure platelet-rich plasma (P-PRP) gel and a leukocyte- and platelet-rich fibrin (L-PRF). Curr Pharm Biotechnol. 2012;13(7):1145–52.
92. Shibli JA, et al. Composition of supra- and subgingival biofilm of subjects with healthy and diseased implants. Clin Oral Implants Res. 2008;19(10):975–82.
93. Ornitz DM, Itoh N. The fibroblast growth factor signaling pathway. Wiley Interdiscip Rev Dev Biol. 2015;4(3):215–66.
94. Kigami R, et al. FGF-2 angiogenesis in bone regeneration within critical-sized bone defects in rat calvaria. Implant Dent. 2013;22(4):422–7.
95. Nagayasu-Tanaka T, et al. FGF-2 promotes initial osseointegration and enhances stability of implants with low primary stability. Clin Oral Implants Res. 2016;28(3):291–7.
96. McCracken M, Lemons JE, Zinn K. Analysis of Ti-6Al-4V implants placed with fibroblast growth factor 1 in rat tibiae. Int J Oral Maxillofac Implants. 2001;16(4):495–502.
97. Ting K, et al. Human NELL-1 expressed in unilateral coronal synostosis. J Bone Miner Res. 1999;14(1):80–9.
98. Cowan CM, et al. Nell-1 induced bone formation within the distracted intermaxillary suture. Bone. 2006;38(1):48–58.
99. Cowan CM, et al. Synergistic effects of Nell-1 and BMP-2 on the osteogenic differentiation of myoblasts. J Bone Miner Res. 2007;22(6):918–30.
100. Aghaloo T, et al. The effect of NELL1 and bone morphogenetic protein-2 on calvarial bone regeneration. J Oral Maxillofac Surg. 2010;68(2):300–8.
101. Grabowski G, Cornett CA. Bone graft and bone graft substitutes in spine surgery: current concepts and controversies. J Am Acad Orthop Surg. 2013;21(1):51–60.
102. Arrington ED, et al. Complications of iliac crest bone graft harvesting. Clin Orthop Relat Res. 1996;329:300–9.

103. Bruder SP, et al. Bone regeneration by implantation of purified, culture-expanded human mesenchymal stem cells. J Orthop Res. 1998;16(2):155–62.
104. Bruder SP, Fink DJ, Caplan AI. Mesenchymal stem cells in bone development, bone repair, and skeletal regeneration therapy. J Cell Biochem. 1994;56(3):283–94.
105. Rush SM. Trinity evolution. Foot Ankle Spec. 2010;3(3):144–7.
106. Vanichkachorn J, et al. A prospective clinical and radiographic 12-month outcome study of patients undergoing single-level anterior cervical discectomy and fusion for symptomatic cervical degenerative disc disease utilizing a novel viable allogeneic, cancellous, bone matrix (trinity evolution) with a comparison to historical controls. Eur Spine J. 2016;25(7):2233–8.
107. Eastlack RK, et al. Osteocel plus cellular allograft in anterior cervical discectomy and fusion: evaluation of clinical and radiographic outcomes from a prospective multicenter study. Spine (Phila Pa 1976). 2014;39(22):E1331–7.
108. Gonshor A, et al. Histologic and histomorphometric evaluation of an allograft stem cell-based matrix sinus augmentation procedure. Int J Oral Maxillofac Implants. 2011;26(1):123–31.

Part III

Immediate Implant Placement and Immediate Provisional Restoration

Advanced Grafting Techniques for Implant Placement in Compromised Sites

7

Bach Le and Joan Pi-Anfruns

Abstract

The loss of teeth can result in up to 50% of alveolar ridge width shrinkage within the first 1–3 years [1]. This bone loss is exacerbated if there are preexisting endodontic pathologies and/or periodontal disease or if the tooth is loss due to trauma. Since prosthetically driven implant placement is only possible when there is an adequate amount of the bone, the presence of significant resorption can pose a considerable clinical challenge. Bone augmentation is often required to create ideal gingival contours and aesthetics.

7.1 Introduction

The loss of teeth can result in up to 50% of alveolar ridge width shrinkage within the first 1–3 years [1]. This bone loss is exacerbated if there are preexisting endodontic pathologies and/or periodontal disease or if the tooth is loss due to trauma. Since prosthetically driven implant placement is only possible when there is an adequate amount of the bone, the presence of significant resorption can pose a considerable clinical challenge. Bone augmentation is often required to create ideal gingival contours and aesthetics.

B. Le (✉)
Department of Oral and Maxillofacial Surgery,
Herman Ostrow School of Dentistry at USC, Los Angeles, CA, USA

Private Practice, Whittier, CA, USA

J. Pi-Anfruns
Division of Diagnostic and Surgical Sciences, Division of Regenerative and Constitutive Sciences, Dental Implant Center, UCLA School of Dentistry, Los Angeles, CA, USA

Todd R. Schoenbaum (ed.), *Implants in the Aesthetic Zone*,
https://doi.org/10.1007/978-3-319-72601-4_7

The high predictability and success of osseointegration have led to a shift in the focus toward achieving ideal long-term aesthetics with peri-implant bone and tissue architecture. Increasing patient demand for natural aesthetic outcomes has redefined the definition of success. Implant success is no longer solely equated with implant survival, yet most studies on implants fail to include criteria for aesthetic success. It is reported that up to 16% of single implant restorations in the aesthetic zone fail for aesthetic reasons [2–4] due to tissue loss or a failure to adequately restore this lost volume [5]. Achieving an ideal aesthetic result in the compromised site is often elusive and, in many cases, not yet possible [6]. The potential for unexpected complications which can compromise the final result always exists with any surgical procedure and should be a part of the initial discussion on expectations. With proper treatment planning and execution, poor outcomes can be avoided.

7.1.1 Aesthetic Risk Assessment in Compromised Sites: FATTT Assessment

Even procedures with a high level of predictability will have aesthetic failures defined by significant tissue recession, long clinical crowns, open gingival embrasures, and/or exposure of the abutment margin. Given the complexity of hard and soft tissue reconstruction, the authors recommend using the following five simple guidelines (FATTT) to help clinicians decrease the risk of an unaesthetic outcome with hard and soft tissue reconstruction (Table 7.1).

7.1.2 Favorable Gingival Level (F)

Because gingival recession is common after prosthetic delivery [7–9], it is critical to assess the preoperative gingival margin height of the tooth or implant site. This margin is usually dictated by the underlying facial bone level. A free gingival margin that lies coronal to the planned restorative margin offers some insurance against recession and is considered more favorable (Fig. 7.1). Ideally, the implant platform should be placed 3 mm below the *planned* gingival margin with an abundance of soft tissue height for prosthetic sculpting to achieve a harmonious gingival margin with the adjacent teeth (Fig. 7.2a–d). In clinical cases where the gingival margin is

Table 7.1 Aesthetic risk assessment (FATTT)

FATTT criteria	Favorable	Non-favorable
Favorable gingival level	Free gingival margin >1 mm coronal to anticipated level	Free gingival margin at or apical to anticipated level
Attachment on adjacent tooth	<5 mm from anticipated contact point	>5 mm from anticipated contact point
Thick/thin biotype	No translucency on probing	Probe visible through gingiva
Thick/thin labial bone	>2 mm of residual labial bone	<1 mm of residual labial bone
Tooth shape	Square	Triangular

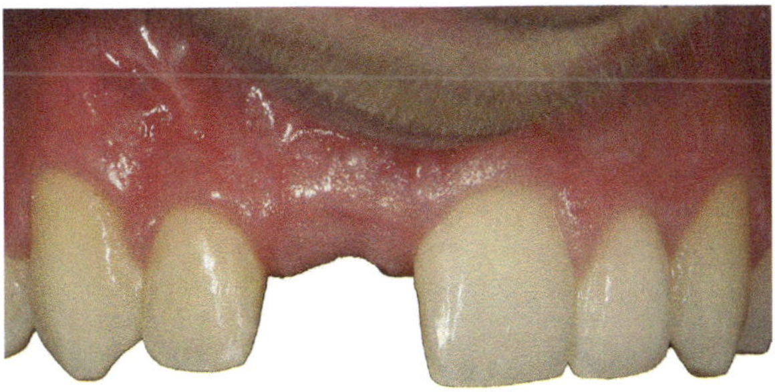

Fig. 7.1 (**a**) A free gingival margin that lies coronal to the planned restorative margin offers some insurance against recession and is considered more favorable

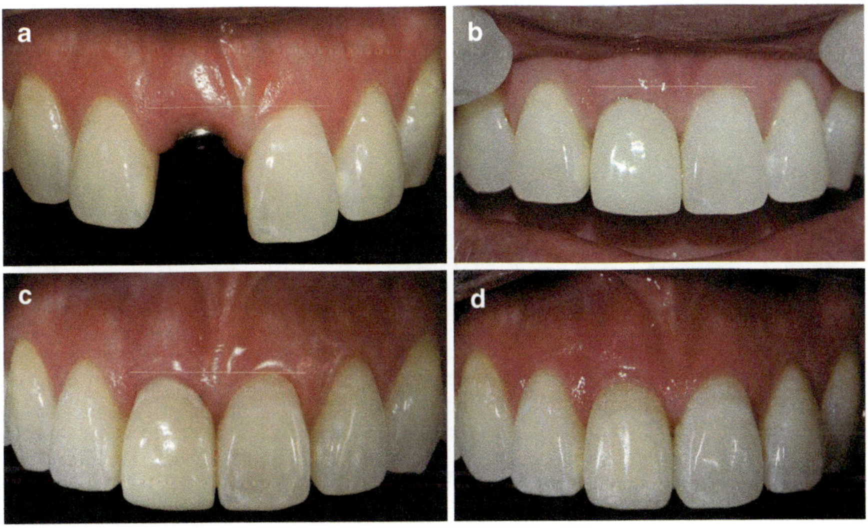

Fig. 7.2 (**a**–**d**) A favorable gingival margin level and an abundance of soft tissue thickness should exist for prosthetic sculpting to achieve a harmonious gingival margin with the adjacent teeth. Ideally, the implant platform should be at least 3 mm below the *planned* gingival margin

in an unfavorable position, bone augmentation with coronal tissue advancement (open-book flap design) (Figs. 7.3a–c and 7.4a–i) or slow orthodontic extrusion may bring the gingival margin and bone into a more coronal level prior to implant placement [10, 11] and should, therefore, be considered.

7.1.3 Attachment on the Adjacent Tooth (A)

The development of papilla adjacent to the implant is a critical part of dental implant therapy. This will result in a more natural, youthful-looking dental restoration, which is critical in the aesthetic zone. Predictable papilla formation is dependent on the gingival biotype and the proximal bone height of the adjacent teeth rather than the tooth to be extracted (Fig. 7.5a–b) [12, 13].

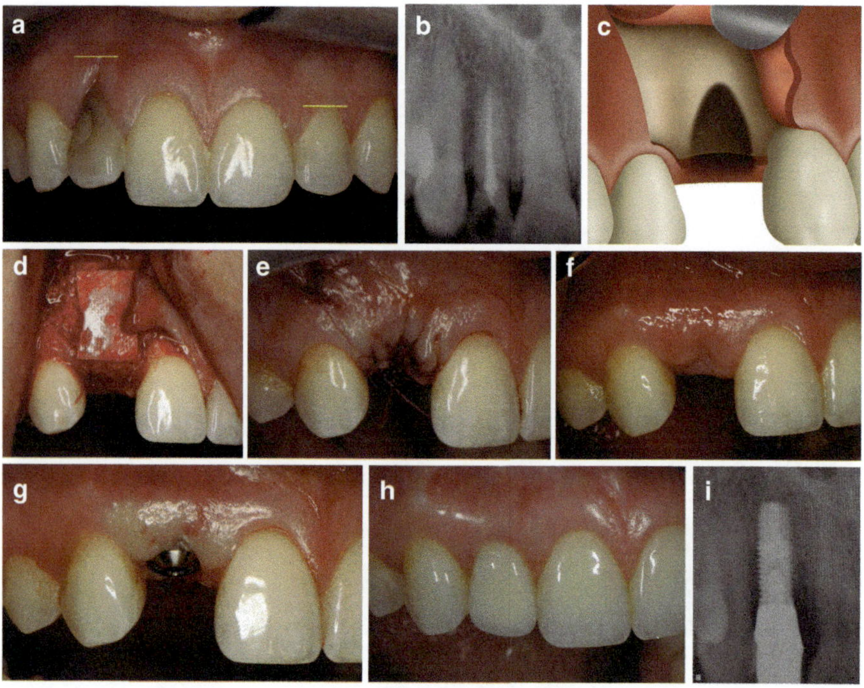

Fig. 7.3 (**a–i**) Management of extraction defect with labial wall defect with loss of labial attached tissue using the open-book flap. (**a–b**) Failing right maxillary lateral incisor with loss of labial attached tissue (**c–d**) open-book flap incision design. Mineralized cancellous allograft placement with overcorrection and cross-link collagen membrane coverage. (**e**) Soft tissue closure; note slight exposure of the cross-link collagen membrane left to heal by secondary intention. Keratinized tissue is expected to fill the exposed area because it is surrounded by the remaining keratinized tissue due to strategic repositioning using the open-book flap. (**f–g**) Healing at 4 months postoperative showing significant increase in the width of keratinized tissue (bone-driven tissue transformation—BTT). Implant placement is performed using a flapless approach to minimize disruption of the soft tissue maturation and minimize bone resorption. (**h–i**) Final restoration at 3 years with corresponding radiograph

The presence of intercrestal bone is a predictable indicator of whether papilla regeneration is plausible [14–17]. The distance between the contact point between the crowns and the proximal bone crest influences the papilla fill. One study on natural dentition [16] reported that when this distance was ≤5 mm, complete papilla fill was always found, while unpredictable papilla formation was seen in sites when this distance was greater than 5 mm [16]. When treatment planning immediate implants, sounding depths of greater than 5 mm from the anticipated contact point may result in a "black triangle" caused by the absence of papillary tissue, as well as other undesirable aesthetic results. Because it is difficult to predictably graft the bone to gain adequate papillary attachment, this limitation should be anticipated so that patient expectations can be appropriately addressed. For optimal aesthetic outcomes, consideration must be given to options to increase interproximal bone height, including slow orthodontic extrusion and/or extraction of the affected teeth with GBR and restoring the dental implant with an adjacent pontic (i.e., cantilever bridge).

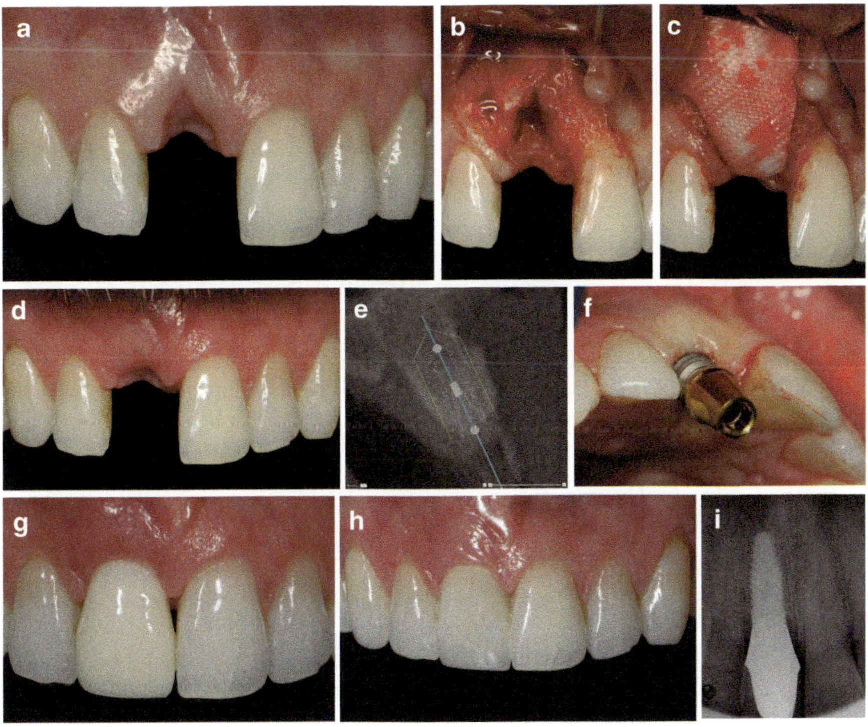

Fig. 7.4 (**a**–**i**) Single-tooth alveolar defects where the gingival margin is in an unfavorable position are usually associated with a low alveolar crest and require bone augmentation to correct the gingival margin level to a favorable position. (**b**–**c**) Coronal tissue advancement (open-book flap design) using guided bone regeneration with overcorrection of the alveolar ridge to achieve ideal contours. (**d**) Clinical healing at 4 months postoperative showing an increase in the width of keratinized tissue and thickening of the soft tissue (bone-driven tissue transformation—BTT). (**e**) Cross-sectional CT image at 4 months postoperative shows alveolar ridge width with adequate crestal bone for implant placement. (f) Implant placement is performed using a flapless approach to minimize disruption of the soft tissue maturation and minimize bone resorption. (**g**) Immediate non-load provisional restoration. (**h**–**i**) Final restoration at 3 years

Furthermore, thick gingival tissue can tolerate more bone loss on the adjacent tooth and still maintain papilla compared to thinner biotypes [15, 18]. Careful treatment planning is therefore needed for patients with thinner biotypes when regenerating papilla.

7.1.4 Thick Biotype (T)

Patients exhibit differences in their gingival phenotypes, often termed "gingival biotypes" [19] (Table 7.2). Most patients will fall into two categories: slender teeth with thin gingiva and scalloped periodontium or square teeth with thick gingiva and blunted periodontium [19, 20] (Fig. 7.6a–b). In a study of 100 volunteers, De Rouck et al. demonstrated that approximately one-third of the patients exhibited thin biotype, which was usually associated with females. Two-thirds were thicker biotypes

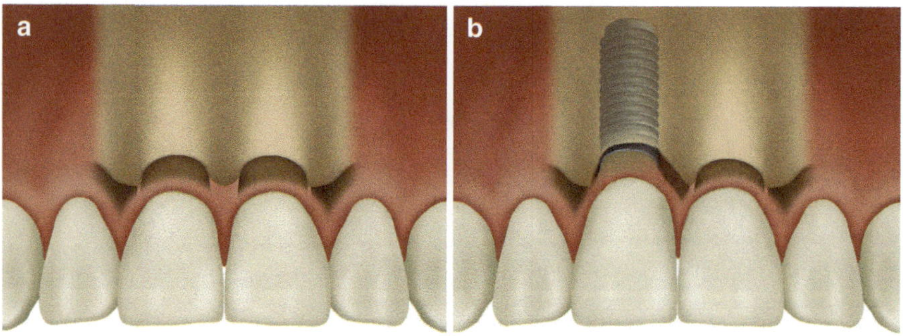

Fig. 7.5 (**a**–**b**) Predictable papilla formation is dependent on the gingival biotype and bony attachment of the adjacent teeth rather than the tooth to be extracted or the proximal bone level of the adjacent implant

Table 7.2 Gingival biotype

	Periodontium	Band of keratinized tissue	Papilla	Tooth shape	Interproximal contact	Associated gender
Thin biotype	Scalloped	Thin	Long and thin papilla	Triangular	Coronal 1/3 of the crown	Females
Thick biotype	Blunted	Thick	Short and wide papilla	Square	Middle 1/3 of the crown	Males

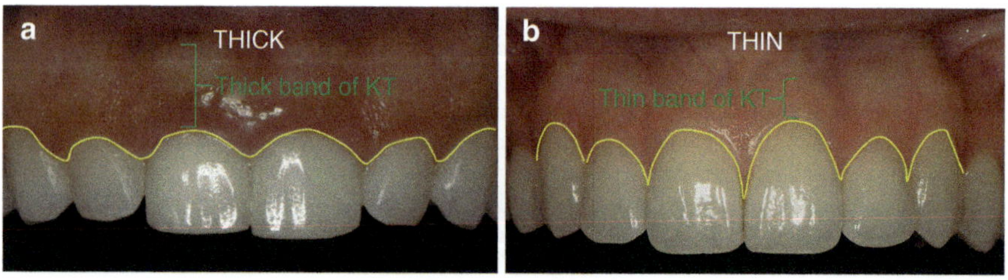

Fig. 7.6 (**a**–**b**) Gingival biotype. Most patients will fall into two categories: slender teeth with thin gingiva and scalloped periodontium or square teeth with thick gingiva and blunted periodontium

usually associated with males (De Rouck, Eghbali, Collys, De Bruyn, & Cosyn). They classified the two biotypes by using the translucency of the gingiva on probing as a marker for thickness: if the probe was visible through the facial gingival tissue, this was considered a thin biotype [20].

Much consideration has been given to the thickness of the gingiva related to implant dentistry. The thinner biotype is more prone to recession and loss of interdental papilla [18, 20–22]. In the aesthetic zone, some clinicians advocate the routine use of connective tissue grafts to transform thin biotypes into thicker tissue for enhanced aesthetic outcomes [12, 23]. If an implant site exhibits a thin biotype, a

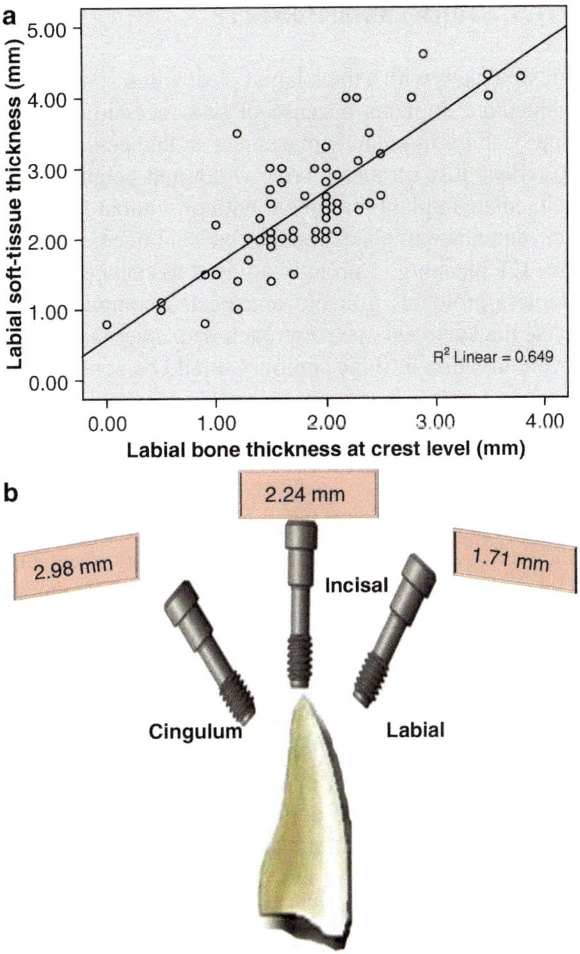

Fig. 7.7 (**a**) Labial soft tissue thickness and labial bone thickness. Linear correlation between labial crestal soft tissue thickness and underlying bone thickness. (**b**) Implant angulation and crestal labial soft tissue thickness—significant differences were detected between crestal labial soft tissue thickness of implants with cingulum and incisal, as well as cingulum and labial angulations. Implants with cingulum angulation had a mean crestal soft tissue thickness of 2.98 mm, while those with incisal and labial angulation had decreased mean tissue thickness of 2.24 and 1.71 mm, respectively

connective tissue graft or bone augmentation should be considered prior to or at the time of implant placement to reduce the risk of recession and graying of the tissue. It is important to note that soft tissue thickness around dental implants can be correlated with other factors not related to the patient's initial biotype. These factors include implant position, angulation, and the presence of labial bone. Le et al. showed a high correlation between labial crestal soft tissue thickness and underlying bone thickness, demonstrating that soft tissue thickness around dental implants can be heavily influenced by the underlying labial bone thickness (Fig. 7.7a) [24]. Le et al. studied the relationship between crestal labial soft tissue thickness and implant buccolingual angulation [25]. The buccolingual angulation was recorded as cingulum, incisally, or labially angled based on the position of the screw access hole of the provisional restoration. Of implants with cingulum, incisal, and labial angulations, 3.4%, 20%, and 53.3%, respectively, had crestal labial soft tissue thickness of <2 mm (Fig. 7.7b).

7.1.5 Thick Labial Bone (T)

Fresh sockets with a thick labial plate will respond more favorably to treatment with immediate implants because of less recession on the facial aspect. The flapless approach for immediate placement should be the preferred technique in these cases to reduce loss of buccal bone width and height. A pilot study in dogs comparing immediate implant placement with or without flap found that the flapless approach for immediate implants reduces buccal bone height loss [26]. The use of preoperative CT planning is strongly advised to evaluate socket dimensions when utilizing flapless protocols to avoid unexpected complications. In sockets with thin labial plate thickness, an open approach with external bone grafting of the socket wall for overcorrection of ridge contours should be considered.

Thick labial bone → immediate implant w/o flap
Thin labial bone → flap w/ bone grafting

7.1.6 Tooth Shape (T)

Bone augmentation with extensive flap elevation can result in some loss of tissue to the teeth adjacent to the graft site. This can result in either loss of papilla height, exposure of existing restorative margins, or leave unaesthetic black triangles in the final restorations. Because it is difficult to regenerate a missing papilla, alteration of the contact point of the adjacent teeth may become necessary to achieve a more symmetric appearance of the final restorations (Fig. 7.8a–i). It is important to inform patients prior to surgical intervention of the possibility that additional costs will be incurred due to the need for additional restorations on the adjacent teeth.

It is important to note that the aesthetic outcomes perceived by the dental professionals and the patients do not always match [27–30]. Kokich et al. compared the aesthetic perception of dentists, orthodontist, and the layperson on various parameters [29]. He did this by altering various parameters and asking each group to judge the aesthetic perception of these altered parameters (teeth length, gingival margin level, papilla height, etc.). According to Kokich, patients consider a discrepancy in gingival margin of more than 2 mm to be unaesthetic, similar to those of general dentists. Conversely, the authors found that while dentists had very low tolerance for any discrepancy in papilla height, most laypersons were not able to differentiate a severely compromised papilla height. Tymstra et al. reported the results of placing two adjacent maxillary implants after autogenous block grafts in ten consecutive patients [6]. The authors reported that in 40% of their cases, there was an absence of the interdental papilla. Interestingly, all the patients in this study reported that their results were "acceptable" or better, supporting the findings of Kokich's study.

7.2 Management of Horizontal Defects

Most post-extraction losses of alveolar ridge dimensions occur in the horizontal (width) rather than the vertical (height) plane (Schropp et al.), particularly in the "aesthetic zone." Even when there is adequate bone to place implants, irregular ridge anatomy that is not corrected can result in an unnatural appearance of the final restoration (Fig. 7.9a–b). Bone augmentation prior to or simultaneously with

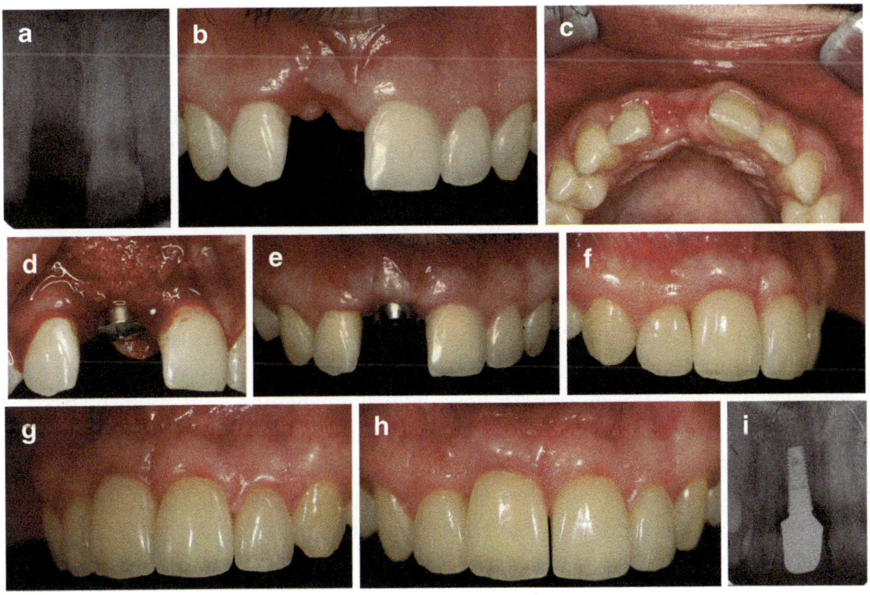

Fig. 7.8 (**a–i**) Because it is difficult to regenerate a missing papilla, alteration of the contact point of the teeth adjacent to a dental implant restoration may be necessary to achieve a more symmetric appearance of the final restorations. (**a–c**) Initial presentation: missing right central incisor with alveolar bone loss, unfavorable gingival margin level, and loss of proximal bone height on adjacent lateral incisor and corresponding short papilla height. (**d**) Simultaneous aesthetic contour augmentation with single-stage implant placement (open-book flap) to coronally reposition the gingival margin level and labial soft tissue contour. No attempt is made to correct the adjacent deficient papilla height. Instead, restorations were planned with alteration of the contact point of the teeth adjacent to a dental implant. (**f–i**) Final restorations at 12 years postoperative showing acceptable aesthetic results, despite the deficient papilla

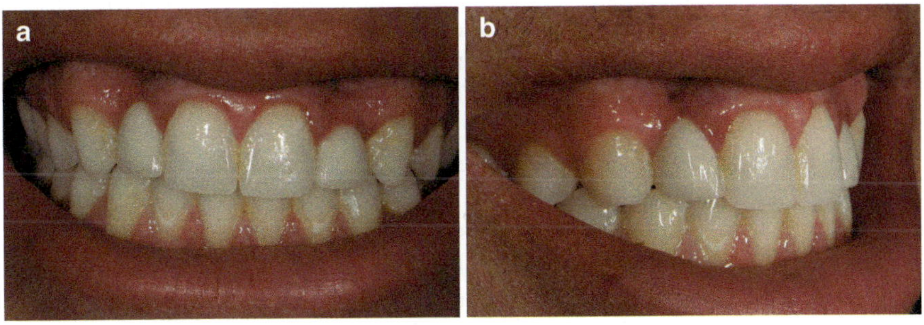

Fig. 7.9 (**a–b**) Even when there is adequate bone to place implants, irregular ridge anatomy that is not corrected can result in an unnatural and unaesthetic soft tissue appearance of the final restoration

implant placement may allow for better implant position. Additionally, the augmented bone will correct ridge contour defects for a more natural-looking restoration and increase facial bone support for long-term peri-implant soft tissue stability [31, 32].

Single-tooth replacement in sites with horizontal defects must follow the same initial guiding principles discussed previously. Important considerations are the level of the gingival margin, as this is dictated by the facial bone level; bone attachment of the adjacent teeth, as this will dictate the presence or absence of final papillary height; and thickness of the tissue biotype (FATTT assessment).

Many techniques have been described for lateral ridge augmentation. These include guided bone regeneration (GBR), ridge expansion/splitting, autogenous onlay block grafting, and connective tissue grafting [33–42].

7.2.1 Particulate Grafting with Guided Bone Regeneration

Particulated bone has been used for horizontal augmentation with good success for mild- to moderate-sized defects [42, 43]. Utilizing the soft tissue matrix theory, meshes, reinforced membranes, screws, dental implants, cortical bone, and the graft itself have been used to maintain this expanded pocket [44–48]. A tenting mechanism to prevent collapse of the soft tissue can be extremely advantageous when augmenting vertical or large horizontal defects.

Block and Degen [35] described a minimally invasive tunneling technique using mineralized particulate allograft to horizontally augment partially edentulous defects for successful implant placement. However, a disadvantage of the tunneling technique is that it can be difficult to position and maintain the graft in a coronal position to augment the peri-implant soft tissue. Additional bone grafting may be necessary at the time of implant placement to address this issue [47]. Maintaining the graft in the crestal area is important in long-term peri-implant soft tissue stability [31, 49].

Ridge augmentation exclusively using particulate grafts in the aesthetic zone is extremely technique-sensitive and operator-dependent. Predictability of lateral ridge augmentation using particulate grafts is largely dependent on the ability to stabilize and maintain the graft or biomaterial at the alveolar crest. Migration or resorption of the graft or biomaterial from the crest often results in soft tissue recession or unaesthetic labial contour defects. Maintaining the stability of this augmented crestal bone becomes more difficult with large ridge defects and long edentulous spans or when there is inadequate basal bone support. The analogy of building a sandcastle applies with the use of particulate grafts for ridge augmentation. When building a sandcastle, a wide base is needed first to support the sand at the highest portion. Without adequate basal bone support, the most coronal portion of the graft often migrates apically. If using only particulate graft for larger width correction, basal bone width can be augmented first using a tunneling approach [35] or an open approach (Fig. 7.10a–n). The remaining defect can be further augmented at the time of implant placement [47, 50–52]. Successful augmentation of the alveolar crest using particulate graft provides an ideal choice for restoring the natural appearance of both the hard and soft tissue architectures of the final restoration. The

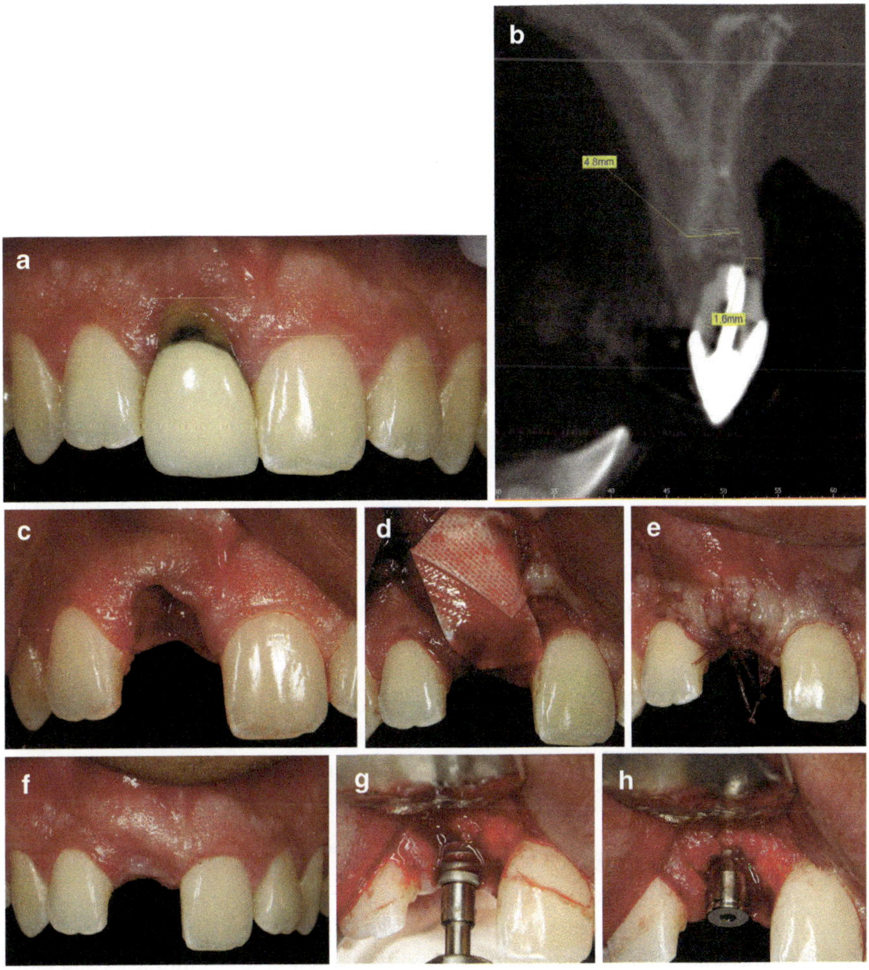

Fig. 7.10 (**a–n**) Predictability of lateral ridge augmentation using particulate grafts is largely dependent on the ability to stabilize and maintain the graft or biomaterial at the alveolar crest (normal crest). Extraction management of a tooth with labial wall defect and loss of labial attached tissue using the open-book flap. (**a–b**) Failing right maxillary central incisor with labial tissue loss. (**c–e**) Open-book flap incision design with placement of mineralized cancellous allograft placement with overcorrection and collagen membrane coverage. (**e**) Soft tissue closure; note slight exposure of membrane left to heal by secondary intention. (**f**) Healing at 4 months postoperative. Note the increase in the band of keratinized tissue (bone-driven tissue transformation—BTT). Although there is adequate bone width for implant placement, an unfavorable gingival margin level exists due to inadequate crestal bone dimension (low crest). (**g–j**) Single-stage implant placement with open-book flap and simultaneous aesthetic contour grafting for coronal repositioning of the gingival margin level and to improve labial soft tissue contour. (**k**) Postoperative healing at 2 months. (**l–n**) Final restoration at 1 year with corresponding radiograph and CT scan

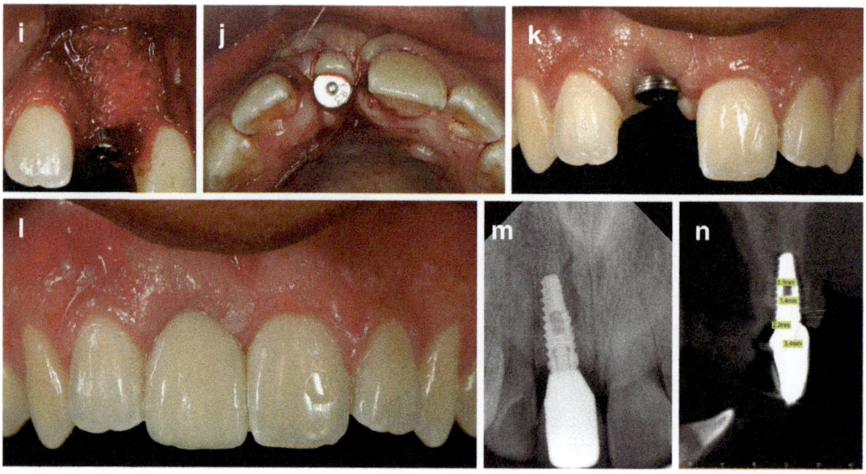

Fig. 7.10 (continued)

soft tissues must receive support from an underlying bony matrix. Using particulate graft at the time of implant placement often negates the need for secondary soft tissue grafting to thicken the soft tissue. Clinical observation of soft tissue thickening and increase in keratinized tissue width has been reported after successful grafting with particulate allograft around previously restored dental implants [53, 54]. This new concept of bone-driven tissue transformation (BTT) may replace the need for soft tissue augmentation in many instances where tissue thickening is needed (Figs. 7.3, 7.4a, and 7.10f).

7.2.1.1 Graft Materials

Various materials have been described for alveolar ridge augmentation. Autogenous bone has long been considered the gold standard for bone grafting due to its biocompatibility and osteogenic properties. Allografts, xenografts, alloplasts, and bone morphogenetic proteins can also be used for grafting socket defects to minimize ridge resorption [39, 55–63]. Cost, ease of use, biocompatibility, bone formation, and resorption are all properties to consider when choosing a graft material. Extensive studies have been performed on xenogenic bone and allogenic bone graft substitutes.

Bovine bone matrix xenograft has shown to delay bone formation when compared to non-grafted control sites [57], and less bone formation has also been observed when bovine bone matrix was compared to autogenous bone in sinus augmentation procedures [64, 65]. Although some have found inhibitory effects, bovine bone matrix has also been reported to preserve the alveolar ridge with adequate bone formation and enable successful implant placement [23, 66, 67]. Bovine bone matrix can be utilized for grafting sockets, if its properties are understood. By allowing adequate time between the grafting procedure and implant placement to pass, sufficient bone formation and graft resorption will allow for successful osseointegration.

Allografts have also been utilized for alveolar ridge augmentation. Histologic analyses of grafted sites have shown adequate bone formation for implant osseointegration [48, 55, 58, 68, 69]. Higher mean bone density has been documented in sites grafted with mineralized allograft with fewer residual particles when compared to bovine bone matrix xenografts and DFDBA [58]. This can also be seen in sinus augmentation procedures [70]. Using mineralized allograft may provide earlier bone formation leading to earlier implant placement and restoration. The biocompatibility of mineralized allograft particles has also been documented [68], and the author's clinical experience suggests that they may tolerate wound exposure better than other bone grafts [48]. Mineross – earlier bone formation & implant placement

7.2.1.2 Particle Size

In selecting particulate graft material, particle size is an important consideration. In a controlled animal study, cortical allograft with particle size between 90 and 300 μm produced rapid healing by direct ossification when placed into critical-sized defects, while particles larger than 300 μm healed slower, and those that were too small were not osseoconductive [71]. Although graft materials of different types and sizes are capable of bone formation when used for socket augmentation, a thorough understanding of the material of choice and its handling properties is important [36] for successful ridge augmentation and subsequent dental implant placement.

7.2.2 Barrier Membranes

Ridge augmentation can be performed with or without barrier membranes [43, 45, 51, 72–74]. A systematic review to determine if the use of barrier membrane in preventing resorption of autologous onlay grafts was inconclusive [74].

Guided tissue regeneration can be performed using resorbable or non-resorbable membranes [43, 45, 72, 73]. Non-resorbable membranes possess predictability in preventing epithelial ingrowth [43, 73]. They are, however, more susceptible to exposure [43, 73, 75, 76] and have higher irritation/infection rates [77] compared to resorbable membranes. Although non-resorbable membranes are associated with higher exposure rates, this does not always equate to graft resorption [43, 72, 73].

Some researchers, however, have reported better results in preserving alveolar ridge dimensions when resorbable membranes were used [76]. This type of membrane is also better tolerated if exposed, and a second surgery is not necessary for membrane removal [43, 76]. Barone et al., in a clinical study on socket augmentation with healing by secondary intention, reported secondary soft tissue healing over grafted sockets did not compromise bone formation and soft tissue level and width of keratinized tissue were improved [78] (see Figs. 7.3 and 7.10).

7.2.3 Single-Stage Implant Placement with Simultaneous Guided Bone Regeneration: "Aesthetic Contour Grafting Technique"

When there is adequate basal bone and the lateral ridge deficiency is mild (<4 mm), implants can be placed simultaneously with the augmentation procedure [50–52]. Le et al. [50] has shown that single-stage implant placement and simultaneous grafting with human mineralized allograft were effective in correcting small- to moderate-sized (3–5 mm) localized horizontal alveolar ridge defects [50]. The likelihood of wound dehiscence, graft exposure and resorption, and subsequent implant thread exposure is increased when larger defects are treated simultaneously. A two-stage, bone augmentation procedure followed by implant placement is recommended for predictable results with large (>5 mm) defects.

7.2.3.1 Surgical Technique (Fig. 7.11a–o)

Two different conservative surgical incisions can be used. In cases with small ridge defects (< 2 mm), a sulcular flap without vertical releasing incisions can be used. In cases with more extensive defects, an open-book flap design is preferred to enhance visualization and access to the graft site. The latter consists of a crestal incision made slightly lingual to the ridge midline to ensure that there is an adequate amount of keratinized tissue present in the flap (Fig. 7.11d–e). This is followed by a distal, curvilinear, vertical incision that follows the gingival margin of the distal tooth. A wide subperiosteal reflection is made to expose two to three times the treatment area, and the papilla is then reflected on the mesial side of the edentulous site. The author prefers the open-book flap when using particulate grafts because the site-specific vertical incision limits excessive flap elevation which promotes graft containment at the alveolar crest. This design also allows for tension-free closure, rotational advancement of the flap for coronal advancement of the gingival margin, and is less invasive.

During implant placement, the implant's restorative platform is positioned to the desire level, and a healing cap is attached to the implant (Fig. 7.11e). The peri-implant soft tissue is released and advanced by scoring the periosteum so that tension-free closure is achieved around the neck of the implant. This is done because moderate graft resorption will occur if there is not an adequate tissue seal around the implant neck or if tension-free closure is not achieved.

To induce bleeding in the graft site, periosteum release is performed as the last step just prior to graft placement. Human mineralized bone allograft is packed into the defect and overcontoured by approximately 20–30% to compensate for anticipated apical migration and resorption of the material (Fig. 7.11f). Prior to surgery, the allograft is hydrated according to the manufacturer's directions and mixed with the patient's blood, which serves as a coagulant. After grafting, the allograft is covered with a resorbable membrane (Fig. 7.11g). The soft tissues are approximated and sutured around the healing abutment (Fig. 7.11h). This creates a tenting effect over the allograft and, together with the healing abutment, helps to develop the labial soft tissue contour.

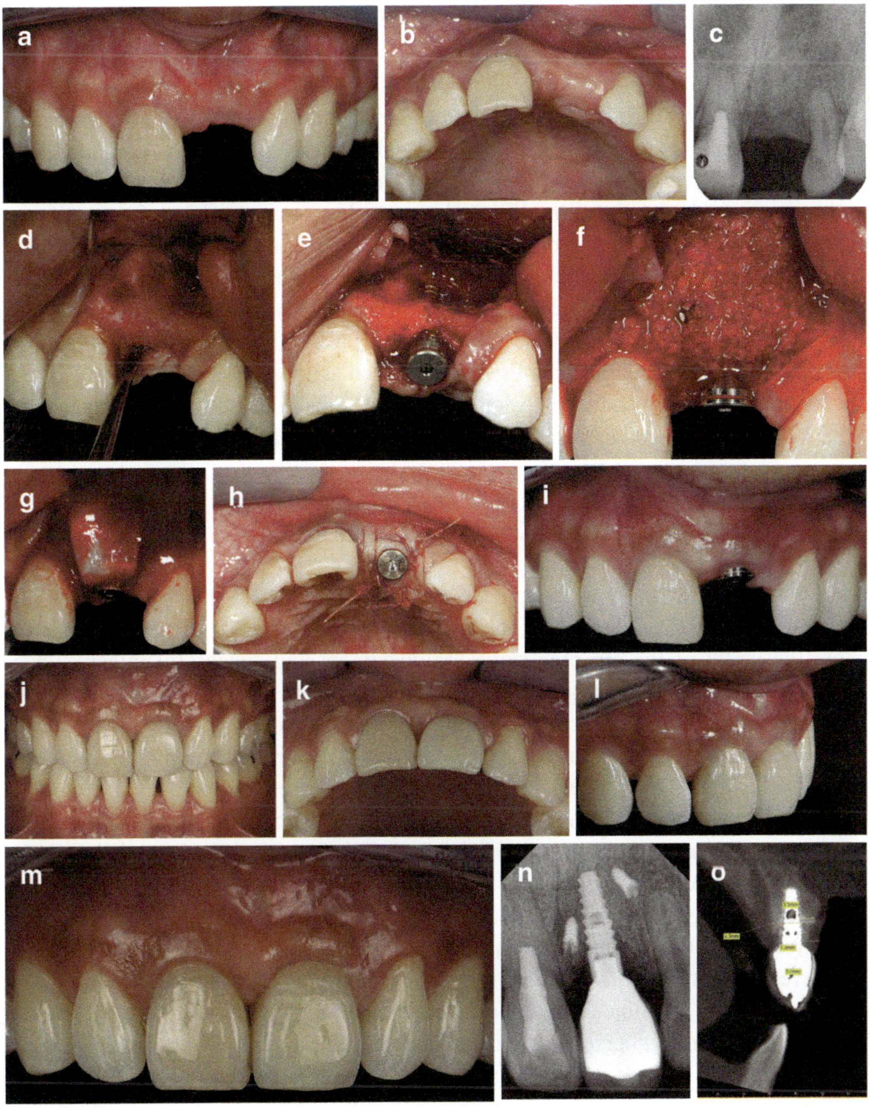

Fig. 7.11 (**a**–**o**) "Aesthetic contour grafting technique." (**a**–**c**) Preoperative defect. (**d**) Incision is made slightly lingual to midline of the crest to capture the available keratinized tissue in the labial flap. (**e**) Implant placement with apical fenestration. (**f**) Tenting screw placed ("screw tent-pole technique) with human mineralized bone allograft is packed into the defect and overcontoured by approximately 20–30%. (**g**) Resorbable collagen membrane is placed over graft material. (**h**) The soft tissues sutured around the healing abutment using a sling suture. (**i**) A 2-month healing. (**j**–**o**) Alveolar ridge form and peri-implant tissue contour at 2-year follow-up. CT image shows stable labial bone and soft tissue thickness (BTT)

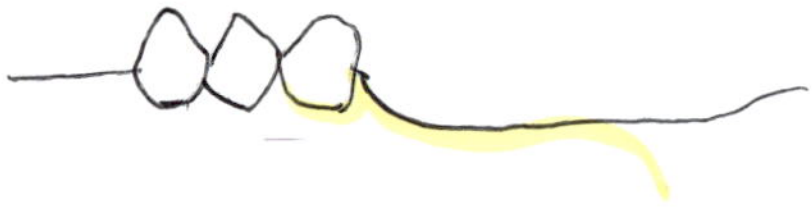

7.2.4 Ridge Expansion and Ridge Splitting

Splitting or spreading the alveolar ridge horizontally can be performed for lateral ridge augmentation [79, 80]. This technique may address mild to moderate deficiencies and may be carried out in conjunction with dental implant placement. Adequate bone height is a prerequisite. Predictably splitting the ridge will be more difficult if the ridge is thinner and/or lacks cancellous bone. This procedure is susceptible to 2 mm of facial bone loss around dental implants when placed simultaneously and without additional bone grafting [80]. The resulting bone loss may jeopardize the aesthetic integrity of the implant and should be used with caution in the aesthetic region. Placing implants after the alveolar ridge has healed may be more predictable. Careful split-thickness flap elevation with maintenance of periosteal blood supply on the buccal cortical segment will minimize crestal bone loss. Treatment planning with three-dimensional cone beam CT scan and the use of a piezotome will help facilitate this procedure.

7.2.5 Autogenous Onlay Grafting

Many clinicians have reported on the use of autogenous bone [36, 44, 81–88], allografts [35, 89], xenografts [90–92], and alloplastic [93, 94] onlay grafts to augment the width of the atrophic ridge for placement and successful integration of endosseous implants. Autogenous bone, considered to be the gold standard for grafting hard tissue defects, can be classified by its embryologic origin. Membranous bones, including the calvarium, ramus, and symphysis, are formed by intramembranous ossification. This process involves embryonic mesenchymal cells differentiating into osteoblasts which can synthesize an osteoid matrix that mineralizes to form hard bone. The bone is also formed by endochondral ossification of cartilage at the epiphyseal surface of long bones. Two examples of endochondral bones used for intraoral grafting are the iliac crest and tibial plateau.

In reviewing the literature on graft survival [95, 96], membranous onlay bone grafts retained greater than 80% of their original volume and had been replaced by new bone, while the iliac (endochondral) bone had undergone 65–88% resorption. In addition to the higher resorption rate of iliac crest grafts, other disadvantages include the high costs of hospitalization, risk of general anesthesia, and morbidity of the procedure [83, 86, 97]. Conversely, the mandibular symphysis and ramus bone appear to undergo less resorption because of the thick cortical layer and their rigid structure [83, 86, 98]. Other advantages of intraoral donor sites include conventional access for surgeons familiar with intraoral anatomy, less anesthesia and reduced operative time due to close proximity of donor and recipient sites, and no cutaneous scars [98–100]. It can also be ideally done as an outpatient surgery thereby decreasing the overall costs of the procedure.

Various intraoral sites have been described for graft donor sites. These include mandibular ramus [36, 81, 82, 101], symphysis [102, 103], maxillary tuberosity [104, 105], maxillary and mandibular tori [106], and osteotomy drill sites [107]. The two most common sites are the mandibular ramus and symphysis. The author prefers the mandibular ramus site over the symphysis due to the high

Table 7.3 Five factors for success with autogenous onlay graft

1. Proper incision and flap design
2. Recipient site preparation
3. Precise graft adaptation
4. Rigid fixation
5. Particulate graft and resorbable membrane coverage

postoperative morbidity associated with the latter. Paresthesia, reported to be as high as 52% at 18 months in one study [108] and 22% at 3 years in another [109], is commonly associated with harvesting from the symphysis [108, 109]. Not only have sensory disturbances been reported, but loss of tooth vitality has also been noted from harvesting the bone from the symphyseal region. Even when a symphysis graft was harvested beyond the commonly recognized safe distance of 5 mm from the root apices, 33% of the teeth still lost vitality [110]. This loss of vitality was likely due to disturbance of the branch of the mandibular incisive canal.

Success with autogenous block onlay grafts requires adherence to five key surgical principles: proper incision design and flap management, adequate recipient site preparation, proper graft adaptation, rigid fixation, and use of particulate graft and membrane (Table 7.3) (Fig. 7.12a–n).

7.2.5.1 Proper Incision and Flap Design

Proper incision design will facilitate tension-free wound closure, which is especially important when a large volume of graft material is used to overcorrect anatomical defects in anticipation of normal graft shrinkage. Bone blocks maintain form and are not prone to apical migration normally seen with particulate grafts. A vertical incision is usually necessary to allow for ease of flap scoring and advancement. Scoring of the periosteum is performed as the last step prior to particulate graft placement to ensure maximum bleeding for angiogenesis. In addition to scoring the periosteum, it is important to perform split-thickness dissection of the flap to surgically expand the soft tissue matrix to create sufficient space for incorporation of graft material.

7.2.5.2 Recipient Site Preparation

This involves decorticating the recipient site to create more walls to incorporate the onlay block graft. Preparing the recipient site also promotes the regional accelerated phenomenon (RAP) [111] to release growth factors and platelets to encourage healing (Fig. 7.12d).

7.2.5.3 Precise Graft Adaptation

Intimate adaptation of the block graft to the prepared recipient site is necessary for graft take (Fig. 7.12e). All sharp edges should be removed to prevent wound dehiscence and graft exposure.

7.2.5.4 Rigid Fixation

Rigid fixation usually requires two screws to prevent rotation of the graft; however, one screw is acceptable if the graft is rigid and well fitted.

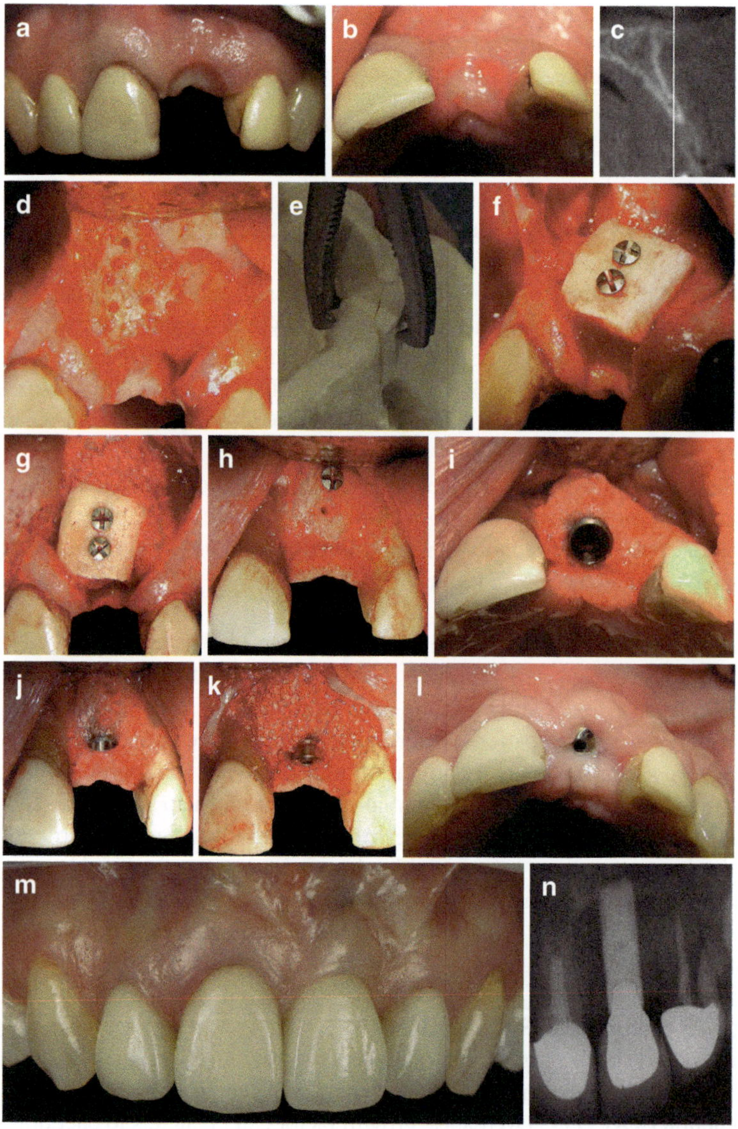

Fig. 7.12 (**a–m**) Autogenous onlay block graft. (**a–b**) Missing left central incisor with moderate horizontal ridge defect. (**c**) Cross-section CT shows a flat one-wall horizontal defect. This single-tooth span defect can be treated with autogenous bone block graft or GBR. The use of particulate bone for bone augmentation in these types of defect configuration is technique-sensitive due to apical migration of the graft. Bone blocks have the advantage of maintaining the form for crestal bone augmentation. (**d**) Recipient site preparation by perforating the recipient bed promotes the regional accelerated phenomenon (RAP). (**e**) Intimate graft adaptations to the recipient site promote graft stability. (**f**) Remove any sharp edges from donor graft to avoid soft tissue dehiscence. (**g**) Covering block graft with particulate mineralized allograft to overcorrect the augmentation in anticipation of graft remodeling and resorption. A resorbable collagen membrane is also placed over the grafted area. (**h–j**) Reentry at 4 months for implant placement. (**k**) Even though an adequate labial thickness of bone was achieved with the bone block, addition aesthetic contour augmentation with mineralized allograft was performed to enhance hard and soft tissue contours. (**l**) Post operative healing of implant site. (**m**, **n**) Clinical follow-up after 15 years shows very stable soft tissue contours

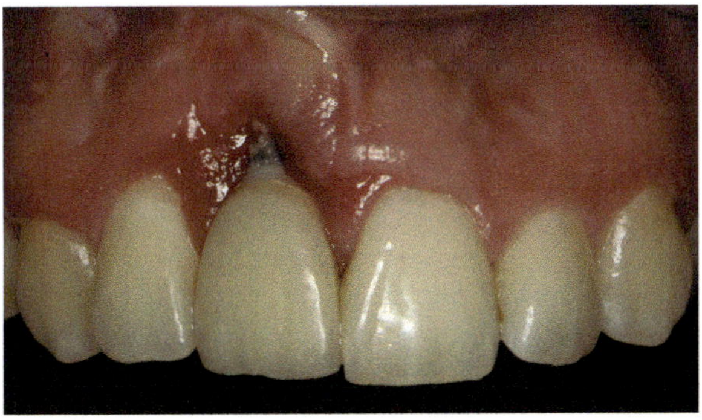

Fig. 7.13 Failed guided tissue regeneration with simultaneous implant placement may lead to exposed implant threads or crown margins

7.2.5.5 Particulate Graft and Resorbable Membrane

Various bone grafts or bone substitutes have been described for use with and without block grafting for guided bone regeneration [33–39, 41, 42, 112]. Autogenous onlay block grafts covered with bovine bone have shown to exhibit less resorption [113]. Le et al. [46] found that when human mineralized allograft was placed over autogenous block graft and covered with a resorbable membrane, bone and soft tissue contours improved with less need for autogenous bone (Fig. 7.12g).

The decision of which technique to employ should be based on the comfort level of the surgeon, as this will dramatically affect the outcome. Failed guided tissue regeneration with simultaneous implant placement may lead to exposed implant threads or crown margins (Fig. 7.13). If done in a two-staged approach, a failure may necessitate additional bone augmentation procedures. Another consideration is the vertical loss of the bone, which is commonly associated with horizontal defects, and the need to employ a technique that can address both problems with minimal surgery.

GBR is more predictable on alveolar ridges with mild to moderate horizontal deficiencies when the defect span is small. GBR techniques become more unreliable and more technique-sensitive as the length of the edentulous span increases. Tenting mechanisms are needed to prevent collapse of the tissue and resorption. Having a wide basal bone below the deficiency also leads to more predictable bone formation using GBR because maintaining this expanded space is more manageable. When mild lateral deficiencies are present, implants can be predictably placed simultaneously with GBR procedures [50]. Ridge splitting/expansion procedures can also correct mild to moderate deficiencies but need adequate height, whereas GBR can simultaneously correct for mild vertical deficiencies.

Moderate to severe lateral deficiencies, as well as long-span edentulous areas, are best treated using a cortical block onlay graft or a combination of onlay block and particulate grafts. Long-span atrophic ridges can be augmented with multiple small cortical bone blocks that are spaced 1 cm apart and covered with human particulate allograft. Bridging the cortical blocks with particulate bone avoids unaesthetic ridge defects between block grafts and minimizes resorption of the particulate allograft volume [46].

7.3 Management of Vertical Defects

Severe vertical alveolar ridge defects are usually three-dimensional and present a difficult challenge to the implant surgeon. Patients with vertical defects usually have concomitant horizontal defects, and these defects must be fully reconstructed in all dimensions to create an aesthetic and functional result. Furthermore, many vertical defects usually have loss of bone attachment to the teeth adjacent to the defect (Fig. 7.14c). In many instances, it is more beneficial to extract these teeth so that a healthy bone attachment level can be attained to graft bone too.

When a vertical defect is not treated, the patient may require an unaesthetic long clinical crown and/or poor crown-to-root ratio, which may negatively affect the longevity of the implant. These defects may be corrected prior to or simultaneous with implant placement, depending on the severity of the defect [114–117].

7.3.1 Short Implants

Short implants have traditionally been associated with higher failure rates [118, 119]. In a review of the literature on implant complications from 1981 to 2001, Goodacre et al. [120] noted a higher failure rate in implants that were shorter than 10 mm (10% versus 3%). With the introduction of roughened surface technologies and improved implant designs, short implants have gained increased interest and now have failure rates similar to implants longer than 10 mm [121–126].

Misch et al. [121] reported a 98.9% survival rate in a 6-year, retrospective, multicentered case series of 74 implants (7–9 mm) placed in the posterior jaws of partially edentulous patients. The authors concluded that short-length implants may be used predictably to support fixed restorations in posterior partial edentulism as long as methods to decrease biomechanical stresses were used. These include eliminating lateral contacts in mandibular excursions and eliminating cantilevers on the prosthesis, placing more implants, increasing the implant diameter, increasing the implant surface area, and splinting the implants together.

7.3.1.1 Does Rough Surface Make a Difference?

A retrospective study by Griffin et al. [127] concluded that the surface of the implants, in addition to biomechanics, may contribute to the predictability of short implants. The authors reported 100% success with short, wide, HA-coated implants that were placed in the posterior maxillas and mandibles and restored by seven different dentists [127]. Biomechanical forces were controlled by avoiding function in lateral excursive movements. Another 5-year retrospective study on rough-surfaced, short implants (BTI, Victoria, Spain) placed into the posterior maxilla and mandible reported only 2 failures out of 532 implants placed [123].

Another meta-analysis on the survival of short implants (≤8 mm) compared to conventional implants (≥10 mm) concluded that the placement of short rough-surfaced implants is not a less efficacious treatment modality compared to the

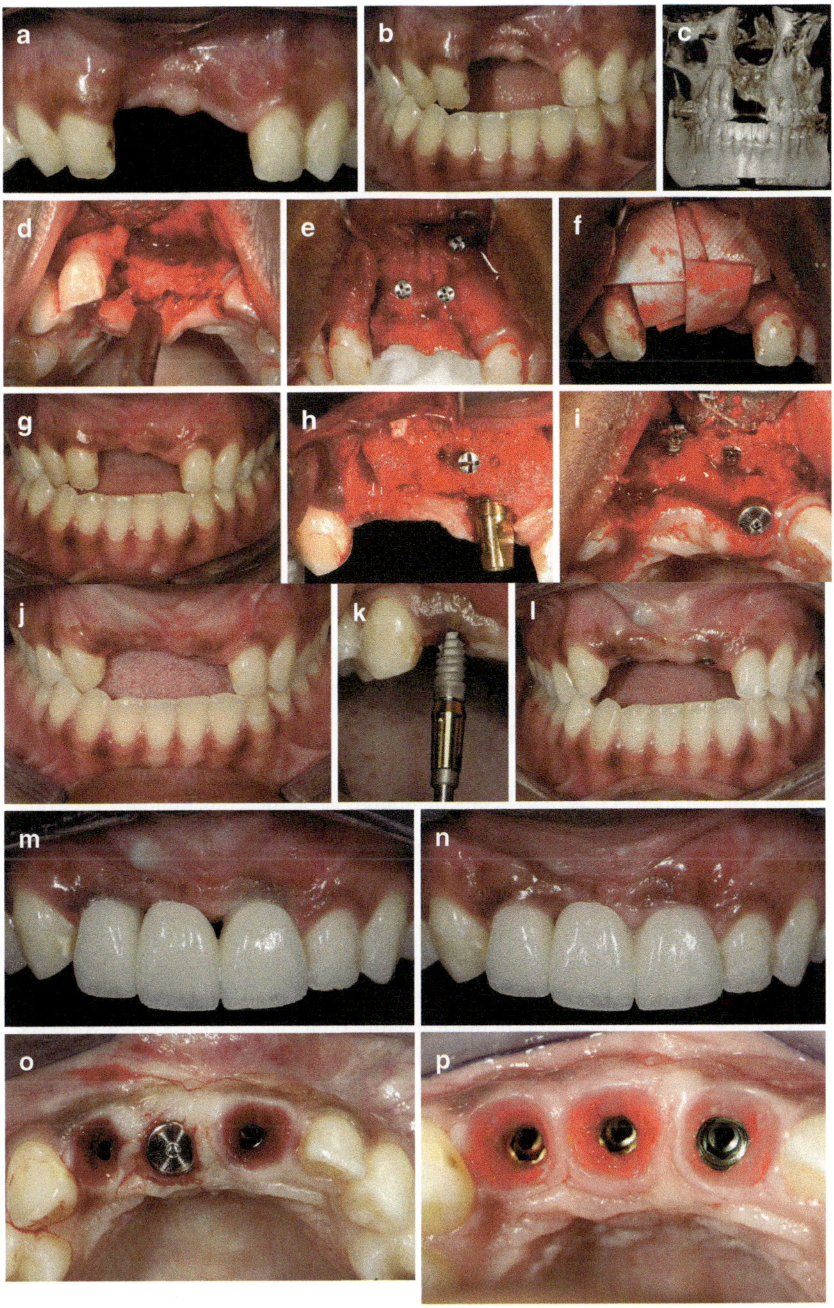

Fig. 7.14 (**a–s**) Vertical defects often have loss of bone attachment to the teeth adjacent to the defect. In many instances, it is more beneficial to extract these teeth so that a healthy bone attachment level can be attained for graft incorporation. Extraction of the lateral incisor was delayed (staged extraction and augmentation protocol) to decrease the span of the defect during initial augmentation. Pontic site development using the screw tent-pole grafting technique was used to optimize vertical tissue height prior to placement of an implant for the right maxillary central

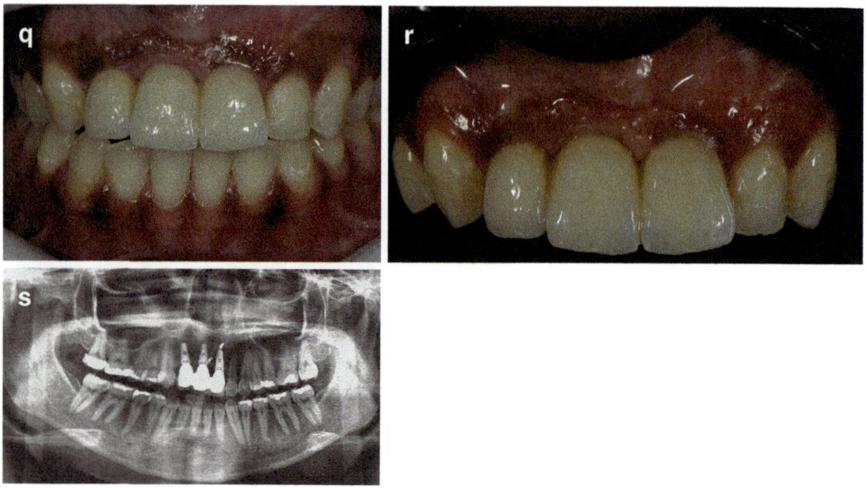

Fig. 7.14 (continued)

placement of conventional rough-surfaced implants for the replacement of missing teeth in either completely or partially edentulous patients [122].

7.3.2 Onlay Block Bone Graft

Autogenous bone graft has long been considered to be the gold standard for grafting severe hard tissue defects. However, reconstruction of large vertical defects often requires a significant amount of autogenous bone, including extraoral sources. Autogenous block grafts have been described to augment vertical defects but may be prone to resorption depending on the type of donor bone [87, 116, 117, 128]. It has also been reported that corticocancellous iliac bone is subject to more resorption when the graft site is not prosthetically loaded [87].

Prerequisites for vertical augmentation using onlay block grafts are a wide recipient bed for adapting a block graft and a healthy bone attachment to the teeth adjacent to the grafted span. 3–5 mm of vertical augmentation can usually be achieved using autogenous block grafts. Larger defects may require two-stage grafting for better outcomes.

7.3.3 Particulate Graft

Particulate grafts lack the structural rigidity of onlay block grafts and are subject to graft migration and displacement. Implants can be placed successfully into these grafted sites; however, resorption must be anticipated during treatment planning as further augmentation procedures may be necessary. Screws, implants, meshes, and reinforced membranes have been used as tenting mechanisms to minimize graft migration, displacement, and resorption [44, 45, 48].

Louis et al. reported on the use of titanium mesh for reconstruction of severely atrophic maxilla or mandible using iliac crest bone graft with a 97% overall graft success rate, although exposure of the titanium mesh was reported to be high (52%) [45]. The obstacles to using iliac crest bone are obvious. In addition to the higher resorption rate of iliac crest grafts, other disadvantages include the high costs of hospitalization, risk of general anesthesia, and morbidity of the procedure [83, 85, 86, 97].

Mineralized particulate allograft can be used similarly with a tenting mechanism for vertical alveolar ridge augmentation [48, 115, 129]. Using particulate allograft and screws, an average of 9.2 mm of vertical height was achieved, and implants were successfully placed [115] (Fig. 7.14a–s). This technique requires a membrane for optimal results and is technique-sensitive. Vertical defects with large spans (two missing teeth or more) have a higher risk of wound dehiscence. Correction of these defects in a two-surgery grafting protocol of smaller increments per graft may reduce the risk of graft dehiscence. Vertical defects of single missing tooth span may be corrected in a one-staged surgery protocol [48]. Usually, failure results from inadequate release of the flap leading to bone graft exposure and resorption. Wound dehiscence can lead to more pronounced bone graft resorption. When using particulate bone, maintaining the soft tissue space is critical. Proper flap design and manipulation is critical to prevent wound dehiscence when using these techniques.

7.3.4 Interpositional Osteotomy

Interpositional osteotomies can also be utilized to vertically augment the alveolar ridge, but its use should be limited to multiple-teeth span vertical defects ranging from 3 to 6 mm [114, 130, 131] (Fig. 7.15a–q). Moderate resorption is also expected using this technique but with minimal resorption around the implants placed into the augmented bone [131]. Le et al. [132] reported the vertical height increase with interpositional osteotomies in the anterior maxilla is directly proportional to the span of the edentulous segment with larger segments achieving the most long-term gains and undergoing the least amount of resorption. Long-term vertical gains in 2-teeth segment were very limited. To minimize resorption, the authors recommend performing this procedure in alveolar ridges with a minimum bone width and height of 10 mm. Bone augmentation is sometimes necessary to achieve these criteria prior to performing interpositional ostetotomy. Overcorrection of the vertical height with the osteotomy is also recommended. In the mandible, transient paresthesia has been reported as a potential unwanted side effect, and 5 mm of the basal bone above the inferior alveolar nerve is necessary to carry out this procedure safely without damage to adjacent structures [130, 131]. The use of larger graft particles compared to smaller particles within the osteotomy has been reported to decrease the amount of resorption seen after osteotomies [133].

Laster et al. [134] described a similar technique in the premaxilla region using particulate bovine bone matrix as an interpositional graft and used dental implants to fixate the bone segment. Gained vertical bone height averaged 5 mm and only required one surgery since the dental implants were placed simultaneously [134]. Placing dental implants in the correct three-dimensional position may be difficult with this technique because ideally positioning the transported native bone may

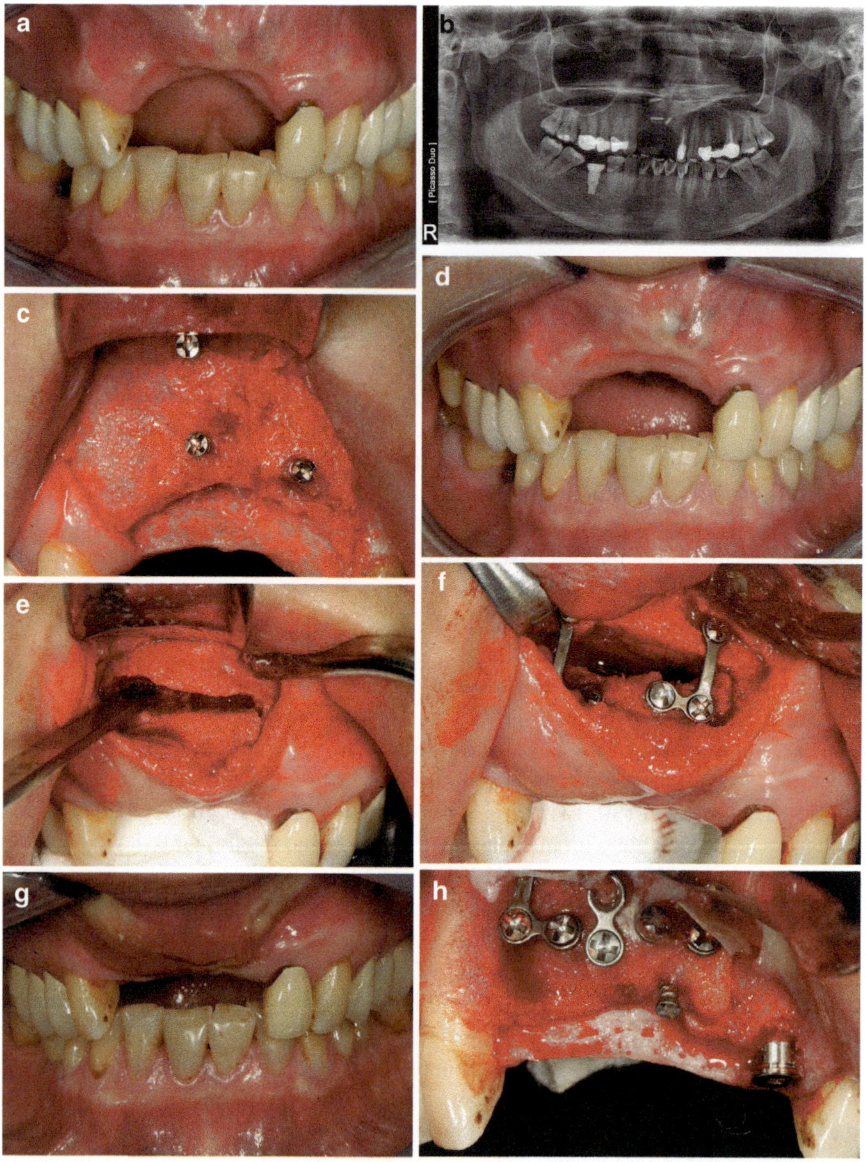

Fig. 7.15 (**a–b**) A severe, multiple-teeth span vertical defect treated using a staged reconstruction. (**c**) Initial staged GBR using the screw tent-pole technique to develop adequate horizontal width. (**c**) The defect site filled with particulate allograft is isolated using a resorbable collagen barrier membrane. (**d**) After 4 months of healing following the initial GBR, ridge width is improved, but ridge height is still deficient. (**e**) Second-stage surgery performed as an osteotomy and down-graft to restore ridge height. (**f**) Segment stabilized with plates. (**g**) Healing after 4 months. (**h–j**) Implants placed at sites # 7 and # 10 with "aesthetic contour grafting" protocol (non-submerged grafting). (**k**) Healing after 2 months showing a lack of attached tissue and vestibular depth. (**l–n**) Vestibuloplasty with free gingival graft from palate to increase the zone of attached tissue. (**o, p**) Final restorations at 3-year follow-up. (**q, r**) Radiograph at 3-year follow-up

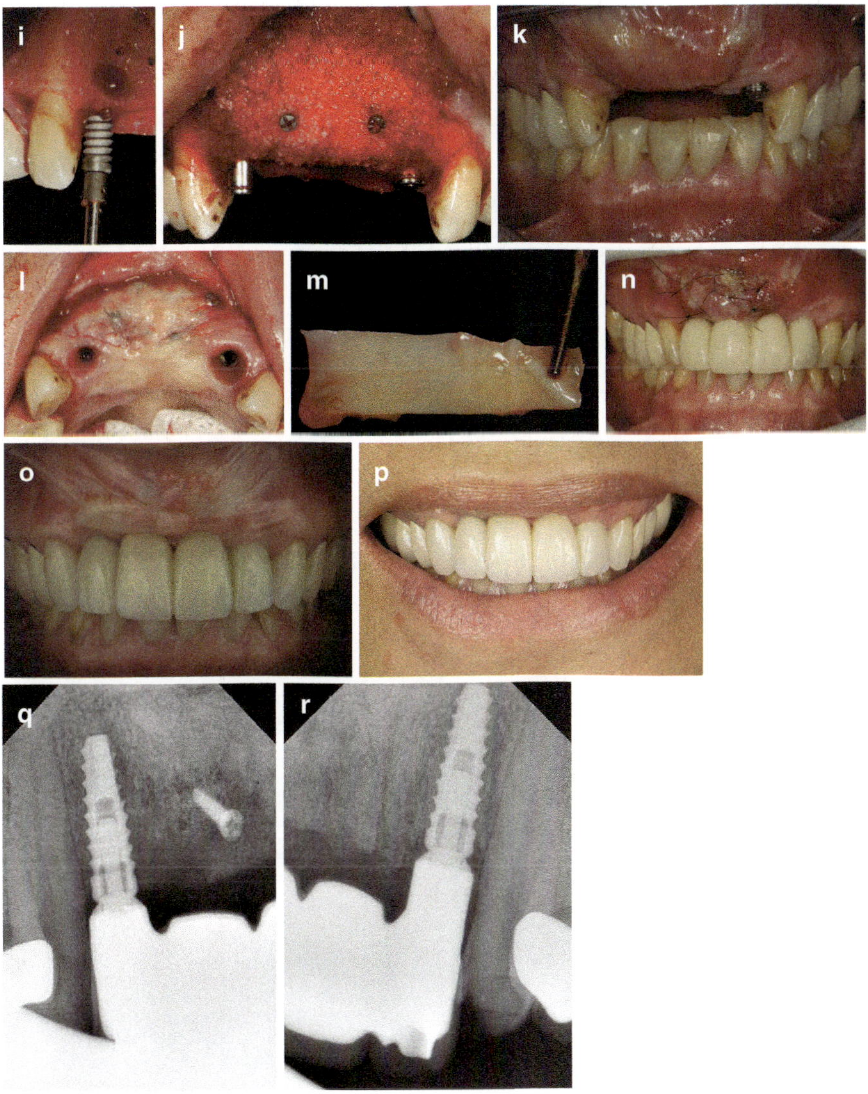

Fig. 7.15 (continued)

not be possible. Careful assessment of the alveolar ridge prior to this procedure and generating a surgical stent may facilitate treatment planning and surgery.

7.3.5 Distraction Osteogenesis

Distraction osteogenesis has been described to address the vertically deficient alveolar ridge but is only recommended for multiple-teeth span (≥4 teeth) severe vertical defects (>6–7 mm) [135–137] (Fig. 7.16a–q). This technique requires a minimal

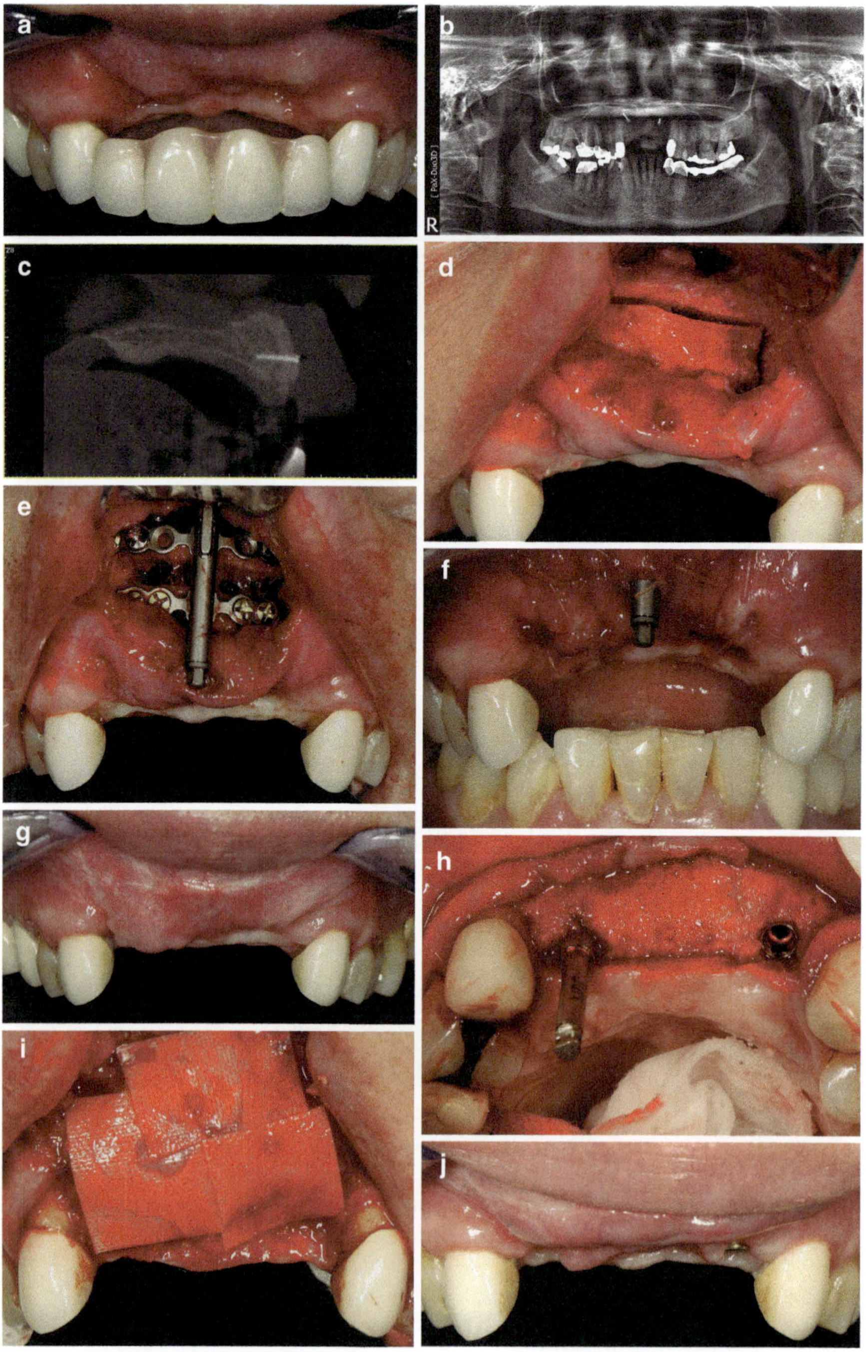

Fig. 7.16 (**a–q**) A severe multiple-teeth span vertical defect treated using a staged reconstruction with initial GBR to increase the alveolar width, followed by distraction osteogenesis to correct the alveolar height, free gingival graft, and implant placement with additional aesthetic contour augmentation

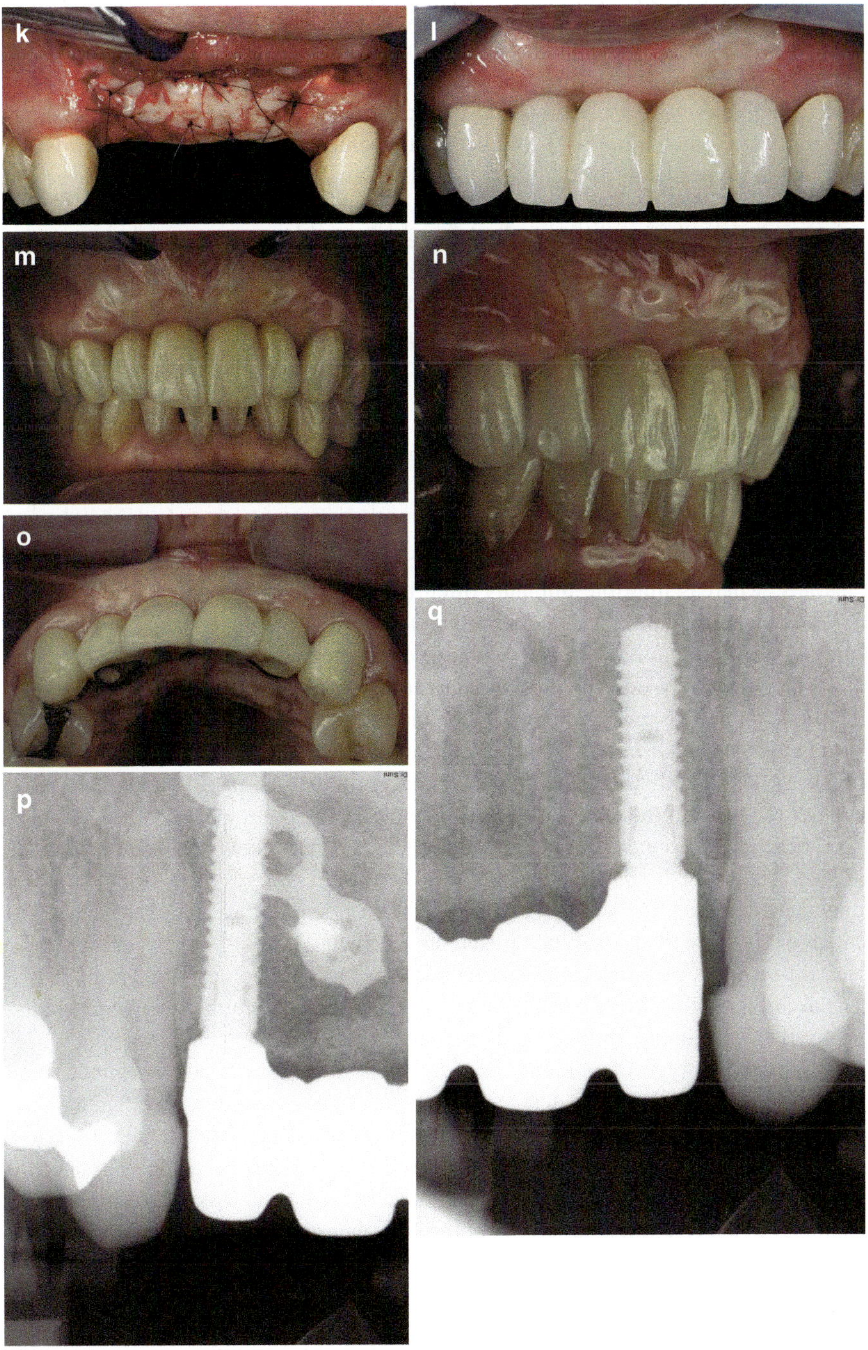

Fig. 7.16 (continued)

amount of the basal bone and frequently requires further augmentation procedures, depending on the available basal bone and the vector at which the bone is distracted. While distraction osteogenesis can be a predictable method for vertical augmentation, complications are common and include moderate resorption requiring additional bone augmentation, lack of buccal augmentation, loss of keratinized tissue, unsatisfactory aesthetic result, and a loss of vestibular depth [138]. The correction of a severe vertical defect in the aesthetic zone often requires multiple different techniques, strategically staged to achieve the ideal hard and soft tissue. Vestibuloplasty with free gingival graft after implant placement is often necessary to increase keratinized tissue attachment and improve aesthetic outcomes. Furthermore, the success of the technique is highly dependent on patient compliance, and hardware costs will have to be factored into the treatment plan.

7.3.6 The Challenge of Multiple Adjacent Implants in Compromised Sites

Single-tooth implant restorations are more likely to have predictable soft tissue anatomy, whereas multiple implants often have compromised soft tissue anatomy [139]. Recreating natural ridge contours in adjacent implants is difficult [140]. The formation of the papilla between two adjacent implants will follow the same principles as previously described. If intercrestal bone is present, the papilla between the implants will be present. However, formation or maintenance of the intercrestal bone height between implants is more difficult to achieve. In a series of 136 interpapillary height measurements between adjacent implants, papilla height from the crest of the bone to the height of the papilla averaged 3.4 mm [16].

Tarnow et al. found that implants demonstrated bone loss on their mesiodistal aspects under loading and that inter-implant bone loss resulted when adjacent implants are close together [17]. Placing implants at least 3 mm apart has been advocated to minimize the loss of intercrestal bone. When adjacent implants are placed at least 3 mm apart, only 0.45 mm of bone loss occurred at the intercrestal region [17]. The use of a pontic should be considered as an alternative treatment when mesiodistal space is inadequate for placement of adjacent implants that are 3 mm apart.

Although the type of implants used by Tarnow et al. was not specified, some advocates of newer implant designs and surfaces have reported significantly less bone loss than older traditional implant designs [141–147]. Additional research is needed to determine if this reported change in bone loss is actually related to implant design or if it simply reflects a change in how bone loss is interpreted. For example, average clinicians have traditionally measured bone changes according to visual assessments of radiographs on light boxes in the office setting. Some researchers have maintained, however, that the only accurate means of assessing bone loss is to monitor the location of marginal bone-to-implant contact (BIC) with the implant surface, which can only be done with special imaging equipment [145–147]. Using this technique, [145–147] if an implant has 1.5 mm of radiographically visible cervical bone loss, but if the microscopic BIC relationship has not changed since the implant was placed, then the implant would be reported as having 0 mm of bone loss.

7.3.6.1 Staged Extraction and Augmentation Protocol

When multiple teeth are indicated for extraction, a staged approach utilizing strategic extractions of selected teeth and fabrication of either a tooth-borne or implant-borne temporary fixed dental prosthesis (FDP) will help to decrease bone loss during healing and maintain the supporting bone and tissue architecture [148, 149]. If multiple grafting procedures are planned for a severe defect, consideration should be given to the timing of extraction to minimize the length of the edentulous span and maximize the outcome of any initial grafting procedure (Fig. 7.14).

7.3.7 Pontic Site Development

The use of a pontic may improve the overall aesthetic outcome when replacing multiple teeth with implants. Some have suggested that the papilla height between pontic and implant can be greater than 5 mm, compared with 3.4 mm with adjacent implants [150] (Fig. 7.14n). Leaving submerged roots or augmenting with a connective tissue graft or a slow resorbing bone graft has been described as techniques to augment the pontic site [150, 151]. However, submerged roots may lead to future problems, and patients should be made aware of potential aesthetic failures if future removal is required. More long-term studies in pontic site development are necessary to assess the longevity of augmentation techniques in conjunction with implant therapy.

Conclusion

Dental implants have unquestionably changed the quality of life of patients with missing teeth. The high survival rate associated with dental implant therapy has quickly led to increasing emphasis on achieving predictable and long-term aesthetics. Prosthetically driven implant placement, along with the restoration and preservation of its supporting bone and tissue architecture, will enhance the aesthetics and success of the dental implant therapy.

References

1. Schropp L, et al. Bone healing and soft tissue contour changes following single-tooth extraction: a clinical and radiographic 12-month prospective study. Int J Periodontics Restorative Dent. 2003;23:313–23.
2. Ekfeldt A, Carlsson GE, Borjesson G. Clinical evaluation of single-tooth restorations supported by osseointegrated implants: a retrospective study. Int J Oral Maxillofac Surg. 1994;9:179–83.
3. Haas R, et al. Branemark single tooth implants: a preliminary report of 76 implants. J Prosthet Dent. 1995;73:274–9.
4. Jemt T, et al. Osseointegrated implants for single tooth replacement: a 1-year report from a multicenter prospective study. Int J Oral Maxillofac Implants. 1991;6:29–36.
5. Oates TW, et al. Long-term changes in soft tissue height on the facial surface of dental implants. Implant Dent. 2002;11:272–9.
6. Tymstra N, Raghoebar GM, Vissink A, Meijer HJA. Dental implant treatment for two adjacent missing teeth in the maxillary aesthetic zone: a comparative pilot study and test of principle. Clin Oral Implants Res. 2011;22(2):207–13.
7. De Rouch T, Collys K, Cosyn J. Immediate single-tooth implants in the anterior maxilla: a 1-year case cohort study on hard and soft tissue response. J Clin Periodontol. 2008;35:649–57.

8. JYK K, et al. Periimplant tissue response following immediate provisional restoration of scalloped implants in the esthetic zone: a one-year pilot prospective multicenter study. J Prosthet Dent. 2007;97(Supplement 1):S109–18.
9. JYK K, Rungcharassaeng K, Lozada J. Immediate placement and provisionalization of maxillary anterior single implants: 1-year prospective study. Int J Oral Maxillofac Implants. 2003;18:31–9.
10. Salama H, Salama M. The role of orthodontic extrusive remodeling in the enhancement of soft and hard tissue profiles prior to implant placement: a systematic approach to the management of extraction site defects. Int J Periodontics Restorative Dent. 1993;13:312–33.
11. Brindis MA, Block MS. Orthodontic tooth extrusion to enhance soft tissue implant esthetics. J Oral Maxillofac Surg. 2009;67(11 Supplement):49–59.
12. JYK K, et al. Facial gingival tissue stability after connective tissue graft with single immediate tooth replacement in the esthetic zone: consecutive case report. J Oral Maxillofac Surg. 2009;67(Supplement 1):40–8.
13. Block MS, et al. Prospective evaluation of immediate and delayed provisional single tooth restorations. J Oral Maxillofac Surg. 2009;67(Supplement 3):89–107.
14. Choquet V, et al. Clinical and radiographic evaluation of the papilla level adjacent to single-tooth dental implants: a retrospective study in the maxillary anterior region. J Periodontol. 2001;72:1364–71.
15. JYK K, et al. Dimensions of peri-implant mucosa: an evaluation of maxillary anterior single implants in humans. J Periodontol. 2003;74:557–62.
16. Tarnow D, et al. Vertical distance from the crest of bone to the height of the interproximal papilla between adjacent implants. J Periodontol. 2003;74:1785–8.
17. Tarnow D, Cho SC, Wallace SS. The effect of inter-implant distance on the height of inter-implant bone crest. J Periodontol. 2000;71:546–9.
18. Chen Stephen T, et al. Immediate implant placement postextraction without flap elevation. J Peridontol. 2009;80:163–72.
19. Seibert J, Lindhe J. Esthetics and periodontal therapy. [book auth.]. In: Lindhe J, editor. Textbook of clinical periodontology. Copenhagen: Munksgaard International Publishing; 1989. p. 477–514.
20. De Rouck T, et al. The gingival biotype revisited: transparency of the periodontal probe through the gingival margin as a method to discriminate thin from thick gingiva. J Clin Periodontol. 2009;36:428–33.
21. Muller HP, Eger T, Schorb A. Gingival dimensions after root coverage with free connective tissue grafts. J Clin Periodontol. 1998;25:424–30.
22. Hammerle CHF, Chen ST, Wilson TG. Consensus statements and recommended clinical procedures regarding the placement of implants in extraction sockets. Int J Oral Maxillofac Implants. 2004;19(Suppl):26–8.
23. Sclar AG. Preserving alveolar ridge anatomy following tooth removal in conjunction with immediate implant placement. Atlas Oral Maxillofac Surg Clin North Am. 1999;7:39–59.
24. Le BT, Borzabadi-Farahani A. Labial bone thickness in area of anterior maxillary implants associated with crestal labial soft tissue thickness. Implant Dent. 2012;21:406–10.
25. Le BT, Borzabadi-Farahani A. Is buccolingual angulation of maxillary anterior implants associated with the crestal labial soft tissue thickness? Int J Oral Maxillofac Surg. 2014;43:874–8.
26. Barros RM, et al. Buccal bone remodeling after immediate implantation with a flap or flapless approach: a pilot study in dogs. Titanium. 2009;1:45–51.
27. Belser UC, Grutter L, Vailati F, Bornstein MM, Weber HP, Buser D. Outcome evaluation of early placed maxillary anterior single-tooth implants using objective esthetic criteria: a cross-sectional, retrospective study in 45 patients with a 2- to 4-year follow-up using pink and white esthetic scores. J Periodontol. 2009;80(1):140–51.
28. Esposito M, Grusovin MG, Worthington HV. Agreement of quantitative subjective. Int J Oral Maxillofac Implants. 2009;24:309–15.
29. Meijndert L, Meijer HJ, Stellingsma K, Stegenga B, Raghoebar GM. Evaluation of aesthetics of implant-supported single-tooth replacements using different bone augmentation procedures: a prospective randomized clinical study. Clin Oral Implant Res. 2007;18(6):715–9.

30. Kokich VO, Kokich VG, Kiyak HA. Perceptions of dental professionals and laypersons to altered dental esthetics: asymmetric and symmetric situations. Am J Orthod Dentalfacail Orthop. 2008;130(2):141–51.
31. Spray JR, et al. The influence of bone thickness on facial marginal bone response: stage 1 placement through stage 2 uncovering. Annal Periodontol. 2000;5:119–28.
32. Takahashi T, et al. Use of endosseous implants for dental reconstruction of patients with grafted alveolar clefts. J Oral Maxillofac Surg. 1997;66:251–5.
33. Hasson O. Lateral ridge augmentation using the pocket technique. J Oral Maxillofac Surg. 2005;63(Supplement 1):26–7.
34. Peleg M. Lateral alveolar ridge augmentation with allogeneic block grafts: observations form a multicenter prospective clinical trial. J Oral Maxillofac Surg. 2005;63(Supplement 1):29.
35. Block M, Degen M. Horizontal ridge augmentation using human mineralized particulate bone: preliminary results. J Oral Maxillofac Surg. 2004;62:67–72.
36. Buser D, et al. Lateral ridge augmentation using autografts and barrier membranes: a clinical study with 40 partially edentulous patients. J Oral Maxillofac Surg. 1996;54:420–32.
37. Raghoebar GM, et al. Augmentation of localized defects of the anterior maxillary ridge with autogenous bone before insertion of implants. J Oral Maxillofac Surg. 1996;54:1180–5.
38. Barone A, et al. Deep-frozen allogeneic onlay bone grafts for reconstruction of atrophic maxillary alveolar ridges: a preliminary study. J Oral Maxillofac Surg. 2009;67:1300–6.
39. Howell TH, et al. A feasibility study evaluating rhBMP-2/absorbable collagen sponge device for local alveolar ridge preservation or augmentation. Int J Periodontics Restorative Dent. 1997;17:124–39.
40. Oda T, et al. Horizontal alveolar distraction of the narrow maxilla ridge for implant placement. J Oral Maxillofac Surg. 2004;62:1530–4.
41. Donovan MG, et al. Maxillary and mandibular reconstruction using calvarial bone grafts and branemark implants: a preliminary report. J Oral Maxillofac Surg. 1994;52:588–94.
42. Peleg M, et al. Maxillary sinus and ridge augmentations using a surface-derived autogenous bone graft. J Oral Maxillofac Surg. 2004;62:1535–44.
43. Llambes F, Silvestre F-J, Caffesse R. Vertical guided bone regeneration with bioabsorbably barrier. J Periodontol. 2007;78:2036–42.
44. Marx RE, Shellenberger T, Wimsatt J, Correa P. Severely resorbed mandible: predictable reconstruction with soft tissue matrix expansion (tent pole) grafts. J Oral Maxillofac Surg. 2002;60:878–88.
45. Louis PJ, et al. Reconstruction of the maxilla and mandible with particulate bone graft and titanium mesh for implant placement. J Oral Maxillofac Surg. 2008;66:235–45.
46. Le B, Burstein J. Cortical tenting grafting technique in the severely atrophic alveolar ridge for implant site preparation. Implant Dent. 2008;17:40–50.
47. Le B, Burstein J. Esthetic grafting for small volume hard and soft tissue contour defects for implant site development. Implant Dent. 2008;17:136–41.
48. Le BT, Rohrer MD, Prassad HS. Screw "tent-pole" grafting technique for reconstruction of large vertical alveolar ridge defects using human mineralized allograft for implant site preparation. J Oral Maxillofac Surg. 2010;68:428–35.
49. Verdugo F, Simonian K, Nowzari H. Periodontla biotype influence on the volume maintenance of only grafts. J Periodontol. 2009;80:816–23.
50. Le BT. Effectiveness of single-staged implant placement with simultaneous grafting using mineralized allograft. J Oral Maxillofac Surg. 2009;67(Supplement 1):57.
51. Hellem S, et al. Implant treatment in combination with lateral augmentation of the alveolar process: a 3-year prospective study. Clin Implant Dent Relat Res. 2003;5:233–40.
52. Le BT, Borzabadi-Farahani A. Simultaneous implant placement & bone grafting with particulate mineralized allograft in sites with buccal wall defects, a 3-year follow-up & review of literature. J Cranio-Maxillofac Surg. 2014;42:552–9.
53. Le B, Borzabadi-Farahani A, Nielsen B. Treatment of labial soft tissue recession around dental implants in the esthetic zone using guided bone regeneration with mineralized allograft: a retrospective clinical case series. J Oral Maxillofac Surg. 2016;74:1552–61.

54. Le B, Borzabadi-Farahani A. Treatment of labial mucosal recession around maxillary anterior implants with tenting screws, particulate allograft and xenogenic membrane: a case report. J Oral Implantol. 2016;10:1563.
55. Block M, Finger I, Lytle R. Human mineralized bone in extraction sites before implant placement: preliminary results. J Am Dent Assoc. 2002;133:1631–8.
56. Elian N, et al. A simplified socket classification and repair technique. Pract Proced Aesthet Dent. 2007;19:99–104.
57. Araujo M, Linder E, Lindhe J. Effect of xenograft on early bone formation in extraction sockets: an experimental study in dog. Clin Oral Implants Res. 2009;20:1–6.
58. Wang H-L, Tsao Y-P. Mineralized bone allograft-plug socket augmentation: rationale and technique. Implant Dent. 2007;16:33–41.
59. Ashman A. Postextraction ridge preservation using a synthetic alloplast. Implant Dent. 2000;9:168–76.
60. Shi B, et al. Alveolar ridge preservation prior to implant placement with surgical-grade calcium sulfate and platelet-rich plasma: a pilot study in a canine model. Int J Oral Maxillofac Implants. 2007;22:656–65.
61. Masago H, et al. Alveolar ridge augmentation using various bone substitutes–a web form of titanium fibers promotes rapid bone development. Kobe J Med Sci. 2007;53:257–63.
62. Trisi P, et al. Histologic effect of pure-phase beta-tricalcium phosphate on bone regeneration in human artificial jawbone defects. Int J Periodontics Restorative Dent. 2003;23:69–77.
63. Fiorellini J, et al. Randomized study evaluating recombinant human bone morphogenetic protein-2 for extraction socket augmentation. J Periodontol. 2005;76:605–13.
64. Simunek A, et al. Deproteinized bovine bone versus beta-tricalcium phosphate in sinus augmentation surgery: a comparative histologic and histomorphometric study. Int J Oral Maxillofac Implants. 2008;23:935–42.
65. Froum S, et al. Extraction sockets and implantation of hydroxyapatites with membrane barriers: a histologic study. Implant Dent. 2004;13:153–64.
66. Araujo M, et al. The influence of Bio-Oss Collagen on healing of an extraction socket: an experimental study in the dog. Int J Periodontics Restorative Dent. 2008;28:123–35.
67. Molly L, et al. Bone formation following implantation of bone biomaterials into extraction sites. J Periodontol. 2008;79:1108–15.
68. Minichetti JC, D'Amore JC, Hong AY. Three-year analysis of tapered screw-vent implants placed into extraction sockets grafted with mineralized bone allograft. J Oral Implantol. 2005;31:283–93.
69. Le BT, Woo I. Alveolar cleft repair in adults using guided bone regeneration with mineralized allograft for dental implant site development: a report of 2 cases. J Oral Maxillofac Surg. 2009;67:1716–22.
70. Froum SJ, et al. Comparison of mineralized cancellous bone allograft (Puros) and anorganic bovine bone matrix (Bio-oss) for sinus augmentation: histomorphometry at 26 to 32 weeks after grafting. Int J Periodontics Restorative Dent. 2006;26:543–51.
71. Malinin TI, Carpenter E, Temple HT. Particulate bone allograft incorporation in regeneration of osseous defects: importance of particle sizes. Open Orthop J. 2007;1:19–24.
72. Simion M, et al. Guided bone regeneration using resorbable and nonresorbable membranes: a comparative histologic study in humans. Int J Oral Maxillofac Implants. 1996;11:735–42.
73. Simion M, et al. Vertical ridge augmentation by expanded-polytetrafluoroethylene membrane and a combination of intraoral autogenous bone graft and deproteinized anorganic bovine bone (Bio Oss). Clin Oral Implants Res. 2007;18:620–9.
74. Gielkens PFM, et al. Is there evidence that barrier membranes prevent bone resorption in autologous bone grafts during the healing period? A systematic review. Int J Oral Maxillofac Implants. 2007;22:390–8.
75. Lekovic V, et al. A bone regenerative approach to alveolar ridge maintenance following tooth extraction. Report of 10 cases. J Periodontol. 1997;68:563–70.
76. Lekovic V, et al. Preservation of alveolar bone in extraction sockets using bioabsorbable membranes. J Periodontol. 1998;69:1044–9.

77. Murphy KG. Postoperative healing complications associated with gore-tex periodontal material. Part II. Effect of complications on regeneration. Int J Periodontics Restorative Dent. 1996;16:463–77.
78. Barone A, et al. Flap versus flapless procedure for ridge preservation in alveolar extraction sockets: a histological evaluation in a randomized clinical trial. Clin Oral Implants Res. 2015;26:806–13.
79. Coatoam GW, Mariotti A. The segmental ridge-split procedure. J Periodontol. 2003;74:757–70.
80. Jensen OT, Cullum DR, Baer D. Marginal bone stability using 3 different flap approaches for alveolar split expansion for dental implants–a 1-year clinical study. J Oral Maxillofac Surg. 2009;67:1921–30.
81. Buser D, et al. Localized ridge augmentation using guided bone regeneration. II. Surgical procedure in the mandible. Int J Periodontics Restorative Dent. 1995;15:11–29.
82. Buser D, et al. Localized ridge augmentation with autografts and barrier membranes. Periodontology. 1999;19:151–63.
83. Misch CM. Comparison of intraoral donor sites for onlay grafting prior to implant placement. Int J Oral Maxillofac Implants. 1997;12:767–76.
84. Rasmusson L, et al. Effects of barrier membranes on bone resorption and implant stability in onlay bone grafts. An experimental study. Clin Oral Implants Res. 1999;10:267–77.
85. Proussaefs P, Lozada J, Rohrer MD. A clinical and histologic evaluation of a block onlay graft in conjunction with autogenous particulate and inorganic bovine material: a case report. Int J Periodontics Restorative Dent. 2002;22:567–73.
86. Misch CM, Misch CE. The repair of localized severe ridge defects for implant placement using mandibular bone grafts. Implant Dent. 1995;4:261–7.
87. Keller EE, Tolman DE, Eckert S. Surgical-prosthodontic reconstruction of advanced maxillary bone compromise with autogenous onlay block grafts and osseointegrated implants: a 12 year study of 32 consecutive patients. Int J Oral Maxillofac Implants. 1999;14:197–209.
88. Thor A. Reconstruction of the anterior maxilla with platelet gel, autogenous bone and titanium mesh: a case report. Clin Implant Dent Relat Res. 2002;4:150–5.
89. Doblin JM, et al. A histologic evaluation of localized ridge augmentation utilizing DFDBA in combination with e-PTFE membranes and stainless steel bone pins in humans. Int J Periodontics Restorative Dent. 1996;16:121–9.
90. Fugazzotto PA. Report of 302 consecutive ridge augmentation procedures: technical considerations and clinical results. Int J Oral Maxillofac Implants. 1998;13:358–68.
91. Araujo MG, et al. Lateral ridge augmentation by the use of grafts comprised of autologous bone or biomaterial. An experiment in the dog. J Clin Periodontol. 2002;29:1122–31.
92. Friedmann A, et al. Histological assessment of augmented jaw bone utilizing a new collagen barrier membrane compared to a standard barrier membrane to protect granular bone substitute material: a randomized clinical trial. Clin Oral Implants Res. 2002;13:587–94.
93. Kent JN, et al. Alveolar ridge augmentation using nonresorbable hydroxyapatite with or without autogenous cancellous bone. J Oral Maxillofac Surg. 1983;41:629–42.
94. Mentag PJ, Kosinski T. Hydroxyapatite-augmented sites as receptors for replacement implants. J Oral Implantol. 1989;15:114–23.
95. Smith JD, Abramson M. Membranous vs. endochondral bone autografts. Arch Otolaryngol. 1974;99:203–5.
96. Zins JE, Whitaker LA. Membranous vs endochondral bone autografts: implications for craniofacial reconstruction. Plast Reconstr Surg. 1983;72:778–85.
97. James JD, Geist ET, Gross BD. Adynamic ileus as a complication of iliac bone removal. J Oral Maxillofac Surg. 1981;39:289–91.
98. Proussaefs P, et al. The use of ramus autogenous block grafts for vertical alveolar ridge augmentation and implant placement: a pilot study. Int J Oral Maxillofac Implants. 2002;17:238–48.
99. Montazem A, et al. The mandibular symphysis as a donor site in maxillofacial bone grafting: a quantitative anatomic study. J Oral Maxillofac Surg. 2000;58:1368–71.

100. Gungormus M, Yavuz MS. The ascending ramus of the mandible as a donor site in maxillofacial bone grafting. J Oral Maxillofac Surg. 2002;60:1316–8.
101. Misch CM. Ridge augmentation using mandibular ramus bone grafts for the placement of dental implants: presentation of a technique. Pract Periodontics Aesthet Dent. 1996;8:127.
102. Pikos MA. Facilitating implant placement with chin graft as donor sites for maxillary bone augmentation. Dent Implantol Updat. 1995;6:89.
103. Widmark G, Andersson B, Ivanoff CJ. Mandibular bone graft in the anterior maxilla for single-tooth implants: presentation of a surgical method. Int J Oral Maxillofac Surg. 1997;26:106.
104. Tolstunov L. Maxillary tuberosity block bone graft: innovative technique and case report. J Oral Maxillofac Surg. 2009;67:1723–9.
105. Raghoebar GM, et al. Maxillary bone grafting for insertion of endosseous implants: results after 12-124 months. Clin Oral Implants Res. 2001;12:279.
106. Proussaefs P. Clinical and histologic evaluation of the use of mandibular tori as donor site for mandibular block grafts: report of three cases. Int J Periodontics Restorative Dent. 2006;26:43.
107. Hassani A, et al. The "crescent" graft: a new design for bone reconstruction in implant dentistry. J Oral Maxillofac Surg. 2009;67:1735–8.
108. Clavero J, Lundgren S. Ramus or chin grafts for maxillary sinus inlay and local onlay augmentation: comparison of donor site morbidity and complications. Clin Implant Dent Relat Res. 2003;5:154–60.
109. Weibull L, et al. Morbidity after chin bone harvesting–a retrospective long-term follow-up study. Clin Implant Dent Relat Res. 2009;11:149–57.
110. Sbordone L, et al. Clinical survey of neurosensory side-effects of mandibular parasymphyseal bone harvesting. Int J Oral Maxillofac Surg. 2009;38:139–45.
111. Frost H. The regional acceleratory phenomenon: a review. Henry Fort Hosp Med J. 1983;31:3–9.
112. Oda T, et al. Horizontal alveolar distraction of the narrow maxillary ridge for implant placement. J Oral Maxillofac Surg. 2004;62:1530–4.
113. Maiorana C, et al. Reduction of autogenous bone graft resorption by means of Bio-Oss coverage: a prospective study. Int J Periodontics Restorative Dent. 2005;25:19–25.
114. Block M, Haggerty C. Interpositional osteotomy for posterior mandible ridge augmentation. J Oral Maxillofac Surg. 2009;67:31–9.
115. Hearne J, Le BT. Screw "tent-pole" grafting technique for vertical augmentation of the severely atrophic alveolar ridge for implant site preparation. J Oral Maxillofac Surg. 2008;66(Supplement 1):86–7.
116. Roccuzzo M, et al. Autogenous bone graft alone or associated with titanium mesh for vertical alveolar ridge augmentation: a controlled clinical trial. Clin Oral Implants Res. 2007;18:286–94.
117. Roccuzzo M, et al. Vertical alveolar ridge augmentation by means of a titanium mesh and autogenous bone grafts. Clin Oral Implants Res. 2004;15:73–81.
118. Weng D, et al. A prospective multicenter clinical trial of 3i machined-surface implants: results after 6 years of follow-up. Int J Oral Maxillofac Implants. 2003;18:417–23.
119. Ivanoff CJ, et al. Influence of variations in implant diameters: a 3- to 5-year retrospective clinical report. Int J Oral Maxillofac Implants. 1999;14:173–80.
120. Goodacre CJ, et al. Clinical complications with implants and implant prostheses. J Prosthet Dent. 2003;90:121–32.
121. Misch CE, et al. Short dental implants in posterior partial edentulism: a multicenter retrospective 6-year case series study. J Periodontol. 2006;77:1340–7.
122. Fourmousis I, Karoussis IK, Bamia C. A systematic review and meta-analysis on the effect of implant length on the survival of rough-surface dental implants. J Periodontol. 2009;80:1700–18.
123. Anitua E, et al. Five-year clinical evaluation of short dental implants placed in posterior areas: a retrospective study. J Periodontol. 2008;79:42–8.

124. Nedir R, et al. Osteotome sinus floor elevation technique without grafting material: 3-year results of a prospective pilot study. Clin Oral Implants Res. 2009;20:701–7.
125. Nedir R, et al. A 7-year life table analysis from a prospective study on ITI implants with special emphasis on the use of short implants. Results from a private practice. Clin Oral Implants Res. 2004;15:150–7.
126. Nedir R, et al. Osteotome sinus floor elevation technique without grafting material and immediate implant placement in atrophic posterior maxilla: report of 2 cases. J Oral Maxillofac Surg. 2009;67:1098–103.
127. Griffin TJ, Cheung WS. The use of short implants in posterior areas with reduced bone height: a retrospective investigation. J Prosthet Dent. 2004;92:139–44.
128. Polini F, et al. Bifunctional sculpturing of the bone graft for 3-dimensional augmentation of the atrophic posterior mandible. J Oral Maxillofac Surg. 2009;67:174–7.
129. Fontana F, et al. Clinical and histologic evaluation of allogeneic bone matrix versus autogenous bone chips associated with titanium-reinforced e-PTFE membrane for vertical ridge augmentation: a prospective pilot study. Int J Oral Maxillofac Implants. 2008;23:1003–12.
130. Jensen O. Alveolar segmental "sandwich" osteotomies for posterior edentulous mandibular sites for dental implants. J Oral Maxillofac Surg. 2006;64:471–5.
131. Jensen OT. Alveolar segmental sandwich osteotomy for anterior maxillary vertical augmentation prior to implant placement. J Oral Maxillofac Surg. 2006;64:290–6.
132. Le B, Mirzaians A, Yip K. Vertical alveolar ridge augmentation in the anterior maxilla and mandible using interpositional osteotomy. Abstract American Association of Oral Maxillofacial Surgeons Annual Meeting, Chicago, IL. Oct 2018.
133. Kheur M, Kheur S, Lakha T, Jambhekar S, Le BT, Jain V. Does graft particle type and size affect ridge dimensional changes after alveolar ridge split procedure? J Oral Maxillofac Surg. 2018;76(4):761–9.
134. Laster Z, Cohen G, Nagler R. A novel technique for vertical bone augmentation in the premaxillary region. J Oral Maxillofac Surg. 2009;67:2669–72.
135. Klug CN, et al. Preprosthetic vertical distraction osteogenesis of the mandible using an L-shaped osteotomy and titanium membranes for guided bone regeneration. J Oral Maxillofac Surg. 2001;59:1302–8.
136. Block MS, Baughman DG. Reconstruction of severe maxillary defects using distraction osteogenesis, bone grafts, and implants. J Oral Maxillofac Surg. 2005;63:291–7.
137. Jensen O, Horiuchi K. Osteoperiosteal flaps and distraction osteogenesis. [book auth.]. In: Fonseca R, editor. Oral and maxillofacial surgery. s.l. New York: Elsevier; 2017.
138. Froum SJ, et al. Distraction osteogenesis for ridge augmentation: prevention and treatment of complications. Thirty case reports. Int J Periodontics Restorative Dent. 2008;28:337–45.
139. Belser UC, et al. Outcome analysis of implant restorations located in the anterior maxilla: a review of the recent literature. Int J Oral Maxillofac Implants. 2004;19(Suppl):30–42.
140. Priest GF. The esthetic challenge of adjacent implants. J Oral Maxillofac Surg. 2007;65(Supplement 1):2–12.
141. Hurzeler M, et al. Peri-implant bone level around implants with platform-switched abutments: preliminary data from a prospective study. J Oral Maxillofac Surg. 2007;65(Supplement 1):33–9.
142. Canullo L, Iurlaro G, Iannello G. Double-blind randomized controlled trial study on post-extraction immediately restored implants using the switching platform concept: soft tissue response. Preliminary report. Clin Oral Implants Res. 2009;20:414–20.
143. Luongo R, et al. Hard and soft tissue responses to the platform-switching technique. Int J Periodontics Restorative Dent. 2008;28:551–7.
144. Baggi L, et al. The influence of implant diameter and length on stress distribution of osseointegrated implants related to crestal bone geometry: a three-dimensional finite element analysis. J Prosthet Dent. 2008;100:422–31.
145. Astrand P, et al. Astra tech and branemark system implants: a 5-year prospective study of marginal bone reactions. Clin Oral Implant Res. 2004;15:413–20.

146. Palmer RM, Palmer PJ, Smith BJ. A 5-year prospective study of Astra single tooth implants. Clin Oral Implants Res. 2000;11:179–82.
147. Rasmusson L, Roos J, Bystedt H. A 10-year follow-up study of titanium dioxide-blasted implants. Clin Implant Dent Relat Res. 2005;7:36–42.
148. Favero G, et al. Role of teeth adjacent to implants installed immediately into extraction sockets: an experimental study in dogs. Clin Oral Implants Res. 2012;23:402–8.
149. Fickl S. Tissue alterations after tooth extraction with and without surgical trauma: a volumetric study in the beagle dog. J Clin Periodontol. 2008;35:356–63.
150. Salama M, et al. Advantages of the root submergence technique for pontic site development in esthetic implant therapy. Int J Periodontics Restorative Dent. 2007;27:521–7.
151. Landsberg CJ. Implementing socket seal surgery as a socket preservation technique for pontic site development: surgical steps revisited–a report of two cases. J Periodontol. 2008;79:945–54.

The Implant-Supported Screw-Retained Provisional Prosthesis: Science, Fabrication, and Design

8

Todd R. Schoenbaum and Perry R. Klokkevold

Abstract

When properly designed and fabricated, the implant-supported screw-retained provisional prosthesis (ISP) is a crucial component for predictable treatment of implants in the aesthetic zone. It helps to support and maintain the peri-implant soft tissues, particularly when used with immediate implant placement. The materials used in its fabrication should be selected to provide biocompatibility, aesthetics, and strength. The ISP is fabricated in the clinic in conjunction with implant placement. Special care must be given to the occlusion to minimize the risk to the implant.

8.1 Rational and Indications for the Use of Immediate Provisional Restorations

The use of a well-designed implant-supported screw-retained provisional prosthesis (ISP) (Fig. 8.1) is *critical* to the success of implant treatment in the aesthetic zone [1–4]. The ISP allows the clinical team (surgeon, restoring dentist, and technician) to accurately shape and define the positions of the teeth and peri-implant soft tissues prior to the fabrication of the definitive prosthesis. It allows the treatment team and the patient sufficient time to evaluate the four key criteria for success: biology/hygiene, aesthetics, function, and phonetics [5]. The ISP is a crucial element for successful treatment of implants in the aesthetic

T. R. Schoenbaum (✉)
Division of Constitutive and Regenerative Sciences, University of California, Los Angeles, CA, USA
e-mail: tschoenb@ucla.edu

P. R. Klokkevold
Section of Periodontics, University of California, Los Angeles, CA, USA

Todd R. Schoenbaum (ed.), *Implants in the Aesthetic Zone*,
https://doi.org/10.1007/978-3-319-72601-4_8

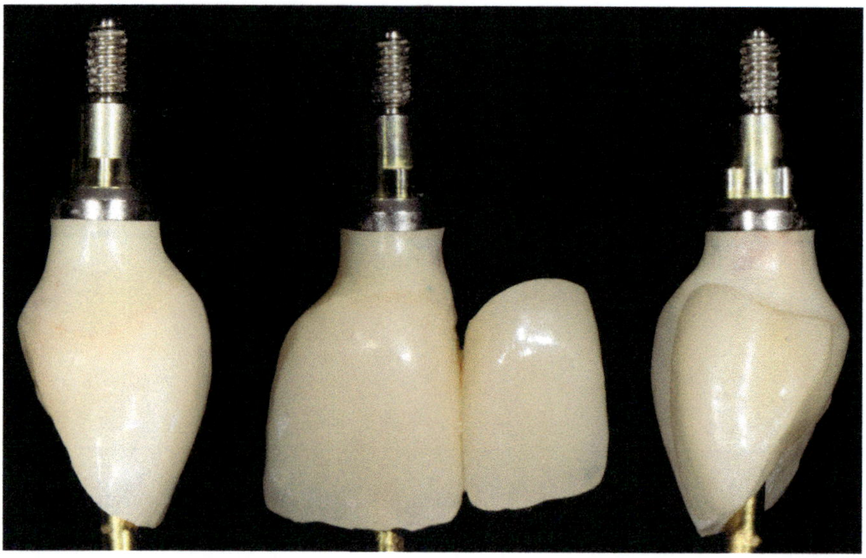

Fig. 8.1 The implant-supported screw-retained provisional prosthesis (ISP) is a critical component for predictable treatment of implants in the aesthetic zone. It is used to preserve and shape the peri-implant soft tissues

zone. It not only maximizes the potential of the peri-implant tissues but allows all involved the opportunity to evaluate the treatment – in situ prior to the fabrication of the definitive prosthesis.

The ISP provides an environment around the implant which encourages maximum tissue volume through the use of appropriate emergence contours and biocompatible materials [6–10]. It will preserve the initial soft tissue architecture and be subsequently modified to appropriately position gingival margins and papilla [2, 7, 8, 11–14]. In areas of significant hard and soft tissue defects, the ISP is used to determine whether or not additional surgical augmentation or pink prosthetic materials are needed to satisfactorily complete the treatment [15–17].

The ISP should be fabricated and delivered at the time of implant placement or stage 2 uncovering [18, 19].

A removable provisional prosthesis is not capable of preserving and shaping the soft tissue with the accuracy and delicacy of one supported by the implant. The movement inherent in a removable provisional restoration may also have a deleterious effect on the potential augmentation and healing of the surgical site. As the peri-implant wound heals, the development of the circumferential connective tissue "ring" will occur against the highly polished surface of the ISP [20]. During the time required for osseointegration, this ring of fibrous tissue will mature and tighten to enhance the seal at implant-abutment junction (IAJ) as described in Chap. 16. This area should be left undisturbed for at least 3 months to ensure minimal remodeling of the peri-implant bone and soft tissue [21, 22]. One study demonstrated histologically that simply removing and replacing healing abutments once a month resulted in nearly 1 mm of bone loss and 1.5 mm of soft tissue loss compared to abutments left in place without removal [21]. The integrity of the peri-implant area is critical to the long-term biological and aesthetic *success* of the implant and prosthesis. Every effort must be made to avoid disturbing the healing and maturation of the tissues during the first 3 months after implant placement.

The ISP can theoretically be fabricated with screw retention or cement retention. This chapter will focus on the use of screw retention [5]. The rationale against the use of a cemented provisional restoration is that most manufacturers make abutments for cemented provisional restorations out of polyether ether ketone (PEEK) which is not as strong or durable as titanium. Breakage of the abutment during the critical integration and maturation phase can greatly compromise the chances for success. The cemented provisional also introduces a margin (where PEEK, cement, and the restorative materials meet) in a subgingival wound space. Even assuming that the clinician was capable of removing all cement, the irregularities at the margin will negatively affect the maturation of the peri-implant tissues [23, 24]. Conversely, the screw-retained provisional can be easily formed and polished to produce surfaces well suited to the healing tissues. In situations where the implants are angled facially, these too can have reasonably aesthetic screw-retained provisional restorations fabricated (Fig. 8.2a–d). This applies even to situations wherein the definitive restoration will be cemented due to angulation concerns. The provisional restoration will be in place during the healing and maturation phase and should be designed with the health of the tissues as the primary concern. Should the

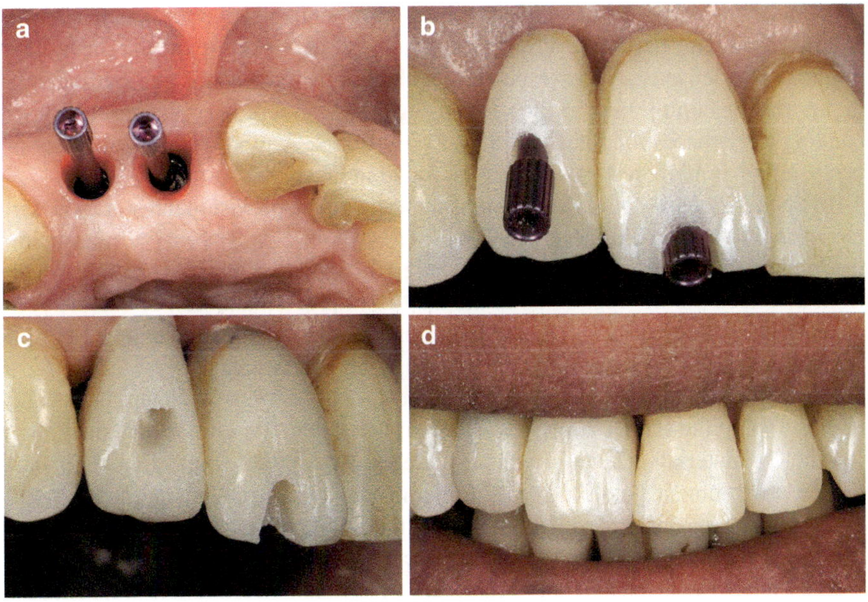

Fig. 8.2 In situations where the implants have been placed such that their straight-line access exits through the facial, the ISP should still be done as a screw-retained restoration. This can be reasonably accomplished and avoids the placement of margins and cement into the healing implant site (**a**–**d**)

definitive prosthesis be cement retained, the abutments will be designed with clearly visible margins, no deeper than 1 mm subgingival [23, 24] as described in Chaps. 12 and 14.

It is challenging to provide definitive criteria for when an implant can be immediately loaded; however available evidence does provide some guidance [18]. For partially edentulous patients, the immediate implant placement and provisional restoration are best utilized for maxillary incisors or premolars or aesthetic zone FDPs. As a single tooth, the canines are a poor candidate for immediate loading due to the large width and length of the root, thus making primary stability of the implant difficult. Additionally, the canine is placed under oblique loads during excursive contact, which are the most problematic for osseointegration. To consider immediate loading, there must be sufficient bone to engage a reasonable portion of the implant. For maxillary incisors, this is found in the palatal bone and at the mesial and distal of the root apex. The amount of the bone that can be engaged depends on the implant length, width, taper, thread design, and anatomy of the remaining bone. The primary stability of the implant in the bone is critical to the success of immediate loading. This stability can be judged by the surgeon using "feel," the torque required to seat the implant, or with a device which reads the implant stability quotient (ISQ). There is no unified agreement on which method is most reliable or what torque or ISQ is required for immediate loading, though recommendations exist [25]. The Immediately loaded provisional must be designed well out of occlusal contact in MIP and throughout the excursive range. This will likely require a tooth that is thinned out palatally and short at the incisal edge. The patient is instructed to not use the provisional tooth for any eating purposes. Patient selection and occlusion are key in this regard, because even with sufficient primary stability, if the immediate implant is loaded excessively (especially with oblique forces), it is at a significantly higher risk of failure. Best available data suggest that there is no increased risk by creating *interproximal* contacts with the provisional. A more detailed analysis of occlusion on implant restorations can be found in Chap. 15.

In Sect. 8.2 below, the technical steps to fabricate the provisional restoration will be described, but should the implant fail to reach sufficient stability at placement, the implant should not be loaded, and an alternative provisional must be fabricated. Both a bonded pontic (Fig. 8.3a, b) and an "Essix provisional" can be rapidly produced at the time of surgery. Neither will preserve and shape the soft tissues as well as the ISP, but nor will they overload a poorly stabilized implant.

The ISP will be fabricated and delivered at the time of implant placement (Fig. 8.4) or at the stage 2 surgery. As such, it will generally require chairside fabrication. The materials selected for the ISP are based on producing the most biocompatible environment possible [6], eliminating the risk of abutment fracture, and producing as reasonably aesthetic result. If the implant was placed in a two-stage approach, an index of the implant position can be made at the stage 1 surgery and used by a laboratory technician to fabricate a provisional restoration in its entirety that will be delivered at the stage 2 uncovering. The technical steps for fabrication of the immediate ISP are described below.

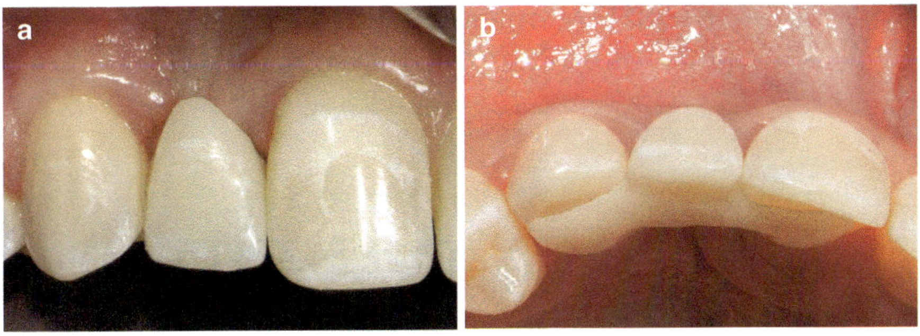

Fig. 8.3 Should the implant fail to reach sufficient stability at placement, it should not be immediately loaded with the ISP. In such scenarios, alternatives for provisionalization include the use of a bonded composite pontic (**a**) or a removable Essix-type retainer. Wings on the pontic as seen here (**b**) facilitate accurate placement and are removed after bonding as needed to establish proper occlusion

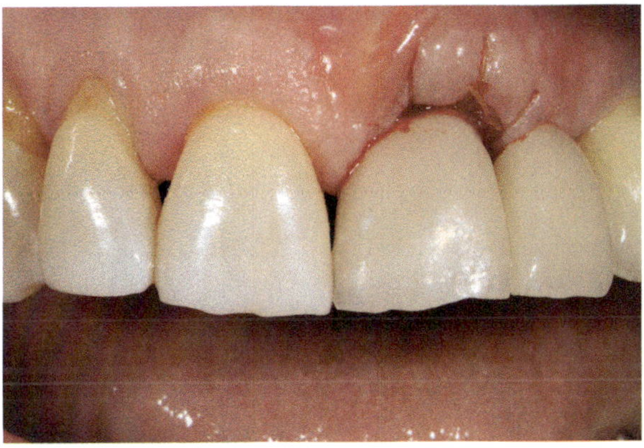

Fig. 8.4 The ISP delivered at the time of surgery should preserve and protect the peri-implant tissues, while leaving space for coronal migration of the papilla and gingival margin

8.2 Fabrication of the Immediate Provisional Prosthesis (ISP)

The implant-supported screw-retained provisional prosthesis (ISP) can be fabricated chairside at the time of implant placement. When done in conjunction with the extraction of the tooth, this procedure is commonly known as "immediate loading." However, it will be designed completely out of occlusion to minimize loading on the implant. Prior to initiating the procedure, impressions must be made of the areas and a shade selected for the crown. Parts for the implant to be used will also need to be ordered in advance. The materials needed are found in Table 8.1.

The preoperative impressions are used by the technician to fabricate the composite provisional shell (Fig. 8.5a–d). This is essentially a crown or a bridge made by the laboratory technician out of composite of the appropriate shade. Acrylic

Table 8.1 Materials needed for fabrication of the ISP

– Provisional shell (made from composite resin)
– Titanium provisional abutment with screw
– Implant analog
– Composite bonding resin
– Light-curing unit
– Flowable composite
– Opaquing resin
– Metal cutting disc
– 30 fluted (red stripe), egg shape carbide (i.e. 7408)
– Composite polishing instruments

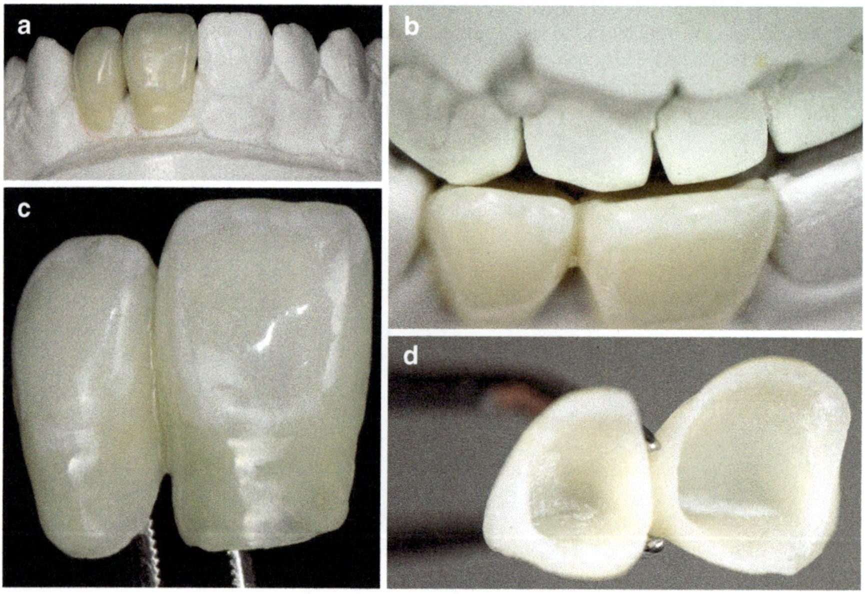

Fig. 8.5 The technician will fabricate composite shells (**a**) prior to the procedure. These are essentially hollow crown forms (**c**, **d**). They should not have the access holes drilled unless a guided surgical approach is utilized. PMMA and other acrylics are a poor alternative due to their inability to bond to composite and difficulty in using acrylic in a surgical site. The shells should be designed out of occlusion (**b**) to minimize forces to the implant when immediately loading

(i.e., PMMA) is a poor alternative for the provisional shell as using acrylic in and around a fresh surgical site is challenging at best. Additionally, connecting an acrylic shell to the abutment with composite resin will typically result in debonding. The internal aspect of the composite shell should be sandblasted and steam cleaned prior to use. Alternatives to the composite shell are the patient's natural tooth or pre-existing crown (Fig. 8.6a–e).

The provisional abutment is a critical component in the fabrication of the ISP (Fig. 8.7a–c). It is responsible for ensuring the integrity of the provisional during the integration and maturation phases. It also makes up the apical area of the restoration which will be in contact with the healing tissues. As such, these requirements are best met only through the use of titanium provisional abutments (as opposed to PEEK). Titanium has a well-proven record for both strength and biocompatibility.

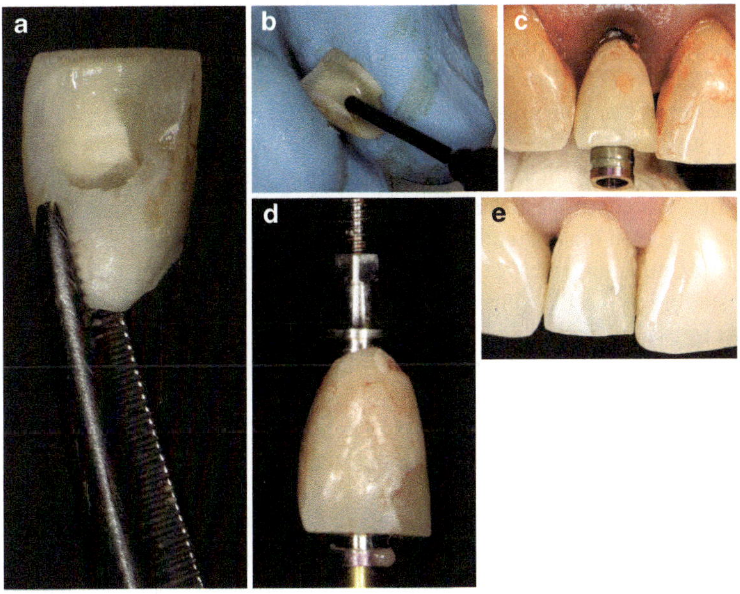

Fig. 8.6 As an alternative to the composite shells, the patient's extracted tooth (**a**) can be transformed into the ISP in a similar manner. After extraction, the root is removed, and the crown carefully hollowed out. It is prepared for bonding (**b**) and connected to the titanium cylinder in situ (**c**). After polymerization, it is removed (**d**) and cleaned and the emergence area filled in with flowable composite. Sufficient space should be left in the gingival embrasures for coronal migration of the papilla (**e**)

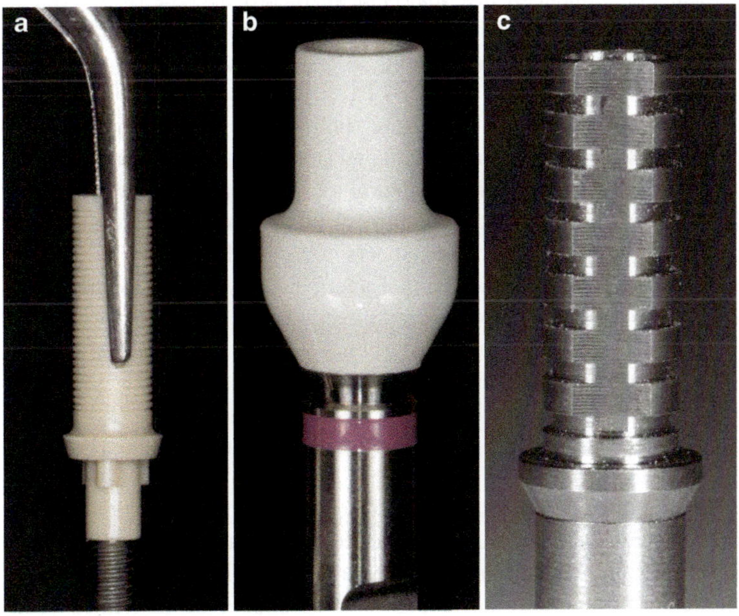

Fig. 8.7 There are various choices for provisional abutment materials. (**a**) PEEK. (**b**) PEEK/titanium, and (**c**) titanium. The full titanium provisional abutment is the best choice due to its proven biocompatibility and resistance to fracture, unlike the PEEK and PEEK/Ti versions

Do not use Ti/Peek

The only rational against titanium provisional abutments is their tendency to decrease the color value of the overlying crowns, though this is easily mitigated as described below. There are a few manufacturers which offer hybrid Ti/PEEK abutment. However, these are grossly overcontoured and only viable for use in extremely large sites of little aesthetic concern. The overcontoured design of the Ti/PEEK abutments will also dramatically reduce the volume of critical peri-implant tissues. Attempting to reduce and reshape the contour of the PEEK portion of these abutments will weaken it and greatly increase the risk for abutment fracture.

Some manufacturers have provisional Ti abutments which are also overcontoured starting at the IAJ (Fig. 8.8a). This design flaw makes the abutments more difficult to use for immediate fabrication, and they push the healing soft tissues away from the IAJ where the protective ring is forming. This may be part of the reason for traditionally designed implants (or abutments) with a flared neck having characteristic bone loss to the first or second thread of the implant body. When present, any flare on the provisional abutment with a diameter greater than that of the implant body should be removed. This is easily done preoperatively in the lab with a stone wheel or carbide bur (Fig. 8.8b, c). The emergence area must be fully polished prior to use. Special care must be taken to ensure that the interface area of the abutment is not damaged. The implant analog is attached to the provisional abutment to protect the implant interface area during shaping and polishing of the emergence area.

A commonly seen difficulty with the ISP fabrication is shade management. It is useful to apply an opaquing composite resin to the retentive area of the abutment prior to use (Fig. 8.9a–d). This material needs to be well polymerized prior to use. It will create an abutment surface that is mechanically and chemically retentive for composite and minimize any chance for the titanium to darken the ISP shade.

Presurgical steps for fabrication of the ISP:

1. The technician fabricates a composite shell for the missing tooth or teeth. The intaglio is hollowed out, sandblasted, and steam cleaned. Alternatively, the shell could be made from the patient's natural tooth or existing crown.
2. Order the titanium provisional abutment and analog. For the single tooth, it should engage the anti-rotational aspects of the implant.
3. Steam clean the titanium provisional abutment, dry, apply opaquing resin in a thin layer to the retentive area, and polymerize.
4. Immediately prior to surgery, apply bonding resin to the retentive area of the abutment, the intaglio of the shell, and polymerize.

Chairside fabrication of the ISP at the time of implant placement:

1. Deliver the implant to the desired position (see Chap. 1), and asses the stability (through torque values, ISQ, or tactile feel). If the surgeon determines sufficient stability for immediate loading, continue below. Should the implant not reach sufficient stability, alternative provisionals should be fabricated (i.e., Essix retainer or bonded pontic).
2. Attach the titanium provisional abutment to the implant (Fig. 8.10). Seating is confirmed visually or radiographically if needed. Use care to ensure that the

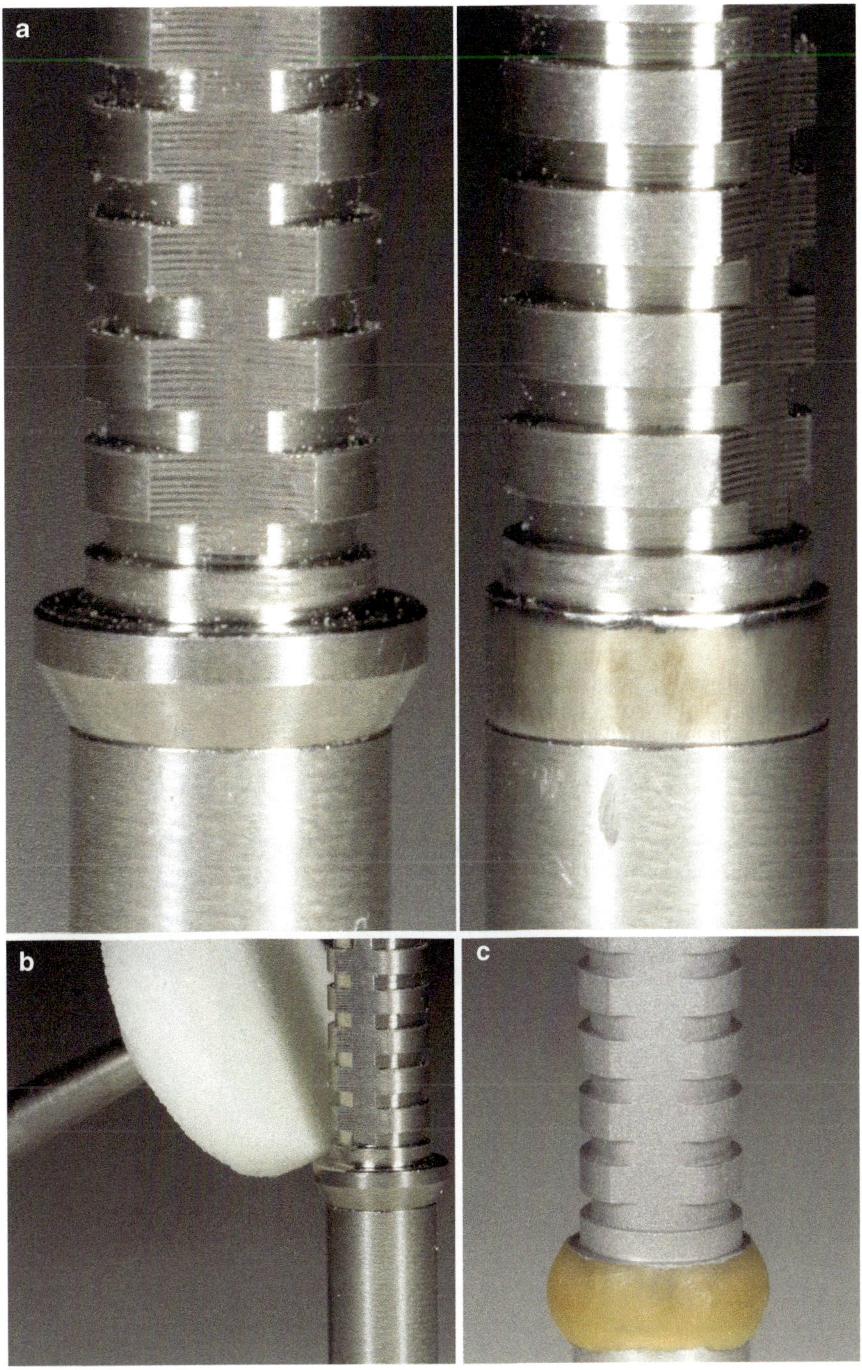

Fig. 8.8 Some manufacturers continue to design the provisional abutments with a flared area at the IAJ (**a**). This is less than ideal due to the pressure it places on the peri-implant tissues. It also takes up valuable space for tissue maturation around the implant. The flared area can be removed with a stone wheel (**b**) or carbide bur. It must be fully polished. The retentive area can also be roughened with HF etch or air abrasion to enhance retention (**c**)

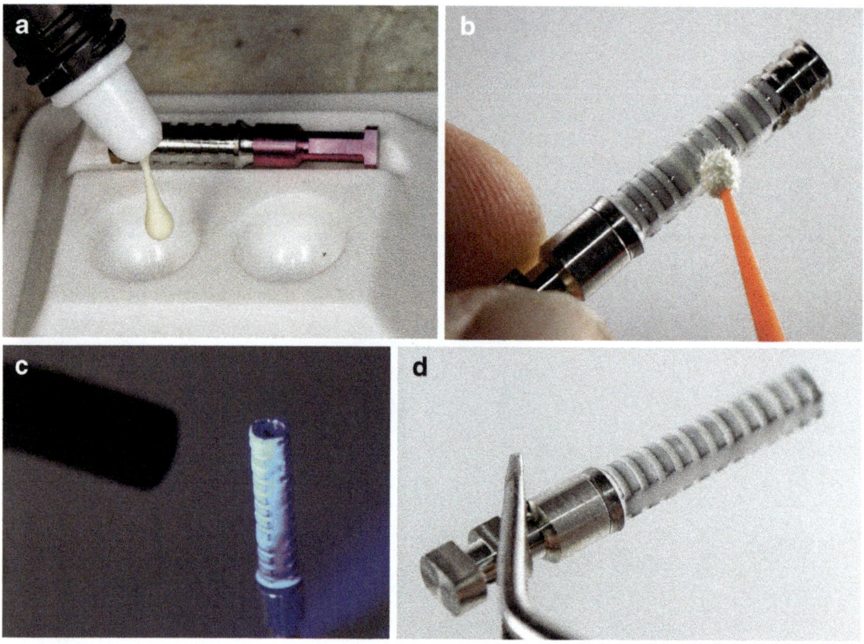

Fig. 8.9 The titanium provisional abutment can cause the ISP to have a gray shade. To prevent this, the abutment is coated with an opaque flowable resin (**a**, **b**): generally shade A1. This is polymerized prior to use (**c**, **d**)

Fig. 8.10 Following placement of the implant and determination of adequate stability, the provisional abutment is carefully placed on the implant. Angulation and the location of the exit through the crown are determined

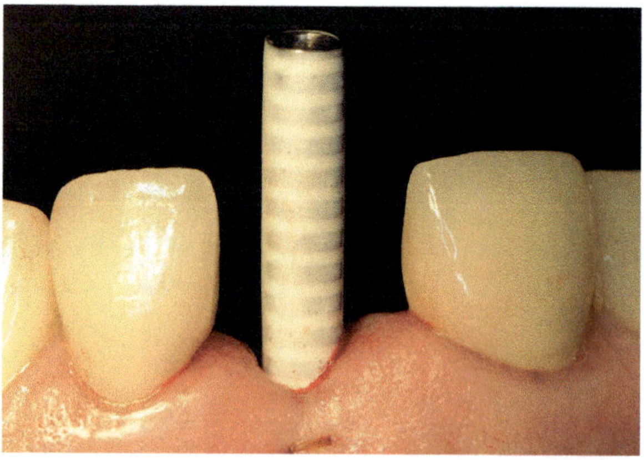

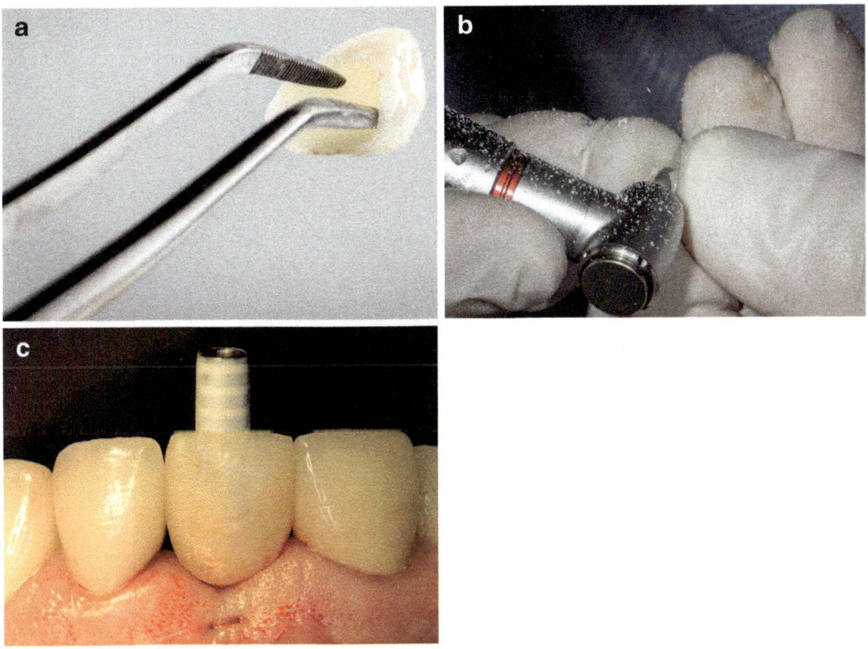

Fig. 8.11 Based on the determined location of the screw access, the composite shell (**a**) is prepared to fit over or around the abutment (**b**). The crown shell is tried in to determine if it fits in the correct location (**c**)

implant position and timing is not altered when placing the abutment or tightening the abutment screw.

3. Adjust the composite provisional shell to fit over or around the abutment (Fig. 8.11a, b). The abutment should *not* be trimmed at this time to maximize its length within the shell for durability (Fig. 8.11c). For lateral incisors, the shell must often be trimmed to resemble a ¾ veneer to fit against the abutment. Special care must be taken to ensure that the shell fits into the precisely correct position in the edentulous space.
4. Clean the abutment and shell of blood and saliva, and add flowable composite to the *coronal* area of each (Fig. 8.12).
5. Place the shell into its correct position and polymerize the composite. Additional composite may need to be added from the palatal to ensure the shell is well connected to the abutment. It is not necessary or desirable at this time to fill in all areas of the shell and emergence areas.
6. Remove the combined abutment/shell as one piece from the implant.
7. In the laboratory, steam clean the abutment, ensuring complete removal of any blood or saliva. Dry, reapply bonding resin, and polymerize.

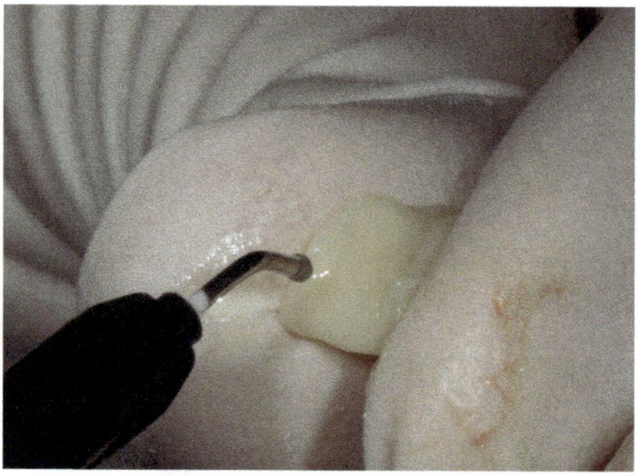

Fig. 8.12 The crown shell (and the abutment) are cleaned of blood and saliva as much as possible. Flowable composite is placed on the coronal half of the crown intaglio. It is then placed on the abutment and polymerized

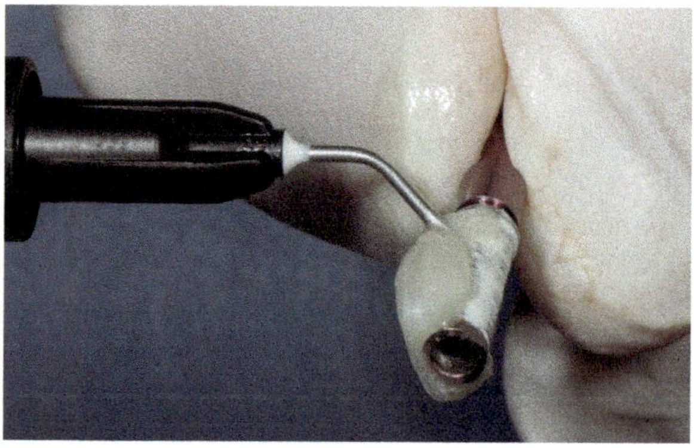

Fig. 8.13 The crown is now connected to the abutment and they are removed together. It is cleaned, bonding agent reapplied, and the emergence areas filled in with flowable composite

8. Carefully apply flowable composite to the emergence area, the intaglio of the shell, and around the palatal area of the titanium cylinder (Fig. 8.13). Polymerize. All gaps and voids should now be filled.
9. Use a metal cutting disc on a lab handpiece, cut off the supra-coronal area of the titanium abutment (Fig. 8.14a, b). A lot of heat and debris will be generated; use caution, and hold the analog with an instrument.
10. Using a large oval 30 flute carbide bur, finish, adjust, and trim the area just cut off (Fig. 8.15).
11. Using the same bur, shape the emergence area such that it is quite narrow near the implant, with a smooth, gentle flare up to the contours of the crown (Fig. 8.16a–c). The emergence should not resemble the removed root in size or

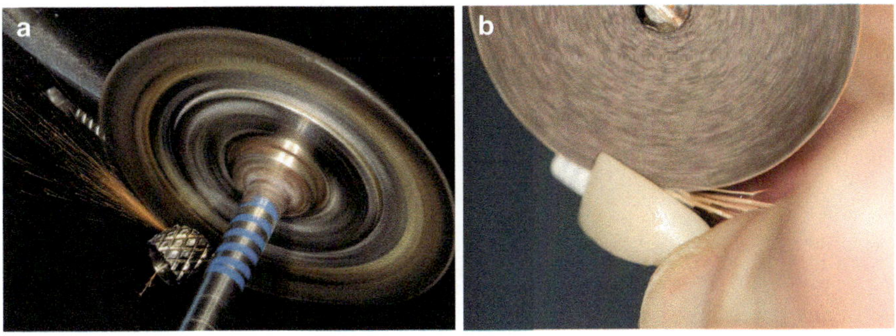

Fig. 8.14 (**a, b**) Using a metal cutting wheel, the portion of the titanium abutment exiting above the crown is removed

Fig. 8.15 A fine oval-shaped carbide bur is used to further refine and adjust the titanium-composite interface. The palatal surface should also be thinned out to ensure the ISP is fully out of occlusion in MIP

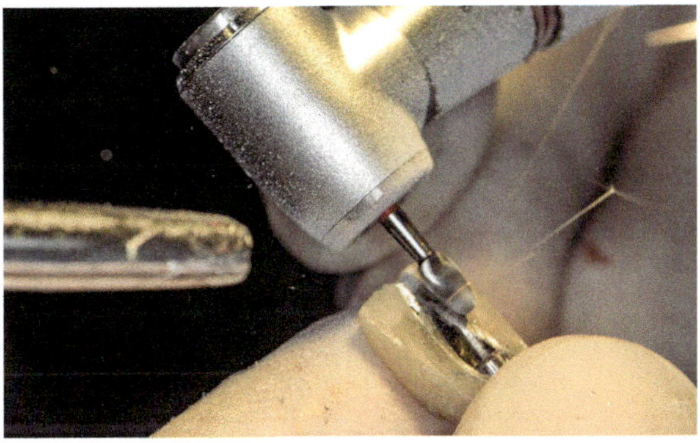

shape, but rather it should be significantly more narrow (see Chap. 11). This concept is derived from the well-proven concept of platform switching [12, 26–30]. Steam clean the ISP.

12. Seat the ISP onto the implant intraorally. First, evaluate the soft tissue: look for any sign of blanching or pressure. These areas will need to be reduced on the emergence area of the ISP. Evaluate the papilla and gingival embrasures: The papilla should not be blanched, and there should be *open* space in the gingival embrasures (Fig. 8.17). This will allow for potential coronal migration of the papilla (see Chap. 9). Lastly, evaluate the occlusion and interproximal contacts: The interproximal contacts should exhibit normal approximation, but there is to be no contact in MIP and throughout the entirety of the excursive range (see Chap. 16). To achieve the latter goal, the

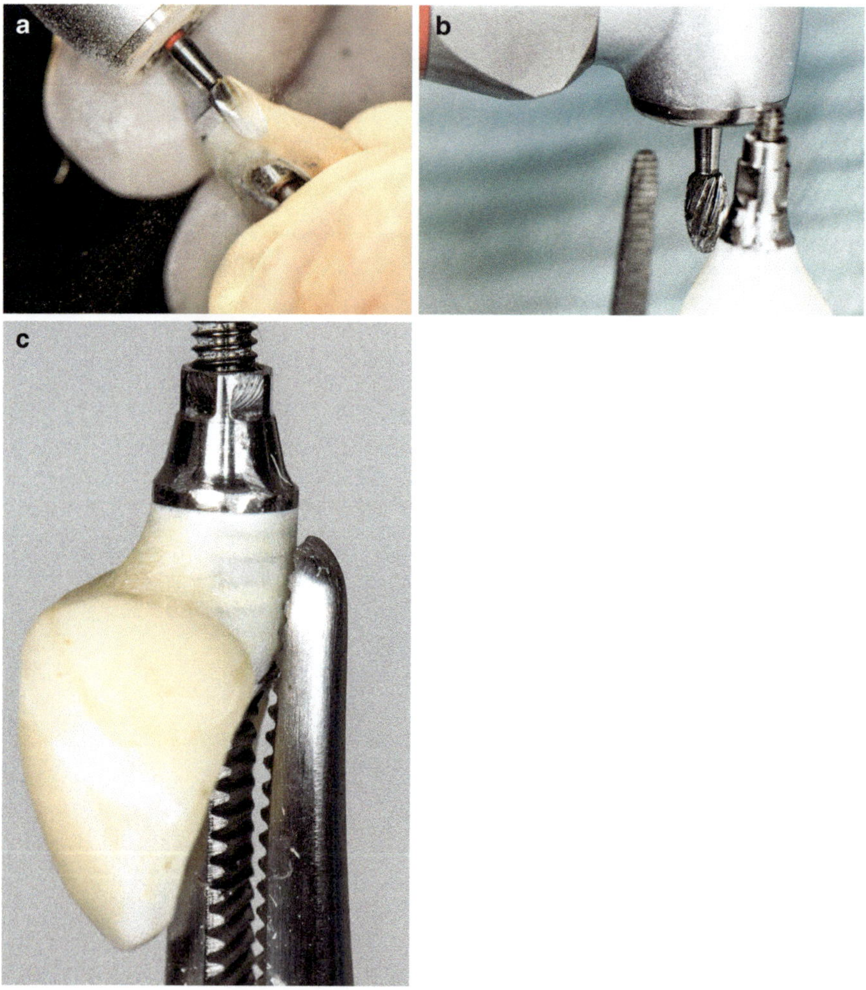

Fig. 8.16 (**a–c**) The fine carbide bur is used to reduce and refined the emergence area. Special attention should be given to ensuring the emergence area is narrow, is fully polished, and has no voids

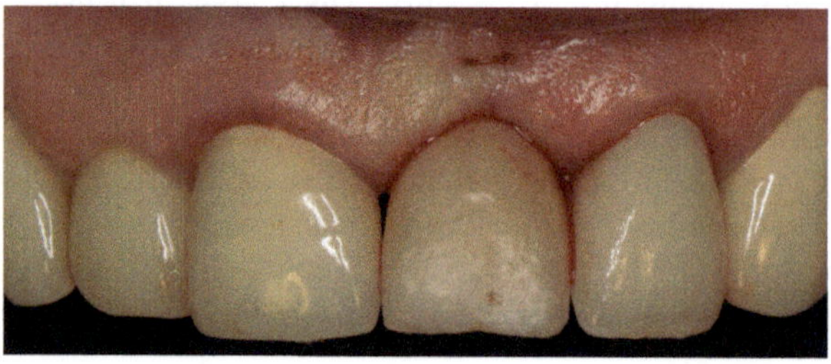

Fig. 8.17 A final check of the ISP on the implant is performed, checking for no blanching of the soft tissues, open gingival embrasures, and no contact in MIP or throughout the excursive range. Any adjustments to the ISP are done outside the mouth, to prevent vibration and forces on the implant

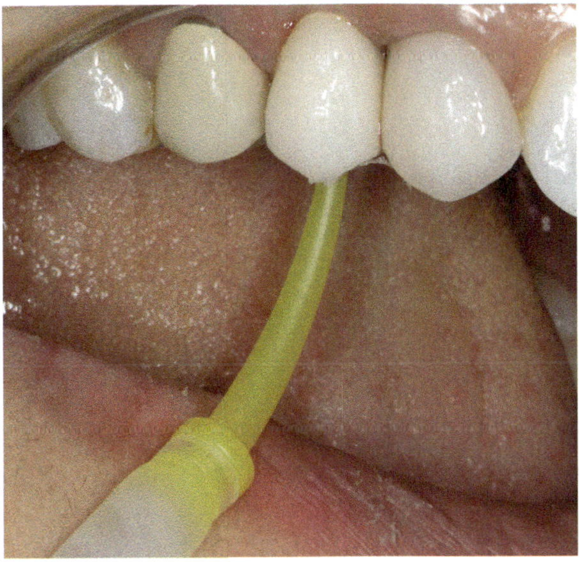

Fig. 8.18 The screw is carefully tightened and the access cleaned with chlorhexidine and filled with clear PVS

ISP may need to be shorter than the length planned for the definitive restorations.

13. Remove the ISP, and adjust emergence, embrasures, and contacts as noted in the previous step. Do not make adjustments to the ISP in a fresh surgical site or when attached to the recently placed implant. Bring all surfaces up to full polish, paying particular attention to the titanium at the base of the ISP, and the composite in the emergence area.
14. Replace the ISP on the implant, and reevaluate the items from step 12. If all is satisfactory, tighten to approximately 10 N cm. Use an anti-torque device (i.e., hemostat) on the crown of the ISP to prevent rotational movement when tightening the screw.
15. Swab the internal aspects of the abutment with chlorhexidine. Fill the screw access hole with PVS impression material (Fig. 8.18) or PTFE tape overlaid with composite [31, 32].

If the implant is placed in a two-stage approach, the ISP should be delivered at the stage 2 appointment. It can be fabricated as above, or an index of the implant position made at the implant placement appointment (Fig. 8.19a) can be used to have the technician fabricate the ISP in the laboratory. This is made during the integration time and ready for delivery at the stage 2 appointment. The lab-fabricated version can be made of PMMA or other acrylic materials, so long as there is >1 mm of titanium at the implant interface (Fig. 8.19b, c). The titanium surface will produce improved healing (compared to composite or acrylic) at the apical area of the sulcus where the connective tissue ring will be forming over the forthcoming weeks.

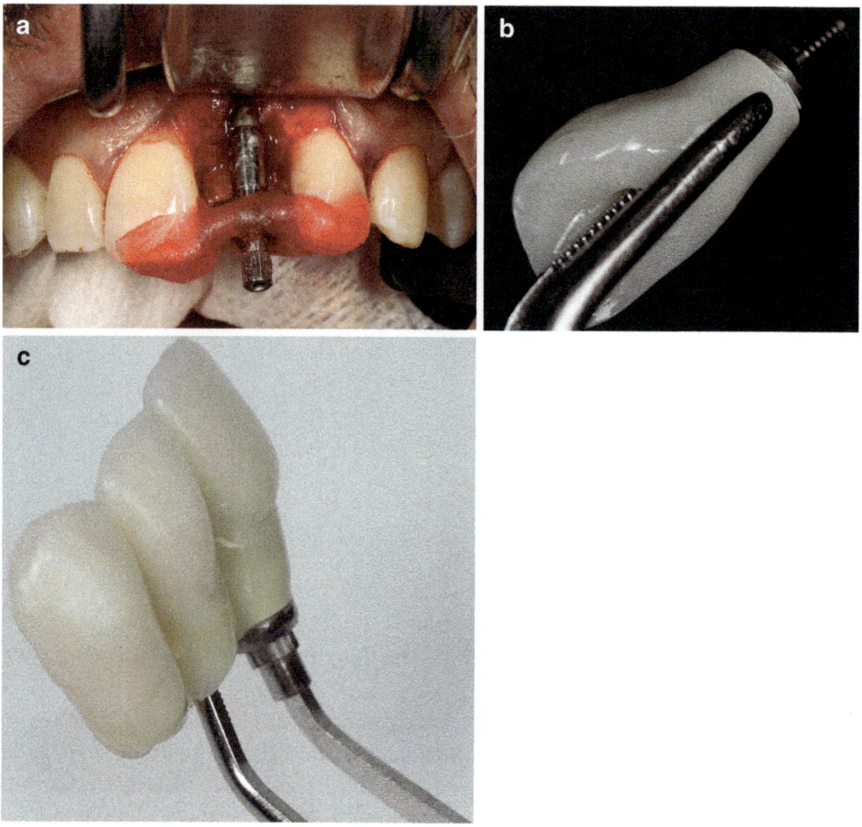

Fig. 8.19 For implants placed in a two-stage approach, an index of the implant position is made at the stage 1 surgery (**a**). The technician uses this to fabricate an ISP to be delivered at the stage 2 surgery (**b**, **c**)

8.3 Summary

The immediately placed ISP is a key component of implant treatment in the aesthetic zone. Its primary role is to preserve, support, and enhance the peri-implant soft tissues. When properly implemented, the ISP can support the papilla and the free gingival margins. It is easier to maintain the soft tissue architecture than it is to recreate it. The materials used in its fabrication are carefully selected to provide biocompatibility (titanium) with strength and aesthetics (composite). The emergence area should be narrow to allow space for soft tissue augmentation, swelling, and maturation (see Chaps. 9 and 11). It must not increase the risk to the implant and thus is kept well out of occlusion and only utilized in patients who will not function on the ISP during osseointegration. It should be stable on the implant and kept in position without removal for 3 months when placed on an immediate implant. Should the peri-implant tissues need minor adjustment, the ISP can be modified to push tissues apically and close open embrasures or undercontoured to allow the tissues to move coronally. Once the treatment team is satisfied with the position of the soft tissues and osseointegration is complete, the impression should be made with a custom impression coping (see Chap. 10). This will provide the technician with a highly accurate model of the soft tissues and produce a predictable definitive restoration.

References

1. Belser UC, Grutter L, Vailati F, Bornstein MM, Weber HP, Buser D. Outcome evaluation of early placed maxillary anterior single-tooth implants using objective esthetic criteria: a cross-sectional, retrospective study in 45 patients with a 2- to 4-year follow-up using pink and white esthetic scores. J Periodontol. 2009;80:140–51.
2. Cosyn J, De Bruyn H, Cleymaet R. Soft tissue preservation and pink aesthetics around single immediate implant restorations: a 1-year prospective study. Clin Implant Dent Relat Res. 2013;15(6):847–57.
3. Kan JY, Rungcharassaeng K, Lozada JL, Zimmerman G. Facial gingival tissue stability following immediate placement and provisionalization of maxillary anterior single implants: a 2-to 8-year follow-up. Int J Oral Maxillofac Implants. 2011;26(1):179–87.
4. Van Nimwegen WG, Goené RJ, Van Daelen AC, Stellingsma K, Raghoebar GM, Meijer HJ. Immediate implant placement and provisionalisation in the aesthetic zone. J Oral Rehabil. 2016;43(10):745–52.
5. Chaar MS, Att W, Strub JR. Prosthetic outcome of cement-retained implant-supported fixed dental restorations: a systematic review. J Oral Rehabil. 2011;38(9):697–711.
6. Abrahamsson I, Berglundh T, Glantz PO, Lindhe J. The mucosal attachment at different abutments. J Clin Periodontol. 1998;25(9):721–7.
7. Schoenbaum TR, Chang YY, Klokkevold PR, Snowden JS. Abutment emergence modification for immediate implant provisional restorations. J Esthet Restor Dent. 2013;25(2):103–7.
8. Schoenbaum TR, Swift EJ. Abutment emergence contours for single-unit implants. J Esthet Restor Dent. 2015;27(1):1–3.
9. Su H, González-Martín O, Weisgold A, Lee E. Considerations of implant abutment and crown contour: critical contour and subcritical contour. Int J Periodontics Restorative Dent. 2010;30(4):335–43.
10. Vela-Nebot X, Rodríguez-Ciurana X, Rodado-Alonso C, Segalà-Torres M. Benefits of an implant platform modification technique to reduce crestal bone resorption. Implant Dent. 2006;15:313–20.
11. Abboud M, Koeck B, Stark H, Wahl G, Paillon R. Immediate loading of single-tooth implants in the posterior region. J Prosthet Dent. 2005;94(2):198.
12. Canullo L, Rasperini G. Preservation of peri-implant soft and hard tissues using platform switching of implants placed in immediate extraction sockets: a proof-of-concept study with 12-to 36-month follow-up. Int J Oral Maxillofac Implants. 2007;22(6):995–1000.
13. De Rouck T, Collys K, Cosyn J. Single-tooth replacement in the anterior maxilla by means of immediate implantation and provisionalization: a review. Int J Oral Maxillofac Implants. 2008;23(5):897–904.
14. Del Fabbro M, Ceresoli V, Taschieri S, Ceci C, Testori T. Immediate loading of postextraction implants in the esthetic area: systematic review of the literature. Clin Implant Dent Relat Res. 2015;17(1):52–70.
15. Kan JY, Rungcharassaeng K, Umezu K, Kois JC. Dimensions of peri-implant mucosa: an evaluation of maxillary anterior single implants in humans. J Periodontol. 2003;74(4):557–62.
16. Tarnow DP, Magner AW, Fletcher P. The effect of the distance from the contact point to the crest of bone on the presence or absence of the interproximal dental papilla. J Periodontol. 1992;63(12):995–6.
17. Urban IA, Klokkevold PR, Takei HH. Papilla reformation at single-tooth implant sites adjacent to teeth with severely compromised periodontal support. Int J Periodontics Restorative Dent. 2017;37(1):9.

18. Sanz-Sánchez I, Sanz-Martín I, Figuero E, Sanz M. Clinical efficacy of immediate implant loading protocols compared to conventional loading depending on the type of the restoration: a systematic review. Clin Oral Implants Res. 2015;26(8):964–82.
19. Slagter KW, Meijer HJ, Bakker NA, Vissink A, Raghoebar GM. Feasibility of immediate placement of single-tooth implants in the aesthetic zone: a 1-year randomized controlled trial. J Clin Periodontol. 2015;42(8):773–82.
20. Rodríguez X, Navajas A, Vela X, Fortuño A, Jimenez J, Nevins M. Arrangement of peri-implant connective tissue fibers around platform-switching implants with conical abutments and its relationship to the underlying bone: a human histologic study. Int J Periodontics Restorative Dent. 2016;36(4):533.
21. Abrahamsson I, Berglundh T, Lindhe J. The mucosal barrier following abutment dis/reconnection. J Clin Periodontol. 1997;24(8):568–72.
22. Rodríguez X, Vela X, Méndez V, Segala M, Calvo-Guirado JL, Tarnow DP. The effect of abutment dis/reconnections on peri-implant bone resorption: a radiologic study of platform-switched and non-platform-switched implants placed in animals. Clin Oral Implants Res. 2013;24(3):305–11.
23. Linkevicius T, Vindasiute E, Puisys A, Linkeviciene L, Maslova N, Puriene A. The influence of the cementation margin position on the amount of undetected cement. A prospective clinical study. Clin Oral Implants Res. 2013;24(1):71–6.
24. Linkevicius T, Vindasiute E, Puisys A, Peciuliene V. The influence of margin location on the amount of undetected cement excess after delivery of cement-retained implant restorations. Clin Oral Implants Res. 2011;22(12):1379–84.
25. Rowan M, Lee D, Pi-Anfruns J, Shiffler P, Aghaloo T, Moy PK. Mechanical versus biological stability of immediate and delayed implant placement using resonance frequency analysis. J Oral Maxillofac Surg. 2015;73(2):253–7.
26. Al-Nsour MM, Chan HL, Wang HL. Effect of the platform-switching technique on preservation of peri-implant marginal bone: a systematic review. Int J Oral Maxillofac Implants. 2012;27(1):128–33.
27. Annibali S, Bignozzi I, Cristalli MP, Graziani F, La Monaca G, Polimeni A. Peri-implant marginal bone level: a systematic review and meta-analysis of studies comparing platform switching versus conventionally restored implants. J Clin Periodontol. 2012;39(11):1097–113.
28. Hürzeler M, Fickl S, Zuhr O, Wachtel HC. Peri-implant bone level around implants with platform-switched abutments: preliminary data from a prospective study. J Oral Maxillofac Surg. 2007;65(7):33–9.
29. Lazzara RJ, Porter SS. Platform switching: a new concept in implant dentistry for controlling postrestorative crestal bone levels. Int J Periodontics Restorative Dent. 2006;26:9–17.
30. Pieri F, Aldini NN, Marchetti C, Corinaldesi G. Influence of implant-abutment interface design on bone and soft tissue levels around immediately placed and restored single-tooth implants: a randomized controlled clinical trial. Int J Oral Maxillofac Implants. 2011;26(1):169–78.
31. Paranjpe A, Jain S, Alibhai KZ, Wadhwani CP, Darveau RP, Johnson JD. In vitro microbiologic evaluation of PTFE and cotton as spacer materials. Quintessence Int. 2012;43(8):703–7.
32. Park SD, Lee Y, Kim YL, Yu SH, Bae JM, Cho HW. Microleakage of different sealing materials in access holes of internal connection implant systems. J Prosthet Dent. 2012;108(3):173–80.

Papilla Management and Development Using Provisional Prosthesis

9

Joseph Y. K. Kan and Kitichai Rungcharassaeng

Abstract

Immediate implant placement and provisionalization (IIPP) has been a viable option for replacing single failing maxillary anterior teeth as it preserves the existing osseous and gingival architecture both facially and interproximally. However, when it involves adjacent anterior implants, inter-implant management becomes exponentially more challenging, especially when replacing a failing tooth adjacent to an existing implant restoration. This article describes different scenarios where management of peri- or inter-implant papilla can be accomplished successfully.

Gargiulo et al. [1] histologically evaluated the dimensions of the gingival sulcus, epithelial attachment and the connective tissue attachment of natural teeth, now collectively known as the dentogingival complex (DGC) [2]. The dimension and stability of the dentogingival complex as well as the changes due to surgical and/or restorative procedures have been extensively investigated [1–6]. The average dimension of the dentogingival complex at the facial aspect has been shown to be 3 mm, while a dimension of 4.5 mm was observed at the interproximal aspect of natural teeth [1–4]. This dimensional difference may be attributed to the presence of adjacent teeth and the size of the gingival embrasure [7–10].

Peri-implant mucosa (PIM), like its natural teeth counterpart (the dentogingival complex), comprises similar histologic components (gingival sulcus, epithelial, and

J. Y. K. Kan (✉)
Department of Restorative Dentistry, Loma Linda University School of Dentistry, Loma Linda, CA, USA

K. Rungcharassaeng
Department of Orthodontics and Dentofacial Orthopedics, Loma Linda University School of Dentistry, Loma Linda, CA, USA

Todd R. Schoenbaum (ed.), *Implants in the Aesthetic Zone*,
https://doi.org/10.1007/978-3-319-72601-4_9

connective tissue attachments) [11–13], but with greater facial dimensions (2.84–3.80 mm) [14–20]. While the dimension of each component may change over time, these changes do not significantly affect the overall dimension [17, 19]. A bone-sounding study on two-stage single implants in the anterior maxilla reported average peri-implant mucosa dimensions of 3.63 mm facially and ~6 mm interproximally [21]. This study also reported the average interproximal dentogingival complex dimension of adjacent teeth to be 4.20 mm [21]. These findings are important as they suggest that, for an anterior single implant, the implant papilla level is dependent on the bone level of the adjacent natural tooth and not on the bone levels at the interproximal surfaces of the implant [21].

The periodontal biotype (thick or thin gingiva) [22, 23] has been implicated in the dimensional change of the periodontal tissue [10, 24, 25]. A thick biotype is resilient and therefore prone to pocket formation (increased DGC dimension), while the thin biotype is friable and thus often subject to gingival recession (decreased DGC dimension) following mechanical and/or surgical manipulation [10, 24, 25]. Likewise, greater peri-implant mucosal dimensions have been reported in the presence of the thick peri-implant biotype as compared to the thin biotype [21]. Table 9.1 shows that while the implant papilla may be maintained at or reestablished to the normal level (4.5 mm from the underlying bone) with the thick biotype, it can seldom be re-created beyond 4 mm with the thin biotype [21].

Achieving optimal gingival aesthetics around anterior single implants is a challenging procedure [7, 26], and maintaining it over time can be an equally demanding task. Despite the high success rates achieved with osseointegrated implants [27], the peri-implant mucosal response is not clearly understood. For anterior single implants, up to 16% of gingival recession has been reported [27]. On the other hand, spontaneous rebound of the receded gingiva had also been observed following a few years of function [28–30]. The peri-implant mucosa changes had been postulated as an attempt to establish a stable biological dimension [31]. An understanding of the dentogingival complex and its implant counterpart (peri-implant mucosa) allows the clinicians to predictably balance the biologic/physiologic requirement and aesthetic demand of single implant restorations in the aesthetic zone.

Table 9.1 Bone-sounding measurements of anterior implant single crowns: a comparison between thick and thin biotypes using independent *t*-test at $\alpha = 0.05$ [21]

	Bone-sounding depth (Mean ± SD mm)			
Site	Overall ($n = 45$)	Thick biotype ($n = 28$)	Thin biotype ($n = 17$)	*p*-value
MT	4.20 ± 0.77	4.46 ± 0.78	3.76 ± 0.53	0.002*
MI	6.17 ± 1.27	6.54 ± 1.05	5.56 ± 1.40	0.011*
F	3.63 ± 0.91	3.79 ± 0.89	3.38 ± 0.91	0.150
DI	5.93 ± 1.21	6.14 ± 1.11	5.59 ± 1.31	0.137
DT	4.20 ± 0.64	4.45 ± 0.57	3.79 ± 0.56	0.001*

MT proximal aspect of tooth mesial to the implant, *MI* mesial aspect of implant, *F* midfacial aspect of implant, *DI* distal aspect of implant, *DT* proximal aspect of tooth distal to the implant
*Statistical significance ($p < 0.05$)

The impending loss of a single tooth in the aesthetic zone in a patient with an otherwise healthy periodontium can be a distressing experience [7, 8, 32, 33]. An inevitable loss of soft and hard tissue after an anterior tooth extraction often results in an aesthetically compromised situation for implant treatment. Various augmentation techniques have been advocated as corrective procedures, but they are time-consuming and not always predictable [28, 34–36]. Therefore, the fundamental concept of site development for anterior single implant is to preserve the existing gingival and osseous tissue of the failing tooth if possible [7]. Since 1998, when Wohrle first demonstrated success with immediate implant placement and provisionalization (IIPP) of single anterior maxillary implants [37], numerous studies have substantiated the viability of such treatment [32, 38–49]. One of the most desirable features of IIPP is its efficacy in optimizing aesthetic success by preserving the existing osseous and gingival architecture facially and proximally [8, 32, 37, 50].

The aesthetic success of IIPP procedures is influenced by a number of factors that can be identified as intrinsic or extrinsic [51]. Intrinsic factors are patient-dependent and include the relationship between hard and soft tissues, gingival biotype, and sagittal root position in the alveolar bone [52, 53]. Extrinsic factors, on the other hand, are clinician-dependent and include 3-D implant position and angulation, as well as contour of the abutment and provisional restoration [8, 52].

Proper diagnosis of the patient's condition is crucial to formulating a suitable treatment plan that can be predictably executed. By recognizing unfavorable conditions, adjunctive procedures can be incorporated to mitigate the compromised situations. The following parameters must be evaluated for an IIPP procedure:

1. *Gingival level* of the failing tooth should be [1] the same as (or more coronal than) that of the contralateral tooth and [2] harmonious with adjacent dentition, as some gingival recession can be expected after the procedure (Fig. 9.1) [32]. Therefore, when the gingival level of the failing tooth is more apical than that of the contralateral tooth, orthodontic forced eruption, if possible, should be implemented prior to IIPP [54].

ortho extrusion prior to implant placement

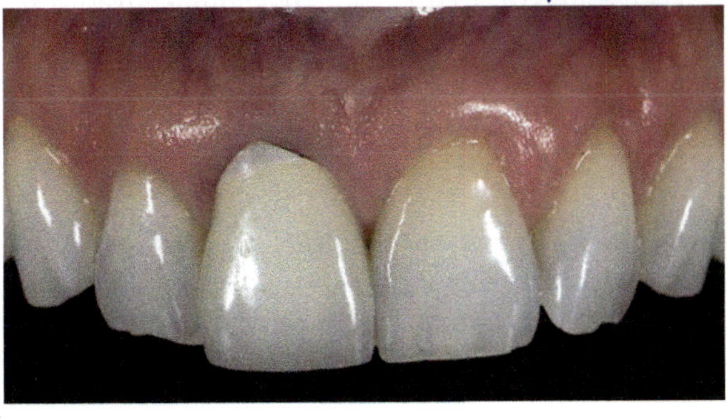

Fig. 9.1 Gingival level of the failing tooth (#8) should be (1) the same as (or more coronal than) that of the contralateral tooth and (2) harmonious with adjacent dentition, as some gingival recession can be expected after the procedure

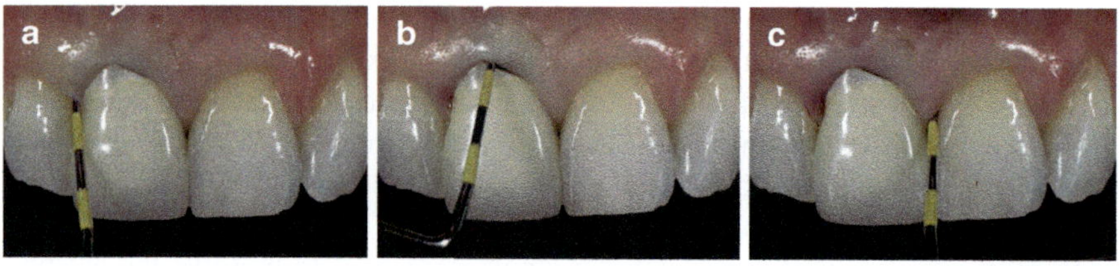

Fig. 9.2 (**a-c**) Osseous-gingival tissue relationship can be evaluated by bone sounding and should measure 3 mm on the facial aspect of the failing tooth and 4.5 mm on the proximal aspect of adjacent teeth

2. *Osseous-gingival tissue relationship* can be evaluated by bone sounding and should measure 3 mm on the facial aspect of the failing tooth and 4.5 mm on the proximal aspect of adjacent teeth (Fig. 9.2). There is a propensity of tissue recession after extraction with or without immediate implant placement in low crest situations, in which bone-sounding measurements are greater than those indicative of an optimal relationship [52]. Depending on the gingival level, orthodontic and/or periodontal treatment can be used to improve the osseous-gingival tissue relationship.
3. *Gingival biotype* can be assessed during bone sounding and categorized according to the visibility of the underlying periodontal probe (SE Probe SD12 Yellow, American Eagle Instruments Inc., Missoula, MT) through the gingival tissue (visible = thin and not visible = thick) (Fig. 9.2) [21, 55]. Higher visibility corresponds to lower level of thickness. Thin gingival biotype, which has been shown to sustain more tissue recession after surgical insults than thick biotype, can be enhanced by using a bilaminar subepithelial connective tissue graft (SCTG) at the time of IIPP [51].
4. *Sagittal root position (SRP)* of the failing tooth in the alveolar bone can be identified via cone-beam computed tomography (CBCT) and can be categorized as one of the four different classes [53] (Fig. 9.3):

    (a) Class I: The root is positioned against the labial cortical plate.
    (b) Class II: The root is centered in the middle of the alveolar housing without engaging either labial or palatal cortical plates at the apical 1/3 of the root.
    (c) Class III: The root is positioned against the palatal cortical plate.
    (d) Class IV: At least 2/3 of the root is engaging both labial and palatal cortical plates.

It is important for clinicians to recognize cases that are favorable for IIPP (Class I SRP), cases that are more technique-sensitive and entail additional attention (Class II and Class III SRP), and cases that are contraindicated for IIPP, requiring hard and/or soft tissue augmentation prior to implant placement (Class IV SRP) [53].

5. *Buccolingual width and inter-radicular mesiodistal width* of the failing tooth determine the diameter of the implant to be used and can be evaluated using CBCT and periapical radiographs (Fig. 9.4) [33].

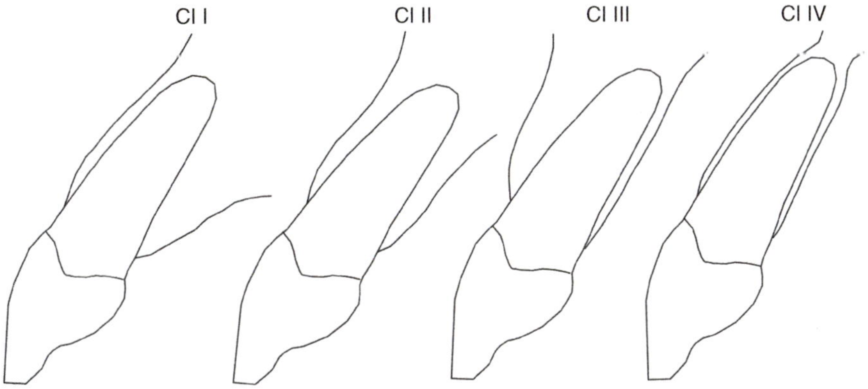

Fig. 9.3 Sagittal root position classification. Class I: The root is positioned against the labial cortical plate. Class II: The root is centered in the middle of the alveolar housing without engaging either labial or palatal cortical plates at the apical 1/3 of the root. Class III: The root is positioned against the palatal cortical plate. Class IV: At least 2/3 of the root is engaging both labial and palatal cortical plates

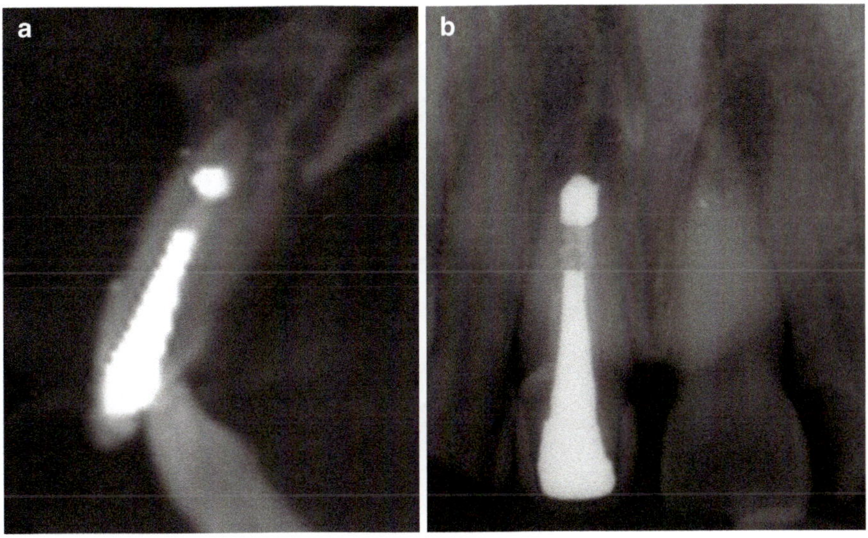

Fig. 9.4 (**a**) CBCT. (**b**) Periapical radiograph of the failing tooth

9.1 Fabrication of Provisional Restoration

Proper diagnostic waxing provides information necessary for treatment planning, especially when adjunctive procedures (orthodontic and/or periodontal intervention) are required. A diagnostic waxing of the failing tooth on the study cast should [1] represent, as closely as possible, the definitive restoration, [2] match the contralateral tooth, and [3] be harmonious with the adjacent dentition. Provisional restoration, as well as implant and soft tissue surgical templates, can be accurately fabricated from a well-executed diagnostic waxing [33].

9.2 Surgical Procedure

Immediate implant placement entails extraction of the failing tooth followed by placement of an osseointegrated implant. The extraction must be minimally traumatic with controlled expansion of the bony socket to avoid soft and/or hard tissue damage. Periotome (Nobel Biocare) can be used to make a sulcular incision with transseptal fiberoctomy that extends apically beyond the marginal bone. This incision separates the tooth from the periodontal tissue, facilitating extraction with minimal damage to the usually thin labial bony plate (Figs. 9.5 and 9.6). The

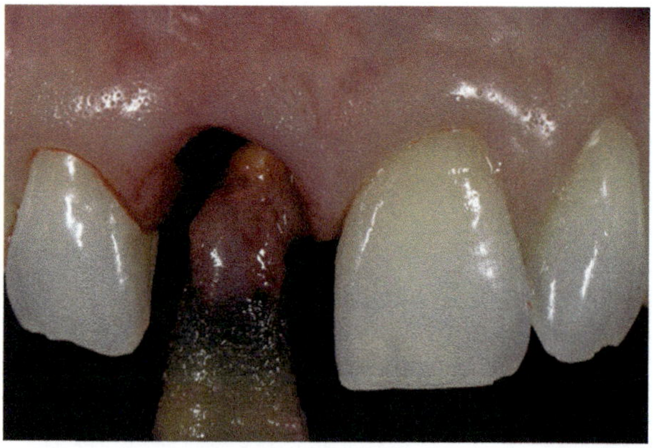

Fig. 9.5 Minimally traumatic extraction of failing tooth #8

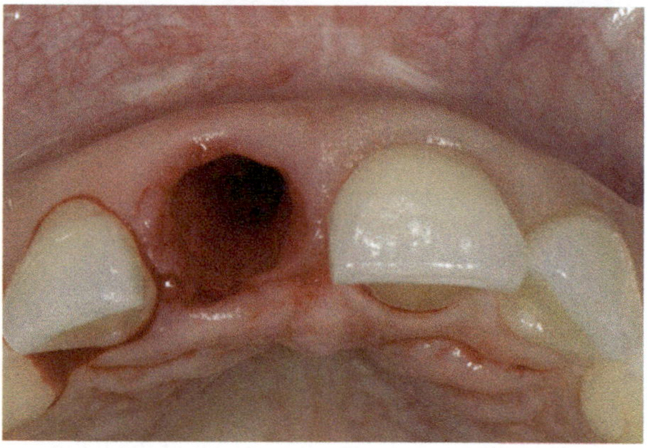

Fig. 9.6 Intact extraction socket

integrity of the labial plate must be verified using a periodontal probe after the extraction. Fenestrations located 5 mm or more apical to the intact facial marginal bone are generally inconsequential to the IIPP procedure, as they can be addressed predictably with grafting.

When a facial osseous dehiscence/defect is detected, the predictability of the IIPP in conjunction with guided bone regeneration (GBR) procedures is determined by the shape/size of the defect [41]. A V-shaped defect, which is isolated only to the midfacial portion of the facial bony plate, responds favorably to IIPP with GBR (Fig. 9.7). On the other hand, significant facial gingival recession after 1 year of function has been reported when IIPP with GBR was attempted on failing teeth with U-shaped (extends to mesial and/or distal aspect of the failing tooth) or UU-shaped (extends to the mesial and distal aspect of the immediately adjacent teeth) defects (Fig. 9.7) [41]. Therefore, a failing tooth with a U-shaped or UU-shaped defect is contraindicated for IIPP [41].

Primary implant stability is the prerequisite for IIPP and is usually achieved by engaging the palatal wall and the bone 4–5 mm beyond the apex of the extraction socket (Fig. 9.8) [8]. Therefore, Class I SRP, with a considerable amount of bone present on the palatal aspect for implant engagement to attain primary stability, is optimal for IIPP. Class IV SRP, with a limited amount of bone for implant engagement, is a contraindication [53]. Class II and III SRP present compromised and/or challenging conditions for IIPP [53]. In Class III SRP, implant stability must rely on its engagement to the available bone on the labial aspect, which can potentially lead to facial fenestration or perforation [53]. In Class II SRP, as available bone on both the palatal and labial aspects is inadequate, the implant stability relies primarily on the amount of available bone beyond the apex of the extraction socket [53].

The final implant position and angulation should be in accordance with the following guidelines:

- Mesiodistally: The implant should be placed at the center of the predetermined mesiodistal width of the final restoration with a minimal distance of 2 mm from the adjacent tooth (Fig. 9.9) [8, 33, 56].

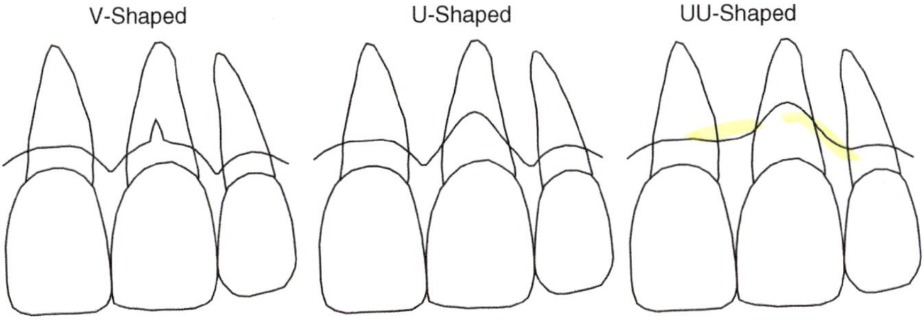

Fig. 9.7 Facial bone defect classification. V-shaped defect: Isolated only to the midfacial portion of the facial bony plate. U-shaped defect: Extends to mesial and/or distal aspect of the failing tooth. UU-shaped defect: Extends to the mesial and distal aspect of the immediately adjacent teeth

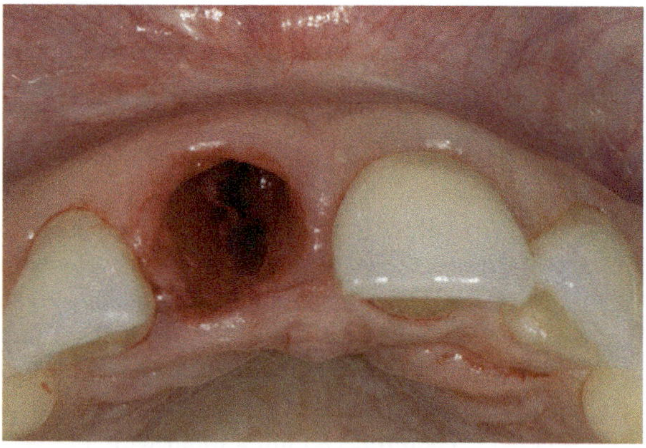

Fig. 9.8 Osteotomy made against the palatal bone for primary implant stability and to avoid potential facial bone damage

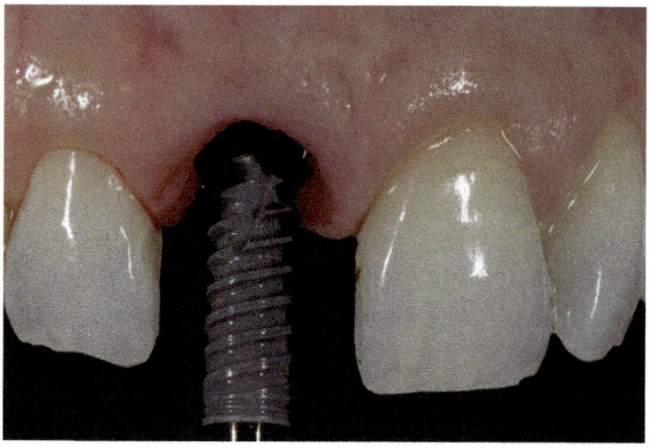

Fig. 9.9 The implant should be placed at the center of the predetermined mesiodistal width of the final restoration with a minimal distance of 2 mm from the adjacent tooth

- Labio-palatally: The implant should be placed along the palatal wall of the extraction socket for primary stability [8]. At the cervical level, the implant should emerge slightly lingual to the predetermined buccolingual width of the final restoration. At the incisal level, the implant should emerge at the incisal edge of the final restoration (Fig. 9.10a) [8, 33]. With this labio-palatal position/placement, a gap of at least 1.5 mm between implant and the buccal bone is maintained and the integrity of the labial bone ensured (Fig. 9.10b) [33].
- Apico-coronally: The implant platform is placed approximately 3 mm apical to the predetermined facial free gingival margin of the final restoration (Fig. 9.11) [8, 33].

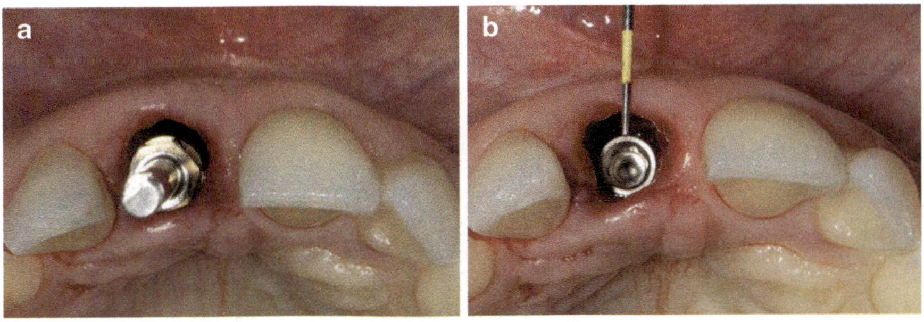

Fig. 9.10 (a) The implant emerging at the incisal edge of the final restoration. (b) A gap of at least 1.5 mm between implant and the buccal bone is maintained to ensure the integrity of the labial bone

Fig. 9.11 The neck of the implant is approximately 3 mm apical to the predetermined facial free gingival margin of the final restoration

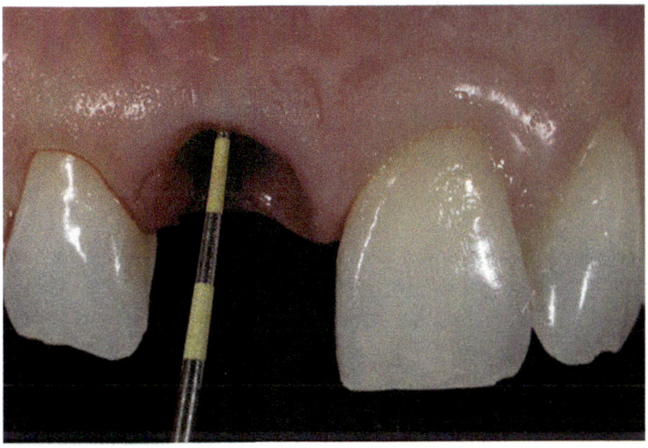

9.2.1 Immediate Provisionalization

For immediate provisionalization, a prefabricated zirconium abutment (Nobel Biocare) or metal temporary abutment is manually prepared extraorally and then hand-tightened onto the implant (Fig. 9.12). The provisional shell is then relined with light-polymerized acrylic resin (Ultradent Products, Inc., South Jordan, UT) to capture the cervical gingival emergence of the extracted tooth and adjusted to clear all centric and eccentric functional contacts.

It has recently been demonstrated that following immediate implant placement in an anterior tooth socket, the facial bony plate would undergo remodeling, characterized by bone fill from the inside of the socket and resorption of the labial bony plate from the outside [57]. Without the bone graft, this usually results in significant horizontal and vertical facial bone loss and, subsequently, facial gingival tissue loss [57–61].

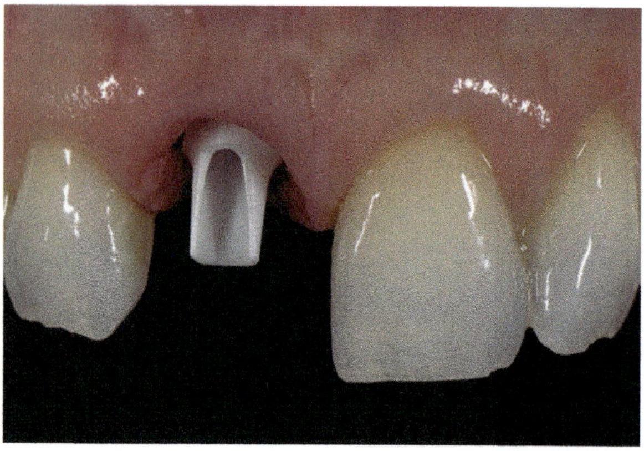

Fig. 9.12 Prefabricated zirconium abutment as provisional abutment

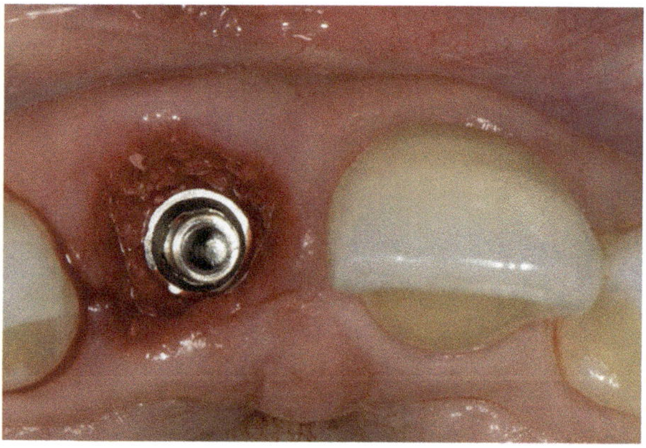

Fig. 9.13 Bone graft material is placed into the gaps between the implant and the bony socket to maintain facial osseous contour

To maintain facial osseous contour, bone graft material (Bio-Oss, Osteohealth, Shirley, NY, and Puros, Zimmer Dental, Carlsbad, CA) is placed into the gaps between the implant and the bony socket (Fig. 9.13). If thin gingival biotype is present, a subepithelial connective tissue graft (SCTG) can be placed subgingivally between the labial free gingival margin and the labial bone to improve the gingival condition (Fig. 9.14) [51]. The cementation of the provisional restoration with provisional cement (Temp-bond, Kerr USA, Romulus, MI) should be performed simultaneously with the SCTG placement (Figs. 9.14 and 9.15a, b).

The amount of cement used should be minimal and mostly isolated at the intaglio incisal and lingual area of the provisional for ease of later cement removal. Light finger pressure must be applied over the grafted site with moist gauze for 5 min to minimize blood clot formation between the graft and its underlying and overlying tissues. A thick blood clot can potentially hinder the

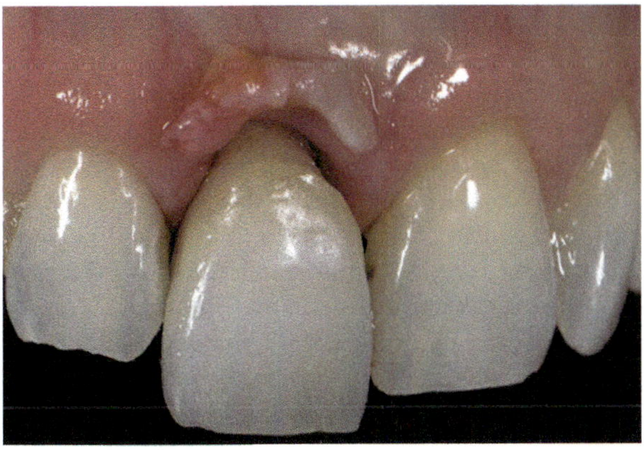

Fig. 9.14 Subepithelial connective tissue graft (SCTG) can be placed simultaneously with cementation of the provisional restoration

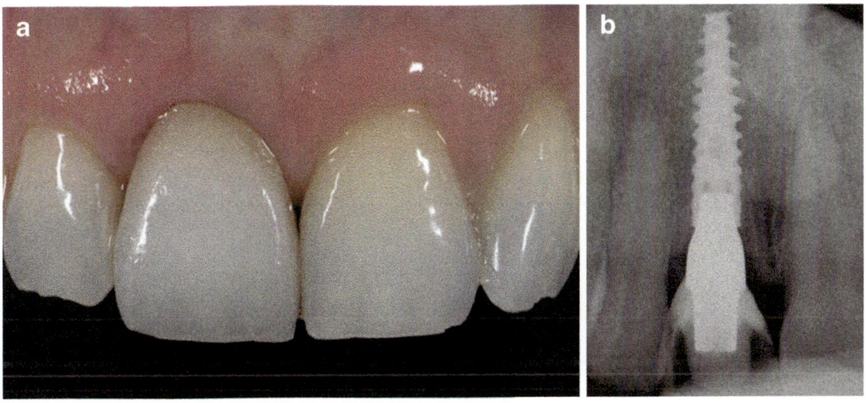

Fig. 9.15 (**a**) Clinical and (**b**) radiographic images of IIPP of #8

anastomosis of new capillary buds from the recipient bed, thus jeopardizing graft survival [62]. The fit of the prosthesis can be ascertained with a periapical radiograph (Fig. 9.15).

9.3 Postoperative Instruction

Appropriate antibiotics and analgesics are prescribed for postoperative use. The patient is instructed not to brush the surgical site but instead rinse gently with 0.12% chlorhexidine gluconate (Peridex, Procter & Gamble, Cincinnati, OH). A liquid diet is required for 2 weeks after the operation, and a soft diet is recommended for the remaining duration of the implant healing phase, which typically lasts 4 months. The patient is also advised against any activity that could irritate the surgical site [8, 33].

2 weeks liquid diet (SCTG + BG)

9.4 Definitive Restoration

The final implant impression is usually made 6 months after the surgery. A customized zirconium/gold alloy abutment (Procera, Nobel Biocare) is fabricated, duplicating the gingival emergence profile of the provisional restoration (Fig. 9.16). The abutment should be tightened onto the implant with the manufacturer's recommended amount of torque, and the fit should be verified with a periapical radiograph. Subsequently, definitive cement (RelyX™ Unicem, 3M ESPE, St. Paul, MN) should be used for the definitive restoration (Figs. 9.17 and 9.18). Follow-up appointments with the patient should occur at 1 month, 3 months, 6 months, 12 months, and annually thereafter in order to ascertain the functional and aesthetic outcome (Fig. 9.18).

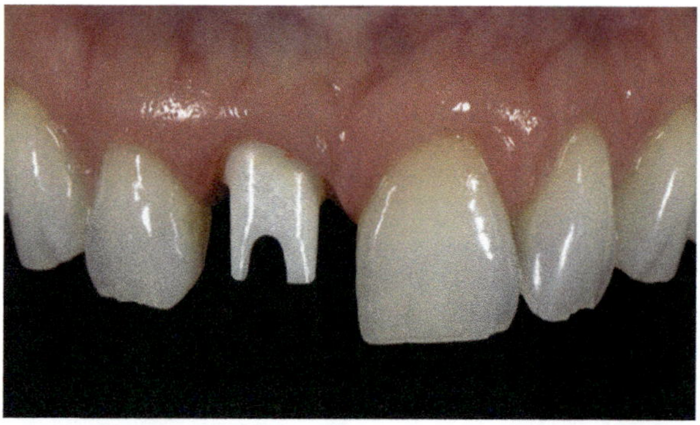

Fig. 9.16 Customized zirconium abutment

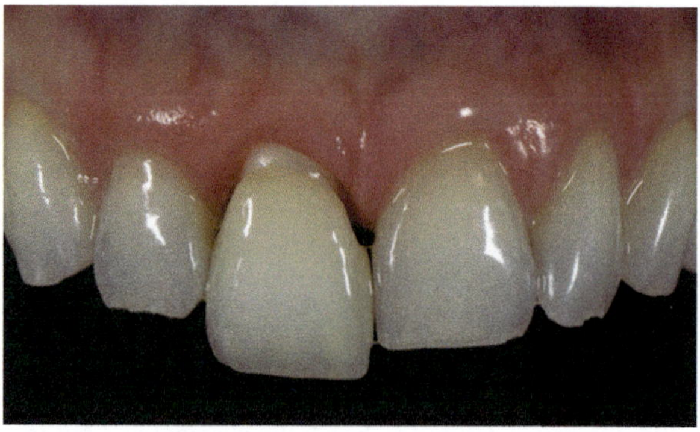

Fig. 9.17 Cementation of an all-ceramic definitive restoration

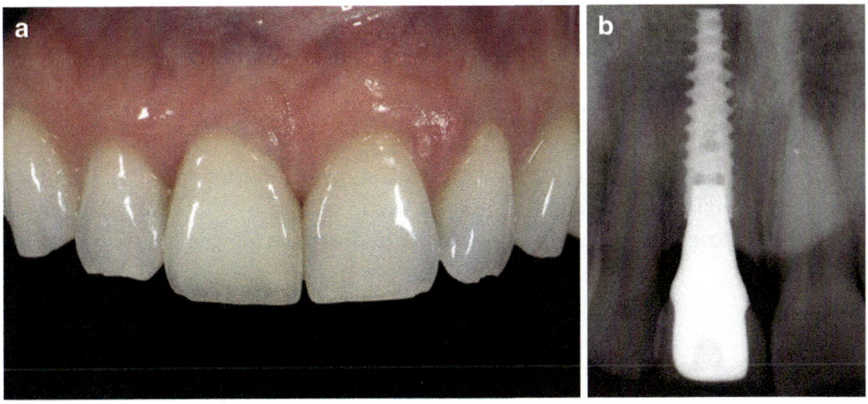

Fig. 9.18 (**a**) Clinical and (**b**) radiographic images of the definitive restoration 12 months after the surgery

9.5 Inter-implant Papilla Preservation: Multiple Failing Anterior Teeth

Replacing multiple adjacent failing teeth presents a much more complex scenario. Simultaneous adjacent teeth removal often results in the flattening of the interproximal osseous scallop and the subsequent collapse of the interproximal papilla from the loss of support. One way to manage it is to approach them as multiple single tooth replacements by alternately performing immediate implant placement and provisionalization procedure one following the osseointegration healing period of the other [63, 64]. This way, the proximal bone on one side of the implant can always be maintained, while the other side is healing. At the same time, the remaining tooth form can be used as guide for implant placement and provisionalization of the other, which would not be possible if both were done simultaneously. This technique also avoids simultaneous extraction of multiple adjacent teeth, which compromises the integrity and stability of the interproximal bone and papilla.

Tarnow et al. reported the importance of the inter-implant distance in maintaining the interproximal bone between two adjacent implants [65]. In their study, two individual and separate angular defects were observed when the distance between two adjacent implants was >3 mm. However, if the two implants are <3 mm apart, the angular defects may cross over creating a horizontal inter-implant crestal bone loss compromising the level of the inter-implant papilla. Therefore, although a distance of 2 mm at the cervical implant level has been suggested as appropriate between an implant and the adjacent teeth [56], a minimal of 3 mm is recommended between adjacent implants [65] to minimize the horizontal bone loss and, hence, the inter-implant papilla loss.

Even with careful execution, facial and or interproximal gingival recession may still occur after immediate implant placement and provisionalization procedures, especially with thin scalloped periodontium. Nevertheless, this tissue discrepancy can sometimes be compensated by altering the gingival emergence of the prosthesis. The facial recession can be minimized by flattening the facial gingival emergence of the implant abutment and/or restoration [26]. On the other hand, interproximal papilla deficit may be compensated by increasing the gingival emergence of the adjacent restorations and/or moving the cervical contact point apically.

9.6 Inter-implant Papilla Preservation: Replacing a Tooth Adjacent to an Implant

Papilla loss is common when replacing multiple adjacent failing teeth with implants in anterior maxillary aesthetic zone [42]. This is due to the fact that the implant platform is positioned based on the facial bone level, and since most available dental implants are uniplanar (flat), the implant platform will be positioned apical to the proximal bone level. In addition, long-term maintenance of the proximal bone coronal to the implant platform has been shown to be more of an exception than the rule [43], even with the use of implants with scalloped [44] or unmatched (platform switch) platform [45]. As a result, the proximal implant marginal bone level is often more apical than that of the adjacent natural teeth ultimately leading to diminished papillary soft tissue, despite stable marginal bone levels of both implant and adjacent tooth. Methods such as alternate immediate implant placement and provisionalization (IIPP) on one failing tooth after the integration of another, proper spacing (at least 3 mm of inter-implant/radicular distance), immediate prosthetic support of the papilla, as well as flapless surgery have been advocated with some degree of success of minimizing, but not preventing, papilla loss [42]. Recently, proximal socket-shield technique utilizes the retained proximal portion of the root in an attempt to preserve the interproximal bone after IIPP, and promising clinical results have been reported [46]. The next section describes the technique of maintaining the inter-implant papilla when replacing a failing tooth adjacent to an implant restoration using proximal socket-shield (PSS) procedure in conjunction with IIPP.

Left maxillary lateral incisor (#10) was failing due to root resorption, and left maxillary central incisor (#9) was a 2-year-old implant restoration (Fig. 9.19, b). After administration of the local anesthesia, the maxillary left lateral incisor (#10) was sectioned (#557 L, Brasseler, Savannah, GA) buccolingually (Fig. 9.20), and the distal half of the root was removed atraumatically without

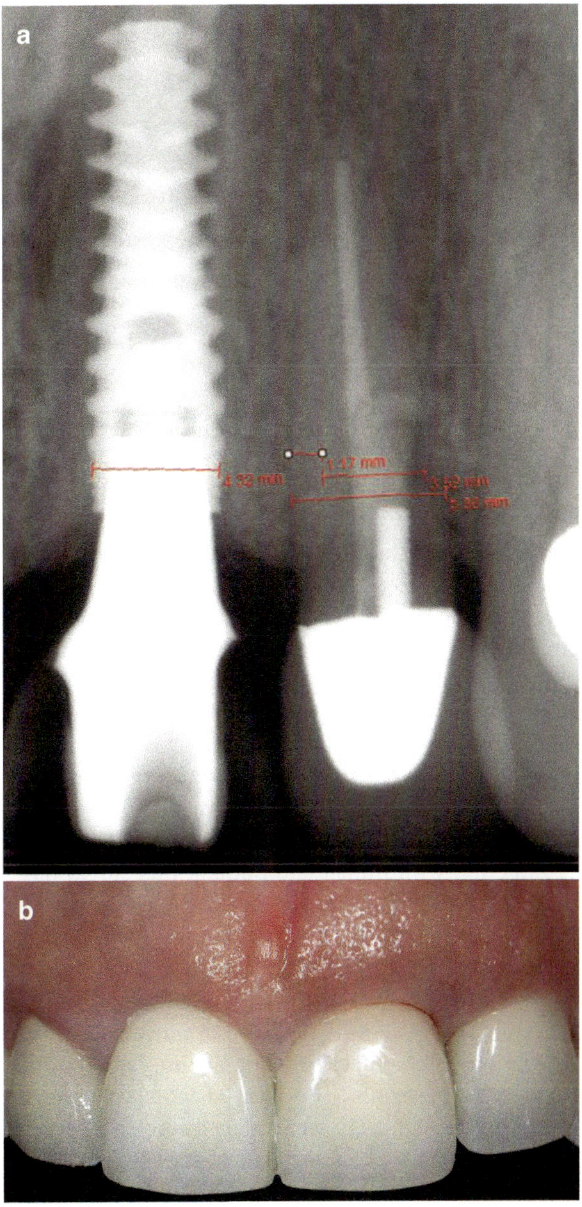

Fig. 9.19 (**a**) Pre-op clinical with failing #10. Note implant had been placed at #9 1 year previously. (**b**) Pre-op image of failing #10

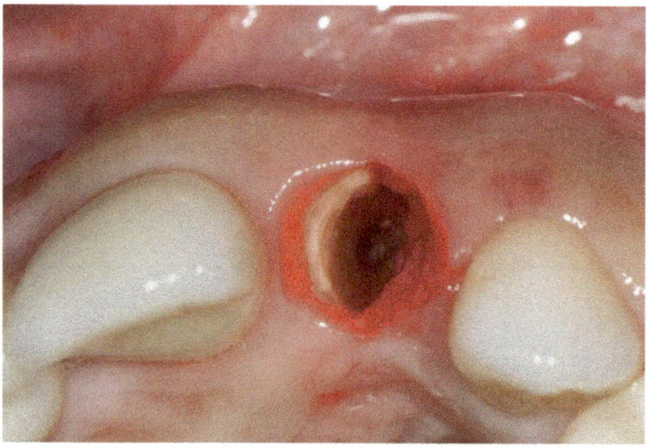

Fig. 9.20 Occlusal view after proximal root shield preparation

- leave root 1mm above marginal bone

flap reflection. The crown portion of the remaining mesial tooth structure was then sectioned horizontally leaving the root with a cervical extension ~1 mm coronal to the mesial marginal bone. The mesial root fragment was prepared creating a 1.5–2 mm uniformly thick C-shaped root fragment spanning from the mesiobuccal to the mesiolingual line angles. After the mesial portion of the tooth socket was debrided and detoxified, sequential implant osteotomy was performed to achieve the proper three-dimensional implant (NobelActive, Nobel Biocare) position in relationship to the mesial root fragment, which might result in contacts between the implant and the mesial root fragment (Figs. 9.21a–c). A histologic study of buccal root fragment retention (socket-shield technique) in conjunction with immediate implant placement has shown that there were connective tissues (a junctional epithelium and the formation of new cementum) interposed between the coronal root fragment and implant, while the more apical portion of the root fragment, which was in direct contact with the tips of the implant threads, was covered by a cellular type of cementum (Hurzeler 2010). These findings seem to suggest the presence of normal peri-implant soft tissue and an intimate contact between the implant and root fragment (Hurzeler 2010). Bone graft materials (Bio-Oss, Osteohealth, Shirley, NY and Puros, Zimmer Dental, Carlsbad, CA) were placed into the gaps between the implant and the bony socket as well as the mesial root fragment. A provisional shell was then relined onto a zirconia abutment and adjusted to clear all centric and eccentric functional contacts.

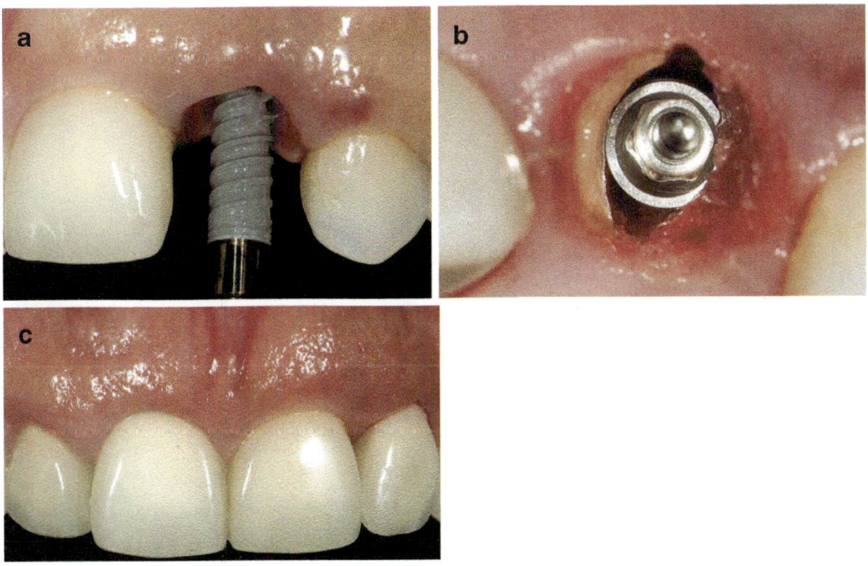

Fig. 9.21 (**a**) Immediate implant placement. (**b**) Occlusal view after implant placed by the proximal root shield. (**c**) Clinical facial view after proximal root shield and immediate implant placement and provisionalization

Appropriate antibiotics and analgesics were prescribed. The patient was instructed not to brush the surgical site but to rinse gently with 0.12% chlorhexidine gluconate (Peridex, Procter & Gamble) and be on a soft diet for 2 weeks. The patient was advised against functioning activities to the implant site for the duration of the implant healing phase (6 months).

The final implant impression was made 6 months after the surgery. The definitive all-ceramic crown (Procera, Nobel Biocare) with a customized zirconia abutment (Procera, Nobel Biocare) was fabricated and cemented. Clinical and radiographic at 3.5 years showed satisfactory aesthetic results with well-maintained inter-implant papilla between #9 and #10 (Fig. 9.22a, b).

The benefits of proximal socket-shield (PSS) procedure with IIPP in maintaining both the bone level and the dentogingival supracrestal fibers have been reported in the literature [47]. Nevertheless, this is a technique-sensitive procedure with limited long-term evidence. Therefore, proper case selection and execution as well as close monitoring in larger-scale studies are needed to substantiate the validity of the procedure.

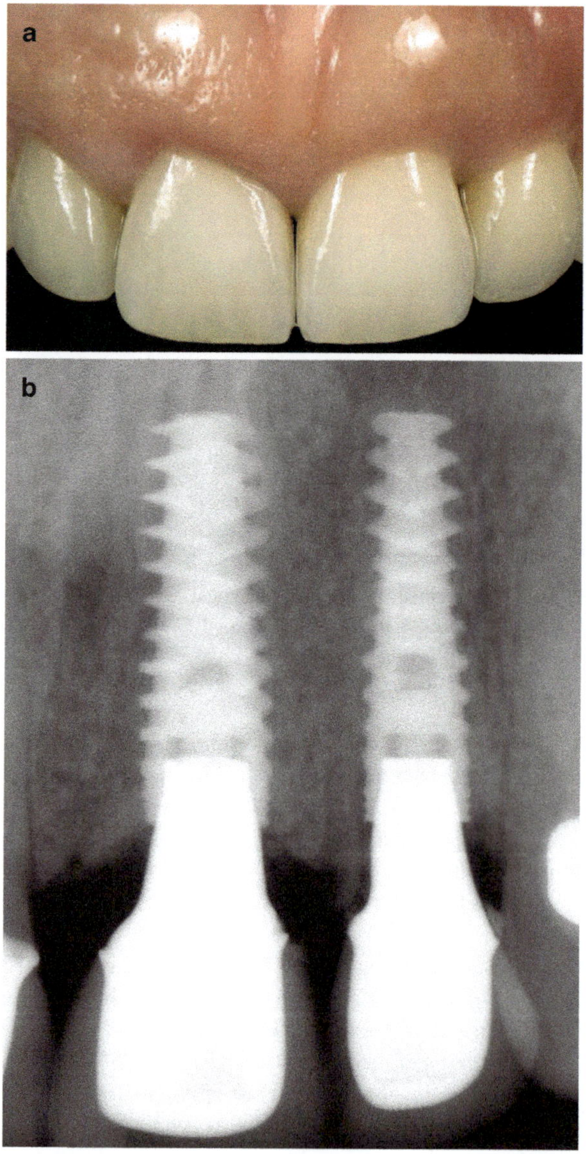

Fig. 9.22 (**a**) Facial clinical view of 4 year follow-up. (**b**) Radiographic of 4 year follow-up

Conclusions

While a well-executed IIPP as well as its adjunctive procedures (alternate IIPP and PSS) of anterior maxillary single implants has been shown to be a predictable treatment modality in maintaining facial and proximal peri-implant tissues, its success depends primarily on careful patient selection, accurate diagnosis, and proper planning. Nonetheless, these are highly technique-sensitive procedures that demand a complete comprehension to deliver a harmonious and functional restoration in the aesthetic zone.

References

1. Gargiulo AW, Wentz FM, Orban B. Dimensions and relations of the dento-gingival junction in humans. J Periodontol. 1961;32:261–7.
2. Kois JC. Altering gingival levels: the restorative connection, part I: biologic variables. J Esthet Dent. 1994;6:3–9.
3. Vacek JS, Gher ME, Assad DA, Richardson AC, Giambarresi LI. The dimension of human dentogingival junction. Int J Periodontics Restorative Dent. 1994;14:155–65.
4. Tarnow DP, Magner AW, Fletcher P. The effect of distance from the contact point to the crest of bone on the presence or absence of the interproximal dental papilla. J Periodontol. 1992;63:995–6.
5. Ingber JS, Rose LF, Coslet JG. The "biologic width": a concept in periodontics and restorative dentistry. Alpha Omegan. 1977;70:62–5.
6. Bragger U, Lauchenauer D, Lang NP. The surgical lengthening of the clinical crown. J Clin Periodontol. 1992;19:58–63.
7. Kan JYK, Rungcharassaeng K. Site development for anterior implant esthetics: the dentulous site. Compend Contin Educ Dent. 2001;22:221–32.
8. Kan JYK, Rungcharassaeng K. Immediate placement and provisionalization of maxillary anterior single implant: a surgical and prosthodontic rationale. Pract Periodontics Aesthet Dent. 2000;12:817–24.
9. Spear FM. Maintenance of the interdental papilla following anterior tooth removal. Pract Periodontics Aesthet Dent. 1999;11:21–8.
10. Kois JC. Predictable single tooth peri-implant esthetics: five diagnostic keys. Compend Contin Educ Dent. 2001;22:199–208.
11. James RA. Peri-implant considerations. Dent Clin N Am. 1980;24:415–20.
12. Hansson HA, Albrektsson T, Branemark PI. Structural aspects of the interface between tissue and titanium implants. J Prosthet Dent. 1983;50:108–13.
13. McKinney RV, Steflik DE, Koth DL. Evidence for a junctional epithelial attachment to ceramic dental implants: a transmission electron microscopic study. J Periodontol. 1985;56:579–91.
14. Buser D, Weber HP, Donath K, Fiorellini JP, Paquette DW, Williams RC. Soft tissue reactions to non-submerged unloaded titanium implants in beagle dogs. J Periodontol. 1992;63:226–36.
15. Abrahamsson I, Berglundh T, Wennstrom J, Lindhe J. The peri-implant hard and soft tissues at different implant systems. A comparative study in dog. Clin Oral Implants Res. 1996;7:212–9.
16. Berglundh T, Lindhe J. Dimension of the periimplant mucosa. Biological width revisited. J Clin Periodontol. 1996;23:971–3.
17. Cochran DL, Hermann JS, Schenk RK, Higginbottom FL, Buser D. Biologic width around titanium implants. A histometric analysis of the implanto-gingival junction around unloaded and loaded nonsubmerged implants in the canine mandible. J Periodontol. 1997;68:186–98.
18. Abrahamsson I, Berglundh T, Moon IS, Lindhe J. Peri-implant tissues at submerged and non-submerged titanium implants. J Clin Periodontol. 1999;26:600–7.
19. Hermann JS, Buser D, Schenk RK, Schoolfield JD, Cochran DL. Biological width around one- and two-piece titanium implants: a histometric evaluation of unloaded nonsubmerged and submerged implants in the canine mandible. Clin Oral Implants Res. 2001;12:559–71.
20. Weber HP, Buser D, Donath K, Fiorellini JP, Doppalapudi V, Paquette DW, Willaims RC. Comparisons of healed tissues adjacent to submerged and nonsubmerged unloaded titanium dental implants. A histometric study in beagle dogs. Clin Oral Implants Res. 1996;7:11–9.

21. Kan JYK, Rungcharassaeng K, Umezu K, Kois JC. Dimensions of peri-implant mucosa: an evaluation of maxillary anterior single implants in human. J Periodontol. 2003;74:563–8.
22. Weisgold AS. Contours of the full crown restoration. Alpha Omegan. 1977;70(3):77–89.
23. Olsson M, Lindhe J. Periodontal characteristics in individuals with varying forms of the upper central incisors. J Clin Periodontol. 1991;18:78–82.
24. Muller HP, Heinecke A, Schaller N, Eger T. Masticatory mucosa in subjects with different periodontal phenotypes. J Clin Periodontol. 2000;27:621–6.
25. Sanavi F, Weisgold AS, Rose LF. Biologic width and its relation to periodontal biotypes. J Esthet Dent. 1998;10:157–63.
26. Phillips K, Kois JC. Aesthetic peri-implant site development: the restorative connection. Dent Clin N Am. 1998;42:57–70.
27. Goodacre CJ, Kan JYK, Rungcharassaeng K. Clinical complications of osseointegrated implants. J Prosthet Dent. 1999;81:537–52.
28. Jemt T. Regeneration of gingival papillae after single-implant treatment. Int J Periodontics Restorative Dent. 1997;17:327–33.
29. Jemt T. Restoring the gingival contour by means of provisional resin crowns after single-implant treatment. Int J Periodontics Restorative Dent. 1999;19:21–9.
30. Cooper L, Felton AD, Kugelberg CF, Ellner S, Chaffee N, Molina AL, Moriarty JD, Paquette D, Palmqvist U. A multicenter 12-month evaluation of single-tooth implants restored 3 weeks after 1-stage surgery. Int J Oral Maxillofac Implants. 2001;16:182–92.
31. Bengazi F, Wennstrom JL, Lekholm U. Recession of the soft tissue margin at oral implants. A 2-year longitudinal prospective study. Clin Oral Implants Res. 1996;7:303–10.
32. Kan JYK, Rungcharassaeng K, Lozada JL. Immediate placement and provisionalization of maxillary anterior single implants: 1-year prospective study. Int J Oral Maxillofac Implants. 2003;18:31–9.
33. Kan JYK, Rungcharassaeng K. Immediate implant placement and provisionalization of maxillary anterior single implants. In: Torabinejad M, Sabeti MA, Goodacre CJ, editors. Principles and practice of single implant and restoration. Missouri: Elsevier Saunders; 2013. p. 119–31.
34. Beagle JR. Surgical reconstruction of the interdental papilla: case report. Int J Periodontics Restorative Dent. 1992;12:145–51.
35. Nemcovsky CE, Moses O, Artzi Z. Interproximal papillae reconstruction in maxillary implants. J Periodontol. 2000;7:308–14.
36. Palacci P. Peri-implant soft tissue management: papilla regeneration technique. In: Palacci P, Ericsson I, Engstrand P, Rangert B, editors. Optimal implant positioning and soft tissue management for the Branemark system. Chicago: Quintessence; 1995. p. 59–70.
37. Wohrle PS. Single-tooth replacement in the aesthetic zone with immediate provisionalization: fourteen consecutive cases reports. Pract Periodontics Aesthet Dent. 1998;10:1107–14.
38. Hui E, Chow J, Li D, Liu J, Wat P, Law H. Immediate provisional for single-tooth implant replacement with Branemark system: preliminary report. Clin Implant Dent Relat Res. 2001;3:79–86.
39. Kan JYK, Rungcharassaeng K, Liddelow G, Henry P, Goodacre CJ. Periimplant tissue response following immediate provisional restoration of scalloped implants in the esthetic zone: a one-year pilot prospective multicenter study. J Prosthet Dent. 2007;97(6 Suppl):S109–18.
40. De Rouck T, Collys K, Cosyn J. Immediate single tooth implants in the anterior maxilla: a 1-year case cohort study on hard and soft tissue response. J Clin Periodontol. 2008;35:649–57.
41. Kan JYK, Rungcharassaeng K, Sclar A, Lozada J. Effects of the facial osseous defect morphology on gingival dynamics after immediate tooth replacement and guided bone regeneration: 1-year results. J Oral Maxillofac Surg. 2007;65(7 Suppl 1):S13–9.
42. Barone A, Rispoli L, Vozza I, Quaranta A, Covani U. Immediate restoration of single implants placed immediately after tooth extraction. J Periodontol. 2006;77:1914–20.
43. Palattella P, Toresllo F, Cordarro L. Two-year prospective clinical comparison of immediate replacement vs. immediate restoration of single tooth in the esthetic zone. Clin Oral Implants Res. 2008;19:1148–53.

44. Norton MR. A short-term clinical evaluation of immediately restorated maxillary TiOblast single-tooth implants. Int J Oral Maxillofac Implants. 2004;19:274–81.
45. Ferrara A, Galli C, Mauro G, Macaluso GM. Immediate provisional restoration of postextraction implants for maxillary single-tooth replacement. Int J Periodontics Restorative Dent. 2006;26:371–7.
46. Tsirlis AT. Clinical evaluation of immediate loaded upper anterior single implants. Implant Dent. 2005;14:94–103.
47. Crespi R, Cappare P, Gherlone E, Romanos G. Immediate versus delayed loading of dental implants placed in fresh extraction sockets in the maxillary esthetic zone: a clinical comparative study. Int J Oral Maxillofac Implants. 2008;23:753–8.
48. Canullo L, Rasperini G. Preservation of peri-implant soft and hard tissues using platform switching of implants placed in immediate extraction sockets: ZA proof-of-concept study with 12- to 26-months follow-up. Int J Oral Maxillofac Implants. 2007;22:995–1000.
49. Groisman M, Frossard WM, Ferreira HM, de Menszes Filho LM, Touati B. Single-tooth implants in the maxillary incisor region with immediate provisionalization: 2-year prospective study. Pract Proced Aesthet Dent. 2003;15:115–22.
50. Garber DA, Salama MA, Salama H. Immediate total replacement. Compend Contin Educ Dent. 2001;22:210–8.
51. Kan JYK, Rungcharassaeng K, Lozada J. Bilaminar subepithelial connective tissue grafts for implant placement and provisionalization in the esthetic zone. J Calif Dent Assoc. 2005;33:865–71.
52. Kois JC, Kan JYK. Predictable peri-implant gingival esthetics: surgical and prosthodontic rationales. Pract Proced Aesthet Dent. 2001;13:711–5.
53. Kan JYK, Roe P, Rungcharassaeng K, Patel R, Waki T, Lozada JL, Zimmerman G. Classification of sagittal root position in relation to the anterior maxillary osseous housing for immediate implant placement: a cone beam computed tomography study. Int J Oral Maxillofac Implants. 2011;26:873–6.
54. Salama H, Salama MA. The role of orthodontic extrusive remodeling in the enhancement of soft and hard tissue profiles prior to implant placement: a systematic approach to the management of extraction sites defects. Int J Periodontics Restorative Dent. 1993;13:312–34.
55. Kan JYK, Morimoto T, Rungcharassaeng K, Roe P, Smith DH. Gingival biotype assessment in the esthetic zone: visual versus direct measurement. Int J Periodontics Restorative Dent. 2010;30:237–43.
56. Esposito M, Ekestubbe A, Grondahl K. Radiological evaluation of marginal bone loss at tooth surfaces facing single Branemark implants. Clin Oral Implants Res. 1993;4:151–7.
57. Araujo MG, Lindhe J. Dimension ridge alterations following tooth extraction. An experimental study in the dog. J Clin Periodontol. 2005;32:212–8.
58. Araujo MG, Sukekava F, Wennstrom JL, Lindhe J. Ridge alterations following implant placement in fresh extraction sockets: an experimental study in the dog. J Clin Periodontol. 2005;32:645–52.
59. Boticelli D, Berglundh T, Lindhe J. Hard-tissue alterations following immediate implant placement in extraction sites. J Clin Periodontol. 2004;31:820–8.
60. Chen ST. Immediate implant placement postextraction without flap elevation. J Periodontol. 2009;80:163–72.
61. Covani U, Cornelini R, Barone A. Bucco-lingual bone remodeling around implants placed into immediate extraction sockets: a case series. J Periodontol. 2003;74:268–73.
62. Nabers J. Free gingival grafts. Periodontics. 1966;4:243–5.
63. Kan JYK, Rungcharassaeng K. Inter-implant papillary preservation in the esthetic zone: a report of 6 consecutive cases. Int J Periodontics Restorative Dent. 2003;23:249–59.
64. Rungcharassaeng K, Kan JY. Aesthetic implant management of multiple adjacent failing anterior maxillary teeth. Pract Proced Aesthet Dent. 2004;16:365–9.
65. Tarnow DP, Cho SC, Wallace SS. The effect of inter-implant distance on the height of inter-implant bone crest. J Periodontol. 2000;71:546–9.

Part IV

Design, Fabrication and Delivery of the Definitive Implant Prosthesis

Enhanced Implant Impression Techniques to Maximize Accuracy

10

Panos Papaspyridakos and Todd R. Schoenbaum

Abstract

Purpose: The purpose of this chapter was to review the scientific literature on implant impression techniques for partially edentulous patients and to propose evidence-based clinical guidelines for implant treatment in the aesthetic zone.

Materials and Methods: Comprehensive review of available literature was conducted in a systematic approach and descriptively analyzed, where applicable.

Results: Based on the available scientific evidence on implant impressions in the aesthetic zone, the customized impression coping technique is recommended for either single implant or multiple implant scenario. Open-tray or closed-tray technique can be successfully used for single implant scenario. The splinted open-tray impression technique is more accurate than non-splinted one and is recommended for multiple implant scenario. Pouring of the impression should be done in low expansion stone with or without soft tissue moulage. Digital implant impressions are gaining popularity and are scientifically validated with a streamlined workflow for single implant scenario.

Conclusion: Aesthetically pleasing implant restorations can be successfully fabricated with the appropriately selected impression technique, depending on the implant scenario.

P. Papaspyridakos (✉)
Division of Postgraduate Prosthodontics, Tufts University School of Dental Medicine, Boston, MA, USA

T. R. Schoenbaum
Division of Constitutive and Regenerative Sciences, University of California, Los Angeles, CA, USA

Todd R. Schoenbaum (ed.), *Implants in the Aesthetic Zone*,
https://doi.org/10.1007/978-3-319-72601-4_10

10.1 Introduction

Oral rehabilitation of partially edentulous patients with micro-textured dental implants is currently a routine procedure, and clinical studies have proven the longitudinal effectiveness of this treatment modality [1]. Due to the fact that dental implants are functionally ankylosed with direct contact to the bone, they lack the inherent mobility of the periodontal ligament, and misfit cannot be tolerated at the implant-abutment interface [2]. The reason is that misfit at the implant-abutment junction of implant fixed dental prostheses (IFDPs) may lead to mechanical strains in the prosthesis and to the transmission of stresses to the alveolar bone and supporting implants after the tightening of all prosthetic screws [2, 3]. Screw loosening and/or fracture, implant fractures, and prosthetic components strain and fracture have been related with prosthesis misfit [4–6].

The clinical fit of an IFDP at the implant-abutment junction is directly dependent on the accuracy of impression technique and cast fabrication [2, 6, 7]. Hence, an accurate implant impression is necessary in order to generate an accurate definitive cast, which is the foundation for the fabrication of an accurately fitting prosthesis. There are several clinical and laboratory variables that affect the accuracy of an implant cast, namely, impression techniques, impression material and die stone properties, pouring techniques, machining tolerance of prosthetic components, implant angulation, and/or depth [8].

10.2 Impression Materials

An accurate impression is incumbent for fabrication of implant prostheses and represents the essential first step. In regard to implant prosthodontics, the impression material must provide adequate rigidity to prevent rotation of the impression coping during the impression taking or implant analog fastening and cast fabrication. The superior mechanical properties of polyether and addition polyvinyl siloxane (PVS) make them the material of choice for implant impressions [9]. In regard to which impression material is better, a systematic review assessed the scientific evidence from ten in vitro studies that compared the accuracy of impression techniques with polyether, PVS, and various other impression materials [8]. The authors reported that the accuracy of implant impressions is not affected by the impression material (polyether and addition PVS) for partially edentulous [8]. Polyether or PVS can be both used for final implant impressions without any difference in the outcomes.

10.3 Impression Techniques

10.3.1 Splinted Versus Non-splinted Impression Techniques

Various implant impression techniques have been used to generate a definitive cast that will ensure the accurate clinical fit of IFDPs. The necessity for rigidly splinting the impression copings has been advocated in several studies, while others have shown no difference.

A systematic review assessed the available evidence for implant impressions in partially edentulous patients, based on 13 in vitro studies comparing the accuracy of splinted vs non-splinted impression techniques [10–23].

Eight in vitro studies reported that the splinted technique was more accurate than the non-splinted technique, three in vitro studies reported that there was no difference, and two in vitro studies reported that the non-splinted was more accurate [8].

Thus, the preponderance of evidence shows that the splinted impression technique was more accurate than the non-splinted conventional impression techniques for partially edentulous patients [8]. Hence, the splinted technique should be the first treatment approach of choice for partially edentulous patients when two or more implants are present.

Regarding the splinting materials used, most of the studies used polymethyl methacrylate (PMMA) autopolymerizing acrylic resin as the splinting material of choice, coupled with dental floss or metal bars. Prefabricated PMMA resin bars, composite resin bars, and visible light-curing acrylic resins were used for splinting as well. An in vitro study showed that the total polymerization shrinkage of Duralay acrylic resin at 1 day was 7.9% and that 80% of the shrinkage occurred within 17 min of mixing at room temperature [24]. That is the reason why sectioning of the acrylic resin splint has been advocated in many studies followed by reconnection with minimal amount of resin to compensate for the polymerization shrinkage. Moreover, the use of new splinting materials like composite resin or visible light polymerizing acrylic resin resulted in better results [8].

Depending on the degree of angulation and implant connection design configuration, variables, such as impression technique (rigid splint vs no splint) and impression material (more rigid vs more elastic), will influence impression accuracy [25]. The removal of rigidly splinted internal connection impression copings may be challenging when the angulation of the implants is extreme (more than 30°). In addition to that, the impression coping design may have an effect on impression accuracy with angulated implants. Some implant designs feature connection types and impression copings with long engaging internal components that do not allow for impression of angulated implants with the traditional engaging copings splinted together. Non-engaging copings can be used alternatively for these implant systems when angulated implants are present and splinting is performed. The number and anteroposterior spread of implants will likely have an additional effect on the ease of removal of the implant impression. Removal of an impression of multiple implants requires flexure of the impression material, whether using the closed- or open-tray impression copings.

10.3.2 Open-Tray Versus Closed-Tray Impression Techniques

The open-tray (pickup or direct) and the closed-tray techniques (transfer or indirect) are the two primary options for taking an implant-level impression.

For partially edentulous patients, the available evidence was evaluated by a systematic review based on 18 in vitro and 1 clinical studies that compared the accuracy with open-tray (direct, pickup) vs closed-tray (indirect, transfer) impression techniques [10, 18–21, 26–37].

Ten in vitro studies reported that the open-tray technique was more accurate than the closed-tray for partially edentulous patients, while seven in vitro studies reported that there was no difference, and one in vitro study reported that the closed-tray was more accurate [8]. Most in vitro studies reported slightly better accuracy with the open-tray technique over the closed-tray one, but the difference was judged as clinically negligible [8]. One clinical study reported that there was no difference between open- and closed-tray techniques [32].

For single implant impressions, two studies compared the accuracy of single implant impressions with open-tray (direct) vs closed-tray (indirect) technique [36, 37]. One study reported that there was no difference, and the other study reported that open-tray was better. It seems that for single implant impressions, both techniques are highly predictable, and the selection of one technique over the other relies on clinician preference and available mouth opening (open-tray techniques require more vertical space).

In conclusion, the open-tray impression technique seems to have similar accuracy to the closed-tray impression technique for partially edentulous patients and two implant-supported three-unit IFDP scenarios [8]. For multiple implants, the open-tray technique has been shown to be more accurate and is the recommended approach [8]. Hence, the open-tray technique should be the first treatment approach of choice for partially edentulous patients when more than two implants are present. Verification of the working cast is recommended as an extra step for accuracy and can be done the day of the final impression for multiple implants.

10.3.3 Digital Impression Techniques

Digital dental technology is currently gaining increasing popularity for application in both fixed prosthodontics and implant dentistry [38–43]. Digital impressions represent cutting-edge technology that allows dentists to create a virtual, computer-generated replica of the hard and soft tissues in the mouth using intraoral optical scanner (IOS) systems.

There are two types of digital impression technology currently available for clinicians to use. One type captures the images as digital photographs (iTero™ and CEREC® Bluecam) that the software "stitches" them together, providing dentists and dental laboratories with a series of images; the other type captures images continuously with video acquisition (3Shape TRIOS®, 3M True Definition™ scanner, CEREC® Omnicam, and E4D NEVO™ scanner). A scan body is connected to the implant in identical fashion as the conventional impression coping, and then an IOS system is used to digitally scan the intraoral situation. Prior to digital scanning, some IOS systems may need powder prior to scanning or not [38–43]. The digital impression is acquired and saved as a Standard Tessellation Language (STL) file in the computer screen while eliminating the intraoral application of impression material which is not pleasant for some patients.

Digital impressions using an IOS eliminate the need for tray selection, dispensing and polymerization of impression materials, disinfection, and shipping to the laboratory, while patient comfort is an additional advantage [8]. The digital impressions are sent and stored electronically, improving efficiency [44, 45]. A conventional impression is captured as negative, making it more difficult to identify mistakes. If mistakes are identified, the dentist will need to take another impression, which means patients must undergo the impression procedure again, resulting in greater inconvenience and a longer appointment, as well as time lost, and added cost and material use for the dentist. On the other hand, a digital impression enables dentists to see the positive image, magnify, and evaluate it carefully. Repeated digital scanning can be made to easily capture a revised impression and improve the previous virtual cast, in case it is deemed not acceptable.

10.3.3.1 Digital Impressions Versus Conventional Impressions for Partially Edentulous Patients

To overcome some of the limitations with conventional impression techniques, intraoral digital scanning was developed. Digital implant impressions are currently gaining popularity; however, limited scientific data are available in terms of accuracy of this technology [8].

For partially edentulous arches with single implant case scenario, an in vitro study with the parallel confocal IOS technology (iTero) reported that the digital impression is equally accurate and efficient with the conventional one [44]. A clinical study with a crossover design and a total of 20 included patients for rehabilitation with two implant single crowns each (2 × 20) was conducted [46]. Each patient received one CAD/CAM zirconia single implant crown with customized titanium abutment (test: digital) and one porcelain fused to metal crown with standardized titanium abutment (control: conventional). Starting with prosthetic treatment, analysis was estimated for clinical and laboratory work steps including measure of costs in Swiss Francs (CHF), productivity rates, and cost minimization for first-line therapy. The results showed that both protocols worked successfully for all test and control crowns. Direct treatment costs were significantly lower for the digital workflow 1815.35 CHF compared to the conventional pathway 2119.65 CHF. Overall, cost minimization analysis exhibited an 18% cost reduction within the digital process. The authors reported that digital workflow was three times more efficient than the conventional one for implant-supported single crowns [46, 47]. Clinical fitting could be achieved with no or minor adjustments within the digital process of intraoral scanning plus CAD/CAM technology [46, 47]. In terms of patient-related parameters, a clinical study with an IOS (Omnicam) versus conventional impressions for implant-supported premolar single crowns reported less fear of repeating the impression, less inconvenience and shortness of breath, and fewer feelings of helplessness during the digital impressions [48]. Another clinical study assessing the patients' preference between digital impressions (iTero) and conventional ones for implant-supported molar single crowns reported that patients preferred the digital pathway with respect to taste effects and their preparatory activities [49].

For partially edentulous arches, an in vitro study compared an IOS system with parallel confocal microscopy technology and image stitching data acquisition (iTero) to a conventional impression with polyvinyl siloxane and found that at 0° and 15° implant divergence, conventional impressions produced definitive casts with a statistically significant higher accuracy. At 30° and 45° of implant divergence there was no significant difference [45]. Another in vitro study compared the accuracy of digital impressions with a blue light active wavefront sampling technology IOS (Lava COS) versus conventional ones for a three-unit posterior mandibular IFDP scenario with two implants [50]. The comparison was done indirectly on the generated casts and the authors reported that the digital impressions produced physical casts that presented with better fit compared with the stone casts [50].

In conclusion, digital implant impressions with IOS are gaining increasing popularity; however, further studies are needed to assess the clinical accuracy of digital vs conventional implant impression techniques for extended applications with multiple implants. The single implant impression and subsequent workflow for the fabrication of single implant crowns should be considered streamlined and scientifically validated [46–48].

10.3.4 Customized Impression Coping Technique

The use of impression copings to generate a definitive implant impression results in a definitive cast in which the soft tissue replica around the implant platform is circular. Therefore, any soft tissue sculpting developed clinically by the provisional restoration is lost. The customized impression coping technique is used to capture the transmucosal part of the peri-implant soft tissue sculpted by a customized provisional restoration and transfer it to an emergence profile cast [51, 52].

The customized impression coping technique has several advantages since it is a fast and cost-effective technique that captures the transmucosal emergence profile to facilitate the fabrication of aesthetic anterior implant restorations. This technique results in an implant restoration that mimics accurately in its emergence profile that of the carefully crafted and customized provisional restoration. A 2-year clinical study showed that the customized impression coping technique may be helpful to reproduce the gingival margin position from the provisional to the definitive restoration. Moreover, the gingival zenith position during the follow-up period seemed to be stable after 2 years of follow-up [52].

There are two indirect techniques for customization of the impression coping. The first technique entails the pickup impression of the actual implant-supported restoration. The pickup impression is poured with soft tissue moulage and stone or only with stone if bone-level type implants have been placed [51, 52]. This leads to the fabrication of an emergence profile cast that is obtained from a pickup impression of the implant-supported provisional restoration. The second indirect technique entails removal of the implant-supported provisional restoration, followed by implant analog connection and dispensing lab putty or impression material around the implant-provisional prosthesis interface [51, 52]. After polymerization of the lab putty or impression material, the implant-supported provisional restoration is removed, and an impression coping is connected to the implant analog. The empty space is filled with acrylic resin or composite resin, and the customized impression coping is fabricated, capturing the transmucosal emergence profile of the provisional crown.

10.4 Factors Affecting Impression Accuracy

10.4.1 Implant Angulation

It has been shown that following tooth extraction in the anterior maxilla, resorption of the alveolar bone volume is 25% during the first year and 40–60% after 3 years [53]. Resorption occurs in a palatal direction, which will lead to palatal placement of the implants if no grafting procedures are performed. If multiple adjacent teeth need to be replaced, there is a high possibility of having angulated implants, both in the mesiodistal and facial-palatal direction.

The effect of implant angulation on the accuracy of implant casts generated with various impression techniques for partially edentulous patients has not been fully investigated yet. Most of the in vitro studies evaluated how to improve the impression accuracy in ideal conditions, with parallel implants, whereas few studies have been carried out to assess the effect of angulated implants on the accuracy of the implant impressions.

Impression distortion may be negatively affected by the implant angulation as well as by the presence of physical undercuts (tooth embrasures, alveolar ridge deformities), as a higher removal strength is needed, affecting the precision of the impressions [8].

The elastomeric impression materials' recovery properties may compensate for the implant angulation and tissue undercuts; however, impression distortion may occur at increased implant angles, yielding to plastic deformation of the impression. The impression removal from internal connection implants is likely to produce a higher level of stress between the impression material and the impression copings, than from external hexagon implants. This stress may hypothetically induce permanent deformation of impression material or movement of the impression copings inside the impression material and cause inaccuracies. No studies were found assessing the effect of internal and external connection on implant impression accuracy. Four in vitro studies reported on comparisons of implant vs abutment/cementable abutment level, and the majority reported better accuracy with the implant-level technique compared to cementable abutment level [8].

For partially edentulous patients, as far as implant angulation is concerned, a systematic review analyzed the available scientific evidence which was based on 1 clinical and 15 in vitro studies [8, 54, 55]. The only clinical study reported no difference on the clinical accuracy between open- and closed-tray impression techniques for partially edentulous patients with two implants and up to 10° angulation, while most in vitro studies reported that with up to 15° angulation, no difference existed between different impression techniques [32].

Nine in vitro studies reported on two implant scenarios with internal or external connections, and the majority reported that angulation more than 20° affected accuracy, but the clinical significance is unknown [8].

10.4.2 Impression Tray

In regard to impressions trays, only one in vitro study compared the effect of custom trays versus stock trays on the accuracy of implant impressions [56]. The investigators reported better outcomes with the rigid custom trays compared with the polycarbonate stock trays. The stock trays used in that study could not produce accurate impressions consistently. On the other hand, a more recent in vitro study reported on the effect of tray on the accuracy of implant impressions. They reported that polyether and PVS can safely be used for the impressions of the edentulous arches with multiple implants and different tray types produce similar accuracy results [57]. In conclusion, there may be benefits when using a custom tray for anterior implant impressions such as ease of tray placement intraorally and uniform amount of impression material, but similar accuracy can be achieved with a stock tray as well.

10.4.3 Other Factors Affecting Accuracy

Other factors that may affect the accuracy of implant impressions are the pouring techniques, machining tolerance, and methodology of accuracy assessment, impression trays and implant depth.

10.4.3.1 Pouring Techniques

In regard to pouring techniques, a few in vitro and two clinical studies have shown that the double pouring technique results in better outcomes [58–60]. The double pouring technique is different than the conventional pouring technique in the following manner. After connection of the implant analogs to the impression copings, low expansion (0.09%) type IV die stone is mixed. First, the stone is mixed manually with distilled water for 15 s to aid the incorporation of the water and then under vacuum, and an initial pour of stone up to the middle of the analogs is carried out. All of the stone mixes are vibrated before and during the pouring [58–60]. After 30 min, the second pour of vacuum-mixed die stone is done. This double pouring technique minimizes the volumetric expansion of the stone and has been shown to lead in more accurate die casts. Another pouring technique includes splinting the implant analogs together prior to pouring [58–60].

10.4.3.2 Machining Tolerance

In regard to the machining tolerance and its effect on accuracy measurements, it has been shown that paired prosthetic components may be rotationally displaced during connection to their respective parts [8]. This displacement cannot be controlled by the clinician and lies within the range of the inherent machining tolerance [61, 62]. Hence, errors occur during connection of impression copings to the implants intraorally and to the implant analogs in the laboratory, respectively. For example, a comparative in vivo study with first-generation prosthetic components of the external connection Branemark system revealed horizontal and vertical discrepancies of component fit with a wide range, while an in vitro study showed that the machining tolerance of the first-generation Branemark components was larger than the currently used components and ranged from 33 to 100 μm [61, 62]. The machining tolerance differs between different implant systems and is an unknown variable in the accuracy measurements.

10.4.3.3 Implant Depth

In regard to the effect of implant depth on accuracy of implant impressions, only three in vitro studies were identified investigating this parameter [63, 64].

The first in vitro study showed that implant depth did not affect the accuracy of implant impressions when impressions were taken with a digital scanner that employs wavefront sampling technology (LAVA C.O.S.) [63]. On the contrary, another in vitro study by the same group showed that impressions of the implants placed at the tissue level were less accurate than implants placed 2 and 4 mm subgingivally, when parallel confocal imaging (iTero) was employed [64].

Another in vitro study showed that when polyether was used, the impression of 4-mm-deep implants with normal impression copings was significantly less accurate than impressions of 0-mm-deep implants [8]. On the contrary, with the PVS, there was no significant difference among the implants with different depths. The results of the above studies were conflicting, and no definitive conclusions may be drawn.

10.4.3.4 Methodology of Accuracy Assessment

The diverse results from some previous in vitro studies may be partially explained by the differences in measurement methodology, machining tolerance, connection designs, and by improvements in dental materials. In regard to the methodology of accuracy assessment and its effect on accuracy measurements, several methods have been employed to measure and quantify the 3-D deviations on the x-, y-, and z-axis between the implant casts produced with different impression techniques including computerized coordinate measuring machine, 3-D photogrammetry, traveling microscope, computerized tomography (CT) scan, and recently optical scanning and digitization [8]. Several studies indirectly assessed the implant impression accuracy by evaluating the fit and/or distortion of fabricated frameworks on the resultant casts with strain gauges and compared the fit and/or distortion of the frameworks on the reference master cast. Other studies indirectly assessed the implant impression accuracy by evaluating the fit of frameworks with microscopes [8]. Lastly, other studies evaluated the accuracy of the implant impressions by measuring inter-implant distances of the working casts in relation to a reference control cast [8]. However, with the advent of 3-D measurement devices, a 2-D assessment of the accuracy cannot be accepted today for scientific purposes. Optical scanning and dedicated software for superimposition of the scanning data sets is currently an efficient and precise technique to measure and compare the 3-D discrepancies at the microscopic level between different groups and thus seems to be the recommended technique for future investigations [8].

10.5 Clinical Recommendations and Case Scenarios

Regarding implant impressions in the anterior aesthetic zone, there are various scenarios.

1. Single implant in the aesthetic zone
2. Two adjacent implants in the aesthetic zone
3. Multiple implants in the aesthetic zone

10.5.1 Single Implant in the Aesthetic Zone

For single implant impression in the aesthetic zone, the customized impression coping technique is recommended, with either a closed-tray or an open-tray approach. The reason is that the shape of the teeth in the CEJ level is triangular and wider compared to the circular impression coping. Capturing the transmucosal part of the provisional implant crown is a crucial step prior to the implant impression and can be done either with a pickup of the provisional or with customized impression copings [65, 66]. In regard to the provisional crown, it has to be highlighted that even though the retention type can be either screw or cement and both yields similar survival rates, screw retention is preferred for the provisionalization phase of the implant treatment in the aesthetic zone [67].

The implant impression after customizing the impression coping is poured either with only in stone without any soft tissue moulage when bone-level type implants have been placed or with stone and soft tissue moulage when bone-level or tissue level implants have been placed. The stone cast without the soft tissue moulage features the customized transmucosal design captured with the customized impression technique and will force the laboratory technician to duplicate this transmucosal part in the final prosthesis without room for error. When the soft tissue moulage technique is used, which is a commonly used technique, attention must be given, so that the laboratory technician will not alter the customized transmucosal part due to the resiliency of the soft tissue moulage. A case is illustrated (Fig. 10.1a–h).

10.5.2 Two Adjacent Implants in the Aesthetic Zone

For impression of two adjacent implants in the aesthetic zone, only the customized impression coping technique is recommended [51, 52, 65]. Pickup impression of the two-unit screw-retained provisional prosthesis may not be possible due to the non-engaging components. If a pickup of the screw-retained prosthesis is done, then the rotation (timing) of the engaging part of the implants will not be captured, rendering the impression erroneous if a cement retained prosthesis or individual units are envisioned.

The aforementioned procedures are used again to fabricate the customized impression copings. Prior to the open-tray impression, the customized impression copings are connected to the implant platforms, and seating is confirmed radiographically. Prefabricated resin bars can be fabricated prior to the impression taking with a previously described technique. Drinking straws are filled with visible light-cured resin (Triad gel) and then light cured, thus creating resin bars of standardized thickness and shape. The resin bars are subsequently removed from the straws and recured. The resin bars are stored for 24 h prior to being used. The prefabricated resin bars are used to splint the impression copings together with the aid of additional light-cured resin (Triad gel). If prefabricated bars are not

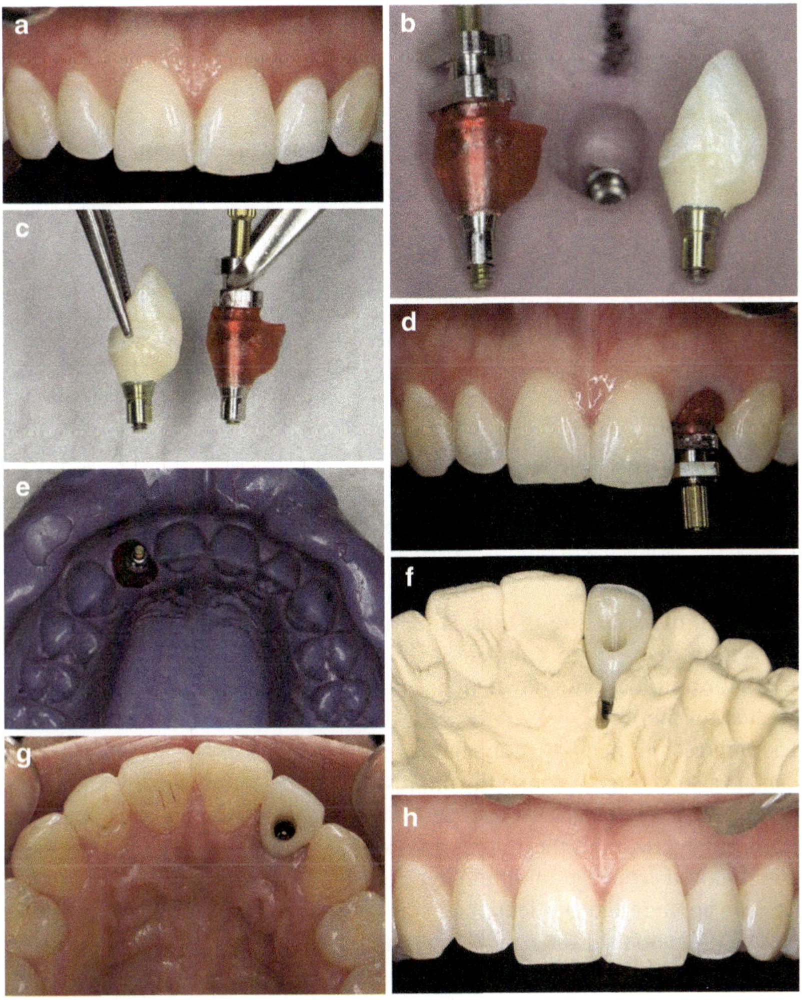

Fig. 10.1 (**a**) Missing maxillary left lateral incisor (#10) was replaced with a dental implant. Peri-implant soft tissue conditioning was done for a period of 3 months with a provisional screw-retained implant single crown, after successful osseointegration. The natural lateral incisor crown is triangular at the CEJ cross section, while the dental implant prosthetic neck is circular. The provisional implant single crown was used to condition the peri-implant soft tissue into the desired shape and emergence profile. (**b**) Customized impression coping duplicating the transmucosal part of the provisional implant single crown. The transmucosal part of the impression coping is fabricated with autopolymerizing acrylic resin with the indirect technique. Note that the buccal aspect is highlighted with black tip pen. Alternatively, the customized impression coping can be fabricated intraorally with light polymerizing resin with the direct technique. (**c**) Customized impression coping duplicating the transmucosal part of the provisional implant single crown. (**d**) Customized impression coping placed intraorally, after removal of the provisional implant single crown. (**e**) Definitive open-tray implant impression with customized impression coping. The implant analog will be screwed into the coping prior to pouring of the impression. (**f**) Working cast poured in low expansion stone without soft tissue moulage. The customized impression coping has captured the transmucosal part of the provisional implant single crown, guiding the laboratory technician to precisely duplicate the transmucosal part into the emergence profile of the final implant single crown. (**g**) Occlusal view of definitive screw-retained implant single crown prior to final insertion. (**h**) Frontal view of definitive screw-retained implant single crown after final insertion

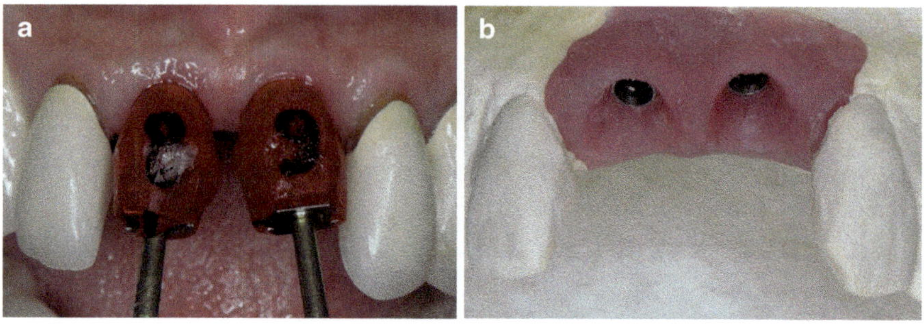

Fig. 10.2 (**a**) Missing right and left central incisors (#8 and 9) were replaced with two dental implants. After successful osseointegration and fixed provisionalization for a 3-month soft tissue conditioning period, the definitive implant impression was taken. Customized impression copings duplicating the transmucosal part of the provisional implant single crowns were used for the definitive implant impression. The customization was done with the indirect technique. (**b**) Working cast poured in stone with soft tissue moulage. The customized impression copings have captured the transmucosal part of the provisional implant single crowns, guiding the laboratory technician to precisely duplicate the transmucosal part into the emergence profile of the final crowns

available and the splinting is done directly intraorally, then the splinting is sectioned with a disk bur to compensate for polymerization thickness and reconnected with minimal amount of light-cured resin (Triad gel). The splint is left untouched for 5 min.

The impression material (polyether or addition PVS) is loaded on the custom tray and is also syringed around the impression copings, followed by placement of the loaded tray on the master cast and appropriate positioning intraorally. After material polymerization, the impression copings are unscrewed, and the impression is removed from the mouth. After connection of the implant analogs to the impression copings and application of soft tissue moulage, low expansion (0.09%) type IV die stone is mixed prior to pouring the impression with stone. All of the stone mixes were vibrated before and during the pouring. The stone casts are allowed to set for 1 h, as per manufacturer's recommendation, before separation from the impressions. Subsequently they are trimmed and finished. A case is illustrated (Fig. 10.2a, b).

10.5.3 Multiple Implants in the Aesthetic Zone

For impression of multiple implants in the aesthetic zone, the customized coping technique is recommended for definitive implant impressions [51, 52, 65]. The aforementioned procedures are used again to fabricate the customized impression copings. Prior to the open-tray impression, the customized impression copings are connected to the implant platforms, and seating is confirmed radiographically. Prefabricated resin bars can be fabricated prior to the impression taking with a previously described technique. Drinking straws are filled with visible light-cured resin (Triad gel) and then light cured, thus creating resin bars of standardized thickness and shape. The resin bars are subsequently removed from the straws and recured. The resin bars are stored for 24 h prior to being used. The prefabricated resin bars are used to splint the impression copings together with the aid of additional light-cured resin (Triad gel). The splint is left untouched for 5 min. The impression material (polyether or addition PVS) is loaded on the custom tray and is also syringed around the impression copings, followed by placement of the loaded tray on the master cast and appropriate positioning intraorally. After material polymerization, the impression copings are unscrewed, and the impression is removed from the mouth. After connection of the implant analogs to the impression copings and application of soft tissue moulage, low expansion (0.09%) type IV die stone is mixed prior to pouring the impression with stone. The use of stone without soft tissue moulage can also be done alternatively, only if bone-level type implants have been placed and small amount of wax is added on the impression coping-analog interface.

First, the stone is mixed manually with distilled water for 15 s to aid the incorporation of the water and then under vacuum, and an initial pour of stone up to the middle of the analogs is carried out. All of the stone mixes are vibrated before and during the pouring. After 30 min, the second pour of vacuum-mixed die stone is done. This double pouring technique minimizes the volumetric expansion of the stone and has been shown to lead in more accurate working casts. A case is illustrated (Fig. 10.3a–f).

10.6 Checklist and Step-by-Step Protocol to Maximize Impression Accuracy

For implant impressions in the aesthetic zone, the customized impression coping technique is recommended. Regarding implant impressions in the anterior aesthetic zone, there are various scenarios.

Clinical scenario	Impression technique	Customized impression coping	Splint or not	Cast verification	Pouring technique
Single implant in the aesthetic zone	Either open or closed tray	Yes	No	No	Stone, with or without soft tissue moulage
Two adjacent single implants in the aesthetic zone	Either open or closed tray	Yes	Yes if splinted restorations No if individual restorations	Yes if splinted restorations No if individual restorations	Stone, with or without soft tissue moulage
Multiple implants in the aesthetic zone	Open tray	Yes	Yes	Yes	Stone, with or without soft tissue moulage

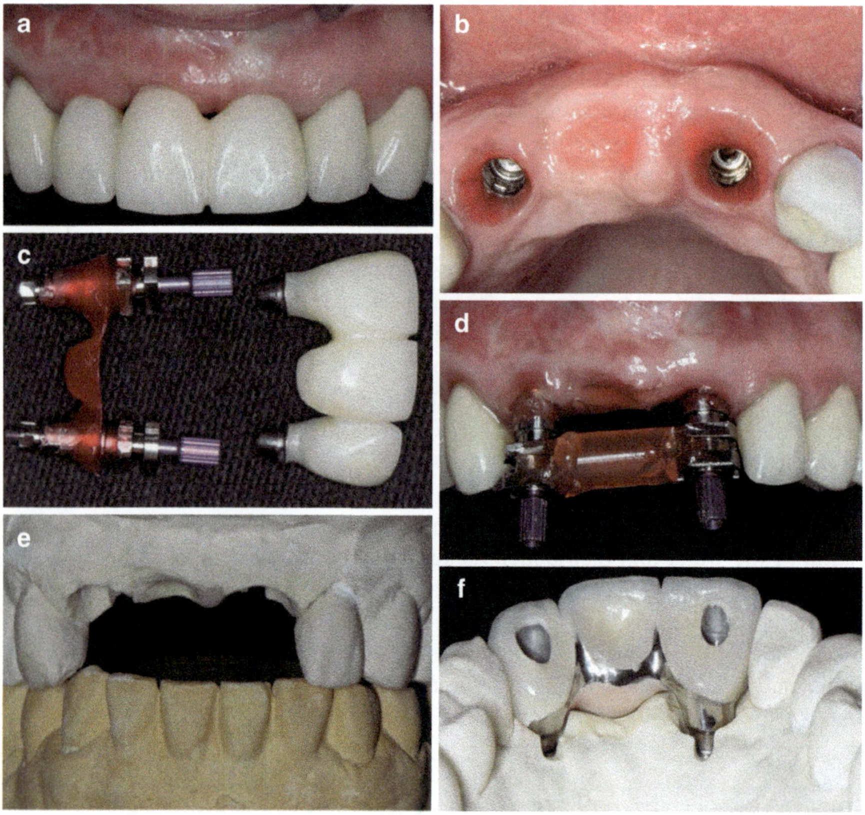

Fig. 10.3 (**a**) Missing right lateral and central incisors and left central incisor (#7, 8, and 9) were replaced with two dental implants for a three-unit implant-supported fixed dental prosthesis (FDP). After successful osseointegration, peri-implant soft tissue conditioning was done for a period of 3 months with a provisional screw-retained FDP. (**b**) Partially edentulous area after peri-implant soft tissue conditioning. (**c**) Customized impression copings duplicating the transmucosal part of the provisional implant FDP. The indirect technique was used for fabrication of the customized copings. (**d**) Customized impression copings placed intraorally, after removal of the provisional implant FDP. Copings are splinted together with prefabricated light polymerized resin bar, in order to enhance the accuracy of the implant impression. Minimal amount of light polymerizing resin was used to lute the prefabricated resin bars to the copings. (**e**) Working cast poured only in stone without soft tissue moulage. The customized impression copings have captured the transmucosal part of the provisional implant FDP, guiding the laboratory technician to precisely duplicate the transmucosal part into the emergence profile of the final FDP. (**f**) Screw-retained final FDP seated on the working cast. The emergence profile and transmucosal contours of the final FDP are a duplicate of the provisional FDP, captured with the customized implant impression. Note the palatal windows to confirm accurate seating of the FDP to the implant prosthetic platforms

References

1. Gallucci GO, Benic GI, Eckert SE, Papaspyridakos P, Schimmel M, Schrott A, Weber HP. Consensus statements and clinical recommendations for implant loading protocols. Int J Oral Maxillofac Implants. 2014;29(Suppl):287–90.
2. Jemt T, Hjalmarsson L. In vitro measurements of precision of fit of implant-supported frameworks. A comparison between "virtual" and "physical" assessments of fit using two different techniques of measurements. Clin Implant Dent Relat Res. 2012;14(Suppl 1):e175–82.
3. de Torres EM, Barbosa GA, Bernardes SR, de Mattos Mda G, Ribeiro RF. Correlation between vertical misfits and stresses transmitted to implants from metal frameworks. J Biomech. 2011;44:1735–9.
4. Duyck J, Naert I. Influence of prosthesis fit and the effect of a luting system on the prosthetic connection preload: an in vitro study. Int J Prosthodont. 2002;15:389–96.
5. Eckert SE, Meraw SJ, Cal E, Ow RK. Analysis of incidence and associated factors with fractured implants: a retrospective study. Int J Oral Maxillofac Implants. 2002;15:662–7.
6. Papaspyridakos P, Chen CJ, Chuang SK, Weber HP, Gallucci GO. A systematic review of biologic and technical complications with fixed implant rehabilitations for edentulous patients. Int J Oral Maxillofac Implants. 2012;27:102–10.
7. Papaspyridakos P, Lal K, White GS, Weber HP, Gallucci GO. Effect of splinted and non-splinted impression techniques on the accuracy of fit of fixed implant prostheses in edentulous patients: a comparative study. Int J Oral Maxillofac Implants. 2011;26:1267–72.
8. Papaspyridakos P, Chen CJ, Gallucci GO, Doukoudakis A, Weber HP, Chronopoulos V. Accuracy of implant impressions for partially and completely edentulous patients: a systematic review. Int J Oral Maxillofac Implants. 2014;29:836–45.
9. Chai J, Takahashi Y, Lautenschlager EP. Clinically relevant mechanical properties of elastomeric impression materials. Int J Prosthodont. 1998;11:219–23.
10. Akca K, Cehreli MC. Accuracy of 2 impression techniques for ITI implants. Int J Oral Maxillofac Implants. 2004;19:517–23.
11. Assuncao WG, et al. Accuracy of impression techniques for implants. Part 1-influence of transfer copings surface abrasion. J Prosthodont. 2008;17:641–7.
12. Assuncao WG, et al. Prosthetic transfer impression accuracy evaluation for osseointegrated implants. Implant Dent. 2008;17:248–56.
13. Assuncao WG, Filho HG, Zaniquelli O. Evaluation of transfer impressions for osseointegrated implants at various angulations. Implant Dent. 2004;13:358–66.
14. Cabral LM, Guedes CG. Comparative analysis of 4 impression techniques for implants. Implant Dent. 2007;16:187–94.
15. Choi JH, et al. Evaluation of the accuracy of implant-level impression techniques for internal-connection implant prostheses in parallel and divergent models. Int J Oral Maxillofac Implants. 2007;22:761–8.
16. Inturregui JA, et al. Evaluation of three impression techniques for osseointegrated oral implants. J Prosthet Dent. 1993;69:503–9.
17. Filho HG, et al. Accuracy of impression techniques for implants. Part 2 - comparison of splinting techniques. J Prosthodont. 2009;18:172–6.
18. Lee HJ, et al. Accuracy of a proposed implant impression technique using abutments and metal framework. J Adv Prosthodont. 2010;2:25–31.
19. Lee YJ, et al. Accuracy of different impression techniques for internal-connection implants. Int J Oral Maxillofac Implants. 2009;24:823–30.
20. Rutkunas V, Sveikata K, Savickas R. Effects of implant angulation, material selection, and impression technique on impression accuracy: a preliminary laboratory study. Int J Prosthodont. 2012;25:512–5.
21. Tarib NA, et al. Evaluation of splinting implant impression techniques: two dimensional analyses. Eur J Prosthodont Restor Dent. 2012;20:35–9.
22. Yamamoto E, et al. Accuracy of four transfer impression techniques for dental implants: a scanning electron microscopic analysis. Int J Oral Maxillofac Implants. 2010;25:1115–24.

23. Al-Abdullah K, et al. An in vitro comparison of the accuracy of implant impressions with coded healing abutments and different implant angulations. J Prosthet Dent. 2013;110:90–100.
24. Mojon P, Oberholzer JP, Meyer JM, Belser UC. Polymerization shrinkage of index and pattern acrylic resins. J Prosthet Dent. 1990;64:684–8.
25. Gracis S, Michalakis K, Vigolo P, Vult von Steyern P, Zwahlen M, Sailer I. Internal vs. external connections for abutments/reconstructions: a systematic review. Clin Oral Implants Res. 2012;23(Suppl 6):202–16.
26. Alikhasi M, et al. Three-dimensional accuracy of implant and abutment level impression techniques: effect on marginal discrepancy. J Oral Implantol. 2011;37:649–57.
27. Carr AB. Comparison of impression techniques for a two-implant 15-degree divergent model. Int J Oral Maxillofac Implants. 1992;7:468–75.
28. Cehreli MC, Akca K. Impression techniques and misfit-induced strains on implant-supported superstructures: an in vitro study. Int J Periodontics Restorative Dent. 2006;26:379–85.
29. Conrad HJ, et al. Accuracy of two impression techniques with angulated implants. J Prosthet Dent. 2007;97:349–56.
30. De La Cruz JE, et al. Verification jig for implant-supported prostheses: a comparison of standard impressions with verification jigs made of different materials. J Prosthet Dent. 2002;88:329–36.
31. Howell KJ, et al. Comparison of the accuracy of Biomet 3i Encode Robocast Technology and conventional implant impression techniques. Int J Oral Maxillofac Implants. 2013;28:228–40.
32. Gallucci GO, Papaspyridakos P, Chen CJ, Kim EG, Brady NJ, Weber HP. Clinical accuracy outcomes of closed-tray and open-tray implant impression techniques for partially edentulous patients. Int J Prosthodont. 2011;24:469–72.
33. Jo SH, et al. Effect of impression coping and implant angulation on the accuracy of implant impressions: an in vitro study. J Adv Prosthodont. 2010;2:128–33.
34. Wegner K, Zenginel M, Rehmann P, Wöstmann B. Effects of implant system, impression technique, and impression material on accuracy of the working cast. Int J Oral Maxillofac Implants. 2013;28:989–95.
35. Wostmann B, Rehmann P, Balkenhol M. Influence of impression technique and material on the accuracy of multiple implant impressions. Int J Prosthodont. 2008;21:299–301.
36. Daoudi MF, Setchell DJ, Searson LJ. A laboratory investigation of the accuracy of two impression techniques for single-tooth implants. Int J Prosthodont. 2001;14:152–8.
37. Daoudi MF, Setchell DJ, Searson LJ. An evaluation of three implant level impression techniques for single tooth implant. Eur J Prosthodont Restor Dent. 2004;12:9–14.
38. Chochlidakis KM, Papaspyridakos P, Geminiani A, Chen CJ, Feng IJ, Ercoli C. Digital versus conventional impressions for fixed prosthodontics: a systematic review and meta-analysis. J Prosthet Dent. 2016;116:184–90.
39. Ender A, Attin T, Mehl A. In vivo precision of conventional and digital methods of obtaining complete-arch dental impressions. J Prosthet Dent. 2016;115:313–20.
40. Papaspyridakos P, Gallucci GO, Chen CJ, Hanssen S, Naert I, Vandenberghe B. Digital versus conventional implant impressions for edentulous patients: accuracy outcomes. Clin Oral Implants Res. 2016;27:465–72.
41. Gherlone E, Cappare P, Vinci R, Ferrini F, Gastaldi G, Crespi R. Conventional versus digital impressions for "all-on-four" restorations. Int J Oral Maxillofac Implants. 2016;31:324–30.
42. Gimenez-Gonzalez B, Hassan B, Ozcan M, Pradies G, et al. J Prosthodont. 2017;26:650. [Epub ahead of print].
43. Vandeweghe S, Vervack V, Dierens M, De Bruyn H. Accuracy of digital impressions of multiple dental implants: an in vitro study. Clin Oral Implants Res. 2017;28:648. [Epub ahead of print].
44. Lee SJ, Betensky RA, Gianneschi GE, Gallucci GO. Accuracy of digital versus conventional implant impressions. Clin Oral Implants Res. 2015;26:715–9.
45. Lin WS, Harris BT, Elathamna EN, Abdel-Azim T, Morton D. Effect of implant divergence on the accuracy of definitive casts created from traditional and digital implant-level impressions: an in vitro comparative study. Int J Oral Maxillofac Implants. 2015;30:102–9.

46. Joda T, Bragger U. Digital vs. conventional implant prosthetic workflows: a cost/time analysis. Clin Oral Implants Res. 2015;26:1430–5.
47. Joda T, Katsoulis J, Brägger U. Clinical fitting and adjustment time for implant-supported crowns comparing digital and conventional workflows. Clin Implant Dent Relat Res. 2016;18:946–54.
48. Schepke U, Meijer HJ, Kerdijk W, Cune MS. Digital versus analog complete-arch impressions for single-unit premolar implant crowns: operating time and patient preference. J Prosthet Dent. 2015;114:403–6.
49. Wismeijer D, Bragger U, Evans C, Kapos T, Kelly JR, Millen C, et al. Consensus statements and recommended clinical procedures regarding restorative materials and techniques for implant dentistry. Int J Oral Maxillofac Implants. 2014;29(Suppl):137–40.
50. Karl M, Graef F, Schubinski P, Taylor T. Effect of intraoral scanning on the passivity of fit of implant-supported fixed dental prostheses. Quintessence Int. 2012;43:555–62.
51. Schoenbaum TR, Han TJ. Direct custom implant impression copings for the preservation of the pontic receptor site architecture. J Prosthet Dent. 2012;107:203–6.
52. Lops D, Bressan E, Cea N, Sbricoli L, Guazzo R, Scanferla M, Romeo E. Reproducibility of buccal gingival profile using a custom pick-up impression technique: a 2-year prospective multicenter study. J Esthet Restor Dent. 2016;28:43–55.
53. Tan WL, Wong TL, Wong MC, Lang NP. A systematic review of post-extractional alveolar hard and soft tissue dimensional changes in humans. Clin Oral Implants Res. 2012;23(Suppl 5):1–21.
54. Jang HK, Kim S, Shim JS, Lee KW, Moon HS. Accuracy of impressions for internal-connection implant prostheses with various divergent angles. Int J Oral Maxillofac Implants. 2011;26:1011–5.
55. Sorrentino R, Gherlone EF, Calesini G, Zarone F. Effect of implant angulation, connection length, and impression material on the dimensional accuracy of implant impressions: an in vitro comparative study. Clin Implant Dent Relat Res. 2010;12(Suppl 1):e63–76.
56. Burns J, Palmer R, Howe L, Wilson R. Accuracy of open tray implant impressions: an in vitro comparison of stock versus custom trays. J Prosthet Dent. 2003;89:250–5.
57. Gökçen-Rohlig B, Ongül D, Sancakli E, Sermet B. Comparative evaluation of the effects of implant position, impression material, and tray type on implant impression accuracy. Implant Dent. 2014;23:283–8.
58. Del'Acqua MA, Arioli-Filho JN, Compagnoni MA, Mollo Fde A Jr. Accuracy of impression and pouring techniques for an implant-supported prosthesis. Int J Oral Maxillofac Implants. 2008;23:226–36.
59. Del'Acqua MA, Chavez AM, Amaral AL, Compagnoni MA, Mollo Fde A Jr. Comparison of impression techniques and materials for an implant-supported prosthesis. Int J Oral Maxillofac Implants. 2010;25:771–6.
60. Papaspyridakos P, Benic GI, Hogsett VL, White GS, Lal K, Gallucci GO. Accuracy of implant casts generated with splinted and non-splinted impression techniques for edentulous patients: an optical scanning study. Clin Oral Implants Res. 2012;23:676–81.
61. Cheshire PD, Hobkirk JA. An in vivo quantitative analysis of the fit of Nobel Biocare implant superstructures. J Oral Rehabil. 1996;23:782–9.
62. Ma T, Nicholls JI, Rubenstein JE. Tolerance measurements of various implant components. Int J Oral Maxillofac Implants. 1997;12:371–5.
63. Gimenez B, Ozcan M, Martinez-Rus F, Pradies G. Accuracy of a digital impression system based on parallel confocal laser technology for implants with consideration of operator experience and implant angulation and depth. Int J Oral Maxillofac Implants. 2014;29:853–62.
64. Gimenez B, Ozcan M, Martinez-Rus F, Pradies G. Accuracy of a digital impression system based on active wavefront sampling technology for implants considering operator experience, implant angulation, and depth. Clin Implant Dent Relat Res. 2015;17(Suppl 1):e54–64.
65. Schoenbaum TR, Swift EJ Jr. Contours for single-unit implants. J Esthet Restor Dent. 2015;27:1–3.

66. Chu SJ, Salama MA, Salama H, Garber DA, Saito H, Sarnachiaro GO, Tarnow DP. The dual-zone therapeutic concept of managing immediate implant placement and provisional restoration in anterior extraction sockets. Compend Contin Educ Dent. 2012;33:524–32.
67. Martin WC, Pollini A, Morton D. The influence of restorative procedures on esthetic outcomes in implant dentistry: a systematic review. Int J Oral Maxillofac Implants. 2014; 29(Suppl):142–54.

Emergence Profile of the Implant Abutment and Its Effects on the Peri-implant Tissues

11

Todd R. Schoenbaum and Sam Alawie

Abstract

The emergence profile is the portion of the implant-abutment-restoration complex that extends from the bone crest to the free gingival margin. Generally this area is made up of the abutment, though in screw-retained restorations, it is part of the restoration as a whole. This area is critical to the long-term health and aesthetics of the rehabilitation in the aesthetic zone. The shape of the emergence profile is responsible for creating and maintaining the soft tissue architecture. This proves especially important in the immediate load treatment scenario. It is critical that the restoring doctor have and understanding of the effects the emergence profile will have on the positioning of the soft tissues. Changes to the emergence profile (particularly during the healing stages) can be strategically used to move the tissues apically or coronally and to shape the papilla.

Following surgical placement of the implant and any additional augmentation, the fine-tuning of the soft tissues (Fig. 11.1) will be largely dependent on the emergence profile of the abutment (Fig. 11.2). In the aesthetic zone, this is a process best accomplished through the use of a proper provisional restoration or custom healing abutment. When sufficient implant stability exists at placement (i.e., ISQ > 65) [1], it is generally easier to preserve and maintain the peri-implant soft tissues with an immediately placed provisional restoration. In cases where implant stability is questionable, the implant should be treated in a two-stage approach or with a custom healing

T. R. Schoenbaum
Division of Constitutive and Regenerative Sciences, University of California, Los Angeles, CA, USA
e-mail: tschoenb@ucla.edu

S. Alawie
Owner/Ceramist Beverly Hills Dental Lab, Beverly Hills, CA, USA

Todd R. Schoenbaum (ed.), *Implants in the Aesthetic Zone*,
https://doi.org/10.1007/978-3-319-72601-4_11

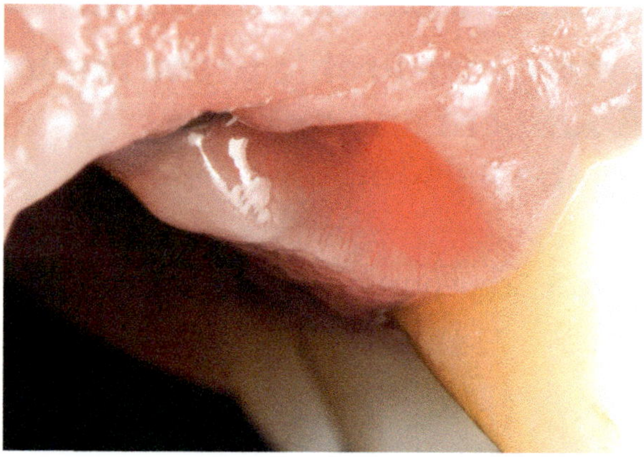

Fig. 11.1 Successful treatment of implants in the aesthetic zone requires proper shaping of the soft tissue with the provisional restorations. The surgical foundation sets the stage for the prosthetic fine-tuning of the gingiva. Inadequate bone and soft tissue cannot be overcome with tissue shaping

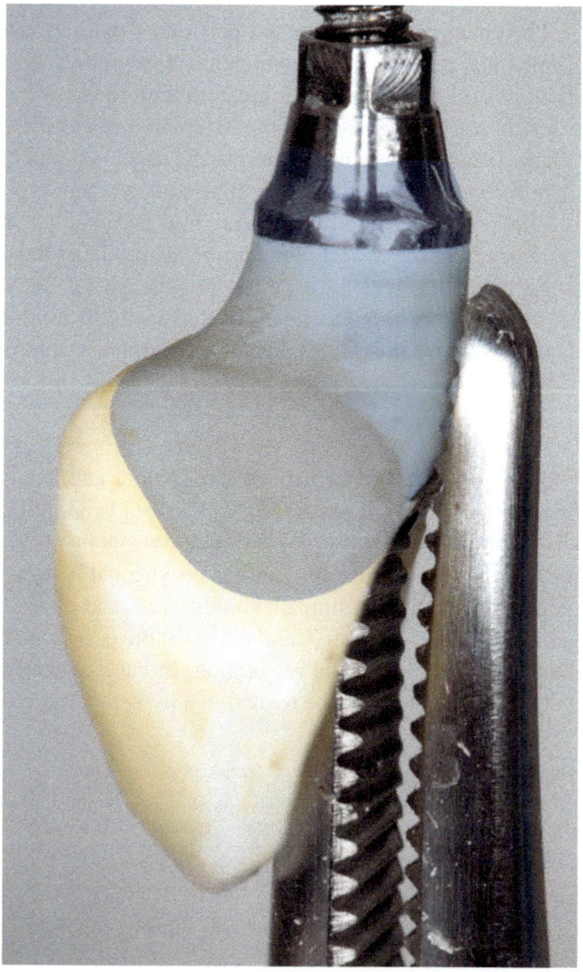

Fig. 11.2 The emergence area of the abutment is defined by the area from the head of the implant to the free gingival margins (here, highlighted in blue). This area is responsible for the final shaping of the peri-implant tissues

abutment. In the latter case, special care must be given to ensure that the removable provisional restoration does not negatively affect the soft tissues during maturation and osseointegration. The shape of the emergence profile can be altered to move the tissues to the desired position (with some genetic and biologic limitations) [2–4]; however, removal and alteration of the abutment should be delayed until at least 3 months after implant placement, and the number of times should be limited [5]. There is solid histological evidence that repeated removal of components from the implant traumatizes the tissues and results in significant loss of bone and soft tissue. This is especially true during the first few months of healing and maturation. Dr. Vela and Dr. Rodriguez provide an in-depth look at this process in the last chapter.

This chapter will focus on the emergence profile of the provisional restoration fabricated and delivered at the time of immediate implant placement to replace a single tooth in the aesthetic zone. Similar concepts should be applied for the use of a custom healing abutment or delivery of a provisional restoration at the stage 2 surgery. More information on the fabrication of provisional restorations can be found in Chap. 8.

11.1 The Peri-implant Tissues: Tooth vs. Implant

Surrounding the natural tooth is a densely collagenous gingiva made up of type 1 collagen. The periodontal gingival fibers are anchored into the cementum on the root surface via Sharpey's fibers, the same mechanism through which the periosteum is attached to the underlying bone. The gingival fibers serve to protect the tooth from the oral environment and provide anchorage for the gingiva. The fibers are categorized by their location and orientation into five groups: gingivodental fibers, transseptal fibers, semicircular fibers, transgingival fibers, and circular fibers. All but the last type (circular fibers) insert *into* the cementum of the tooth root. This is important to note, as the circular fibers are the *only* type present around the dental implant [6–8]. The other fiber types are still present around the implant, but upon encountering the implant surface lacking cementum, they persist in encircling the implant, functionally becoming *circular fibers* [9]. Lacking cementum and any mechanism for proper insertion of the fibers, this leaves the implant more vulnerable to trauma from the oral environment. This also will leave the peri-implant gingiva less stable and more prone to recession.

As the soft tissues mature, the myofibroblasts contract the length of the circular fibers. This contraction will take place over the weeks following surgery [9]. Ultimately, what develops is analogous to an O-ring and serves as the only means of protecting the bone-implant interface. In older flared neck implant designs, the contraction and tightening of the circular fibers moved the "O-ring" apically, taking the bone and soft tissue with it [10]. This results in the typical bone loss to the first thread. The reason the bone is lost to the first thread in older implant designs is likely due to this being the first place on the implant where a tightening O-ring finds a broad base. In more modern implant designs with abutments that are narrower than the implant base, the O-ring tightens at that position, generally resulting in reduced losses of the bone and soft tissue. Further innovation of this concept is described in the last chapter.

The circular fiber O-ring must be disturbed as little as possible. As described by Dr. Abrahamsson's histological study [5], repeated (non-traumatic) disturbances of this area result in significant amounts of bone and soft tissue loss. The effects appear to be most dramatic in the first months following placement.

11.2 Platform Switched Implants and the Narrow Abutment Concept

At a basic level, the "platform-switched" (PS) implant design is one in which the abutment is a narrower diameter than the implant at the interface. Most (though not all) data show that this design maintains peri-implant bone levels better than older designs [11–16]. This works by a few mechanisms (Fig. 11.3). One, the PS implant moves the implant-abutment-junction (IAJ) medially, away from the bone. In nearly every two piece implant ever tested long term, there is a bacterial exudate

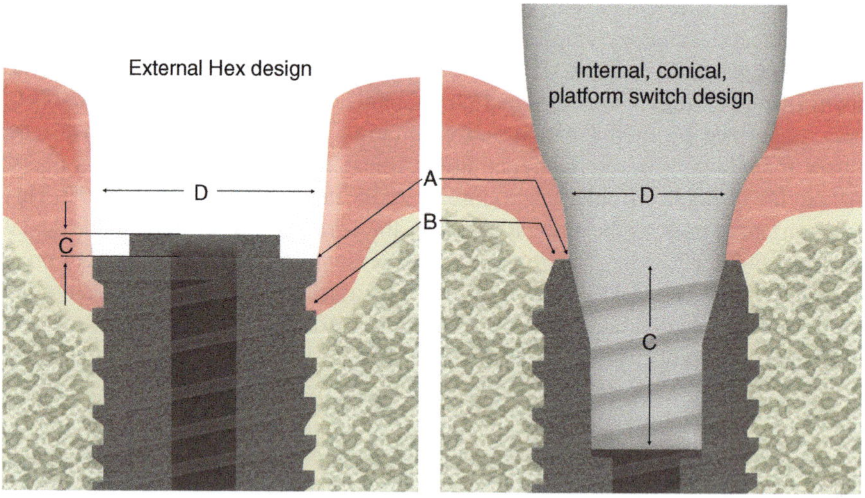

Fig. 11.3 On the left side of this diagram, an older, external hex connection implant is represented; while on the right, an internal, conical, platform-switched connection implant is depicted. The evolution from external hex to the internal conical PS design was brought about in an attempt to reduce bone loss and screw loosening. This implant has the following advantages: (**a**) The implant-abutment-junction (IAJ) is located medially, away from the bone. (**b**) The head of the implant acts like a shelf where the circular peri-implant fibers can tighten without slipping down to the first thread. (**c**) The connection is generally longer and more robust, resulting in less movement and leakage of the abutment over time. (**d**) The emergence area of the abutment is narrower, allowing more room for the bone, peri-implant tissues, and blood supply

that is pumped out from inside the implant at this junction [14, 17]. Moving the IAJ away from the bone may lessen the insult on the bone. Two, the PS implant results in a shelf upon which the gingival fiber O-ring tightens [9, 10]. This is analogous to the first thread in older implant designs but located more coronally and thus allows the bone to be maintained at a higher level. Three, many PS implants were designed in conjunction with more robust connections (compared to the older external hex designs). Some of these connections have a tapered interface which seems to increase the rigidity and durability of the IAJ. This is commonly referred to as a "Morse taper" design, though most implants do not actually have connections that fit any of the 1.5° Morse taper specifications. Nevertheless, the long internal connections seem to produce less leakage at the IAJ compared to the short external hex connections [17, 18]. Lastly, the PS implant, by design, has an abutment that is narrower than the implant. The smooth surface of the titanium (or Zr or Au) abutment is not amenable to bony attachment, so moving this non-integrating surface away from the bone allows the bone to be maintained at a higher position. Conversly, in older style implants the abutment widens directly off the IAJ, which forces the bone to reestablish at a lower position.

The narrowed abutment concept is an attempt to forgo the dimensions of the preexisting root and instead create a peri-implant environment that is more suitable to the unique soft tissue around an implant. PS implants have narrowed abutments by design, but even some non-PS implants can (and should) have the emergence area of the abutment narrowed [3].

The *theoretical* rational for the narrow abutment is that it allows a greater volume of soft tissue to encircle and protect the implant. This greater volume allows more room for the initial blood clot to stabilize, allows more room for postoperative swelling, and allows more room for blood supply of the peri-implant tissues [9, 19]. The above rational is a theory only; we do not yet have the science to explain precisely why narrowed abutment emergence areas generally preserve the bone and soft tissue at higher levels. Though the approach may be evolving (see Chap. 16), currently suggested emergence designs should start narrow out of the implant and progress through a "wine glass" shape as they approach their widest dimension at the gingival margin. This design allows the additional subgingival space for soft tissues and blood supply while providing proper support of the prosthesis.

If a cement-retained crown is to be used, the margins of the abutment should be placed no deeper than 1 mm subgingival [20, 21] as explained in Chap. 12. If a screw-retained restoration is to be used, the technician must pay special attention to the emergence area. It is quite common to see less experienced or less attentive technicians create restorations that are grossly overcontoured in the emergence area (Fig. 11.4). This makes delivery of the restoration difficult and may require additional surgical procedures to complete. It also puts extreme pressure on the peri-implant tissues. In the short term, this pressure causes blanching and is uncomfortable; in the long term, it results in unnecessary apical migration of the bone and gingiva. These subtle changes in the emergence shapes can be skillfully used to fine-tune the position of the soft tissue in the aesthetic zone.

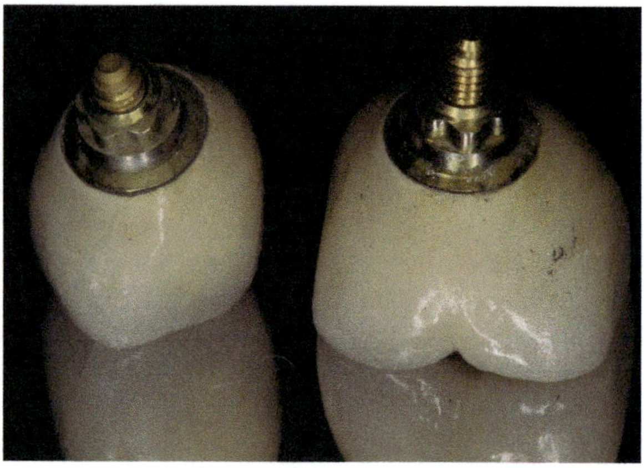

Fig. 11.4 It is not uncommon to see restorations that are overcontoured directly from the head of the implant. This will generally result in migration of the bone and soft tissues to a more apical position

11.3 Fine-Tuning Soft Tissue Position Through Alterations to the Emergence Profile

The process of manipulating and moving the peri-implant soft tissues can be accomplished to a certain degree through the modification of the emergence profile of the abutment. This is a procedure best accomplished during the provisional stage as the definitive titanium, zirconia, or gold alloy abutment is not easily modified once it has been fabricated. The composite or acrylic provisional abutment on the other hand can be easily shaped or added to.

Before we address the particular techniques of tissue shaping with the emergence modification, we need to understand that the final position of the soft tissues are only *partially* shaped by the provisional restoration [22]. The other major factors are implant position/size/type, existing dimensions of the bone and gingiva, and patient genetics. Studies that have taken a cross section of the population and examined their papilla lengths have shown that papilla height ultimately falls on a bell curve [23]. And not unlike the height of our bodies, some patients are short and some are tall, while most fall in the middle. We cannot change the patient's genetics, and by the time the patient is seen for restoration, it may be too late to change many of the other factors as well. As explained in Chap. 1, a collaborative treatment planning approach will increase the overall success and predictability. Challenges with implant position/type, bone and gingival dimensions, etc. should all be addressed prior to initiating definitive restorative treatment. With that being said, we can use the emergence area of the provisional restoration to enhance the gingival position, overall outcome, and to serve as a blueprint for the definitive abutment (Fig. 11.5).

On a basic level, the abutment emergence profile can be overcontoured (Fig. 11.6a) or undercontoured (Fig. 11.6b). Overcontouring places pressure on the soft tissue and will push it apically. Undercontouring will allow space for the soft tissue to drape or migrate coronally. It is the latter effect which is most desirable around implants especially for the papilla. But, as previously mentioned, the extent to which it will move coronally is somewhat dependent on genetics and the success of previous surgical procedures (Fig. 11.7a–d).

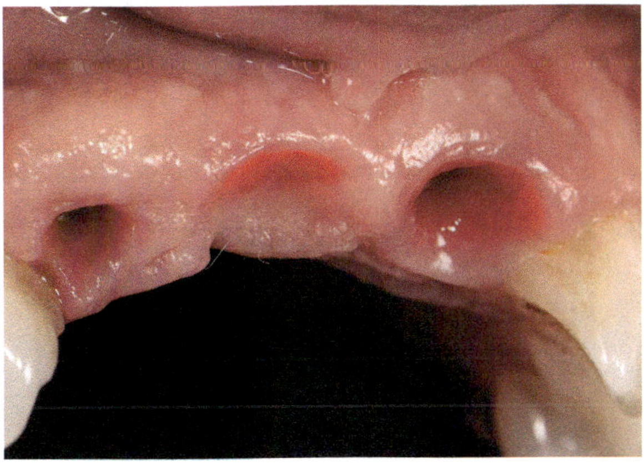

Fig. 11.5 Here a provisional three-unit FDP on two implants has been used to shape the peri-implant tissues and pontic site. It was left in place for at least 6 weeks (Surgery by Dr. Joan Pi-Anfruns)

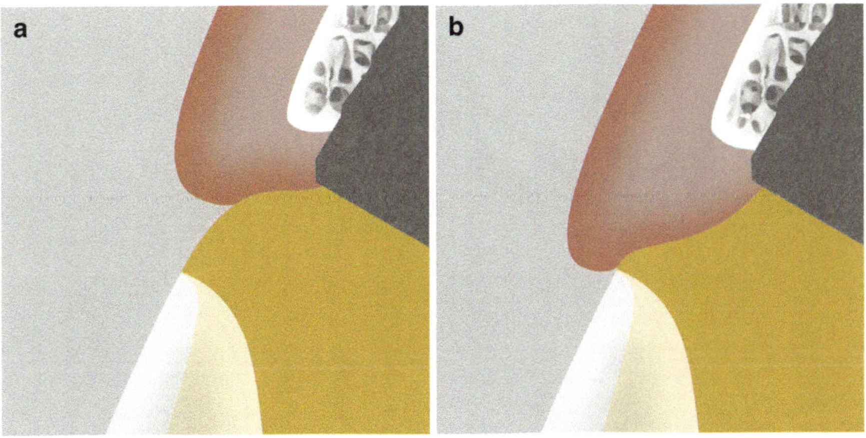

Fig. 11.6 (**a**) Overcontouring the facial area of the emergence will push the tissues apically. This can be useful to elongate the appearance of a tooth. However, this emergence profile should be avoided in the initial healing stages. (**b**) In the immediate implant placement and provisionalization, the facial surface should be significantly undercountoured to allow for swelling, blood supply, and apical migration of the peri-implant tissues. This will generally provide for an excess of tissue, which is advantageous around implants

Overcontouring is useful in two applications: to move and shape the gingival zenith apically to match the contralateral positions and to close gingival embrasure spaces. Around implants in the aesthetic zone, one of the most difficult challenges continues to be deficient papilla. It is not uncommon to hear of the papilla being like a "water balloon" that if compressed at its base will force the tip of it to move coronally. There are a few issues with this idea for our current discussion. This concept comes from manipulation of papilla between natural teeth. As explained early in this chapter, there is no cementum for the soft tissues to insert into to support a

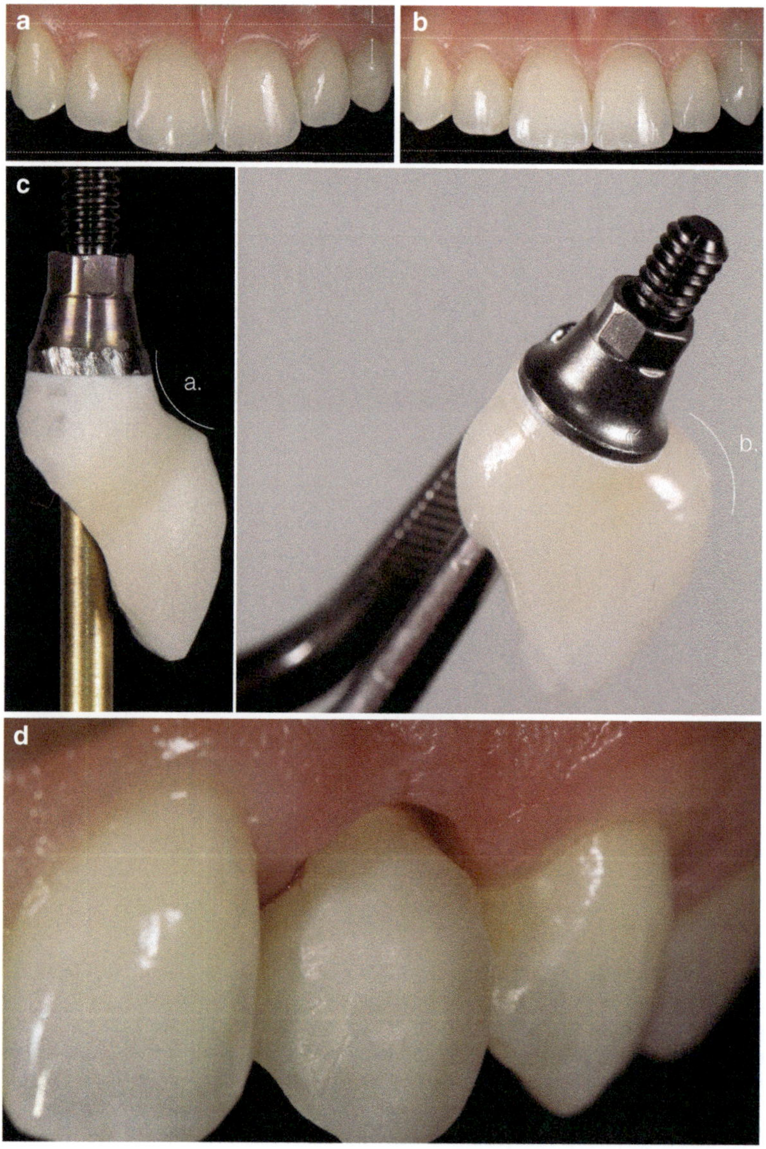

Fig. 11.7 (**a**) This patient has had an implant and provisional restoration placed on the upper left canine. Notice the coronal positioning of the gingival zenith due to the undercountoured emergence profile on the provisional. (**b**) Here the definitive restoration is being tried in. Note that it has been purposefully designed with an overcontoured surface on the facial to push the tissues apically and extend the visual length of the canine. The blanching occurs during the initial tightening of the restoration and should subside over the course of the appointment. No anesthesia is required for this procedure, but care must be taken to progress slowly. (**c**) On the left, we can see the undercontoured facial emergence of the provisional designed to increase tissue volumes. On the right, we can see the overcontoured facial design of the definitive restoration, used to push tissue apically. (**d**) After being in position for 15 min, the overcontoured definitive restoration was removed for additional staining. The provisional was put back into position. Note the significant amount of tissue movement from the change in contour

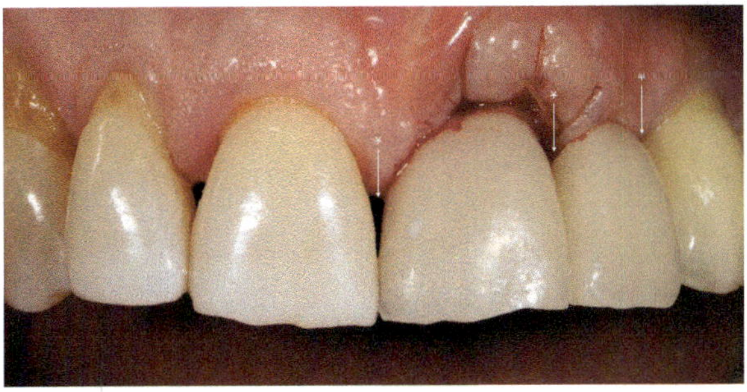

Fig. 11.8 When fabricating the emergence of the provisional restoration, the gingival embrasures should be left open to allow for the papilla to migrate coronally. Every patient does not have the same papilla length, and we must allow for their unique papillary phenotype to reveal itself. If the embrasure is closed off prematurely, the length of the papilla will be stunted

higher position, only more titanium or zirconia. There is no long epithelial attachment on these materials, as there is on clean cementum. The compression of the papilla adjacent to an implant may provide increased length in the very short term (i.e., postop photos), but the increased pressure and contours are more likely to result in decreased blood supply (blanching) and recession over the long term. Again, a large part of where the papilla are or will be is dependent on factors outside the realm of the prosthesis. Dr. Joe Kan has described much of the science behind the peri-implant papilla in Chap. 9.

In the author's *opinion*, peri-implant papilla are best managed by allowing space in the gingival embrasure during the period following implant placement and provisionalization (Fig. 11.8). This allows time for the papilla to mature and migrate coronally to the greatest extent possible given the patient genetics and the hard and soft tissue foundation. The ultimate length of the papilla is not universal but could be represented by a bell curve (Fig. 11.9). Some patients will have papilla that migrate quite far, perhaps up to 7 mm from the crest of the bone, while others will have papilla no longer than 2 or 3 mm [23, 24]. The open gingival embrasure of the provisional restoration allows the clinician to see which part of the bell curve this particular patient falls on. The undercontoured emergence profile maximizes the amount of room for blood supply and postoperative swelling without traumatizing the tissues.

Following osseointegration and maturation of the gingiva, the soft tissue positions are evaluated. This should be performed at 12–16 weeks after placement of the implant and provisional restoration. If the papilla failed to fully fill the gingival embrasure, the remaining space (if desired) can be filled by the definitive prosthesis and perhaps a small restoration on the adjacent teeth. At this point, the position of the gingival margin and zenith are evaluated. If modification is desired, the provisional is removed and composite resin added to the areas where apical movement of the gingiva is desired. This procedure is adapted from the similar procedure used with traditional gingivectomies, to hold the tissues back while they mature. The number of times the provisional restoration is removed and modified should be limited. Repeated removal of components at the implant level has been

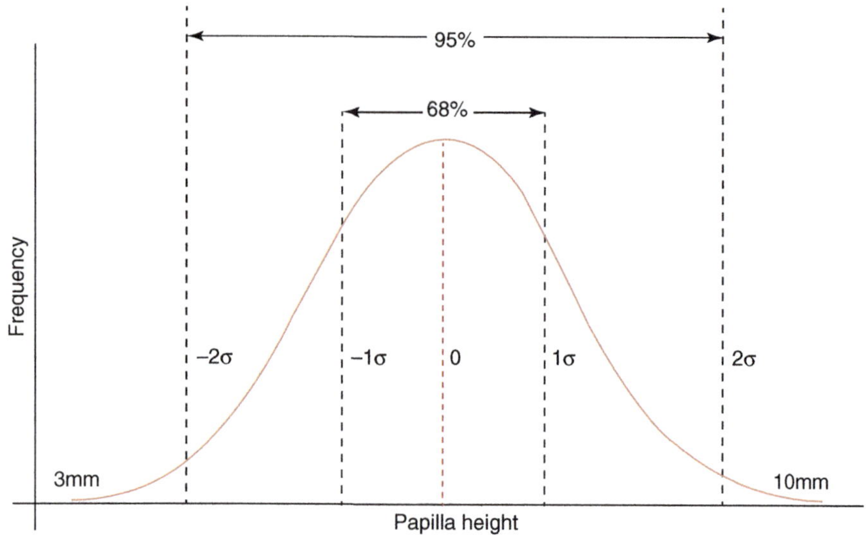

Fig. 11.9 Like most physiologic measurements, the length of the papilla falls along a typical bell curve. Some patients have very short papilla, no matter the surgeon, materials, emergence profiles, etc. Some patients may have papilla of 7 or more millimeters in length. Most evidence has shown that papilla between natural teeth are at least a 5 mm, while those around *reasonably* placed single implants average about 4 mm

shown to result in additional loss of bone and soft tissue, the exact opposite effect of what we are trying to accomplish. As such, removal and modification should not be performed in the first 3 months following implant placement, and it should be done at most once.

After the provisional restoration is modified and replaced, it should remain in place, undisturbed for 6 weeks. This allows sufficient time for the peri-implant soft tissue "O-ring" to develop and mature. It will continue to do so even after 6 weeks, but most of the change has occurred by then. At the 6-week reevaluation, final photos and impressions are made. The use of a custom impression coping (as described by Dr. Papaspyridakos in Chap. 10) should be used to ensure that the laboratory technician has an exact replica of the soft tissue in the patient's mouth.

11.4 Summary

Understanding the physiological effects of the emergence zone allows the clinician to carefully tune the definitive positions of the peri-implant soft tissues. The emergence profile of the abutment can be overcontoured to move tissue apically or undercontoured to allow tissue to move coronally. As described in this chapter, the clinician must carefully employ these concepts at the right time to achieve the best possible results. It should also be clearly understood that this technique is for "fine-tuning." Serious deficiencies of bone or soft tissue must be resolved surgically or with pink prosthetic materials.

References

1. Rowan M, Lee D, Pi-Anfruns J, Shiffler P, Aghaloo T, Moy PK. Mechanical versus biological stability of immediate and delayed implant placement using resonance frequency analysis. J Oral Maxillofac Surg. 2015;73(2):253–7.
2. De Rouck T, Collys K, Wyn I, Cosyn J. Instant provisionalization of immediate single-tooth implants is essential to optimize esthetic treatment outcome. Clin Oral Implants Res. 2009;20:566–70.
3. Schoenbaum TR, Chang YY, Klokkevold PR, Snowden JS. Abutment modification for immediate implant provisional restorations. J Esthet Restor Dent. 2013;25:103–7.
4. Schoenbaum TR, Swift EJ. Abutment emergence contours for single-unit implants. J Esthet Restor Dent. 2015;27(1):1–3.
5. Abrahamsson I, Berglundh T, Lindhe J. The mucosal barrier following abutment dis/reconnection. J Clin Periodontol. 1997;24(8):568–72.
6. Berglundh T, Lindhe J, Ericsson I, Marinello CP, Liljenberg B, Thornsen P. The soft tissue barrier at implants and teeth. Clin Oral Implants Res. 1991;2(2):81–90.
7. Lindhe J, Berglundh T, Ericsson I, Liljenberg B, Marinello C. Experimental breakdown of peri-implant and periodontal tissues. A study in the beagle dog. Clin Oral Implants Res. 1992;3(1):9–16.
8. Piattelli A, Scarano A, Piattelli M, Bertolai R, Panzoni E. Histologic aspects of the bone and soft tissues surrounding three titanium non-submerged plasma-sprayed implants retrieved at autopsy: a case report. J Periodontol. 1997;68(7):694–700.
9. Rodríguez X, Navajas A, Vela X, Fortuño A, Jimenez J, Nevins M. Arrangement of peri-implant connective tissue fibers around platform-switching implants with conical abutments and its relationship to the underlying bone: a human histologic study. Int J Periodontics Restorative Dent. 2016;36(4):533–40.
10. Rompen E, Raepsaet N, Domken O, Touati B, Dooren EV. Soft tissue stability at the facial aspect of gingivally converging abutments in the esthetic zone: a pilot clinical study. J Prosthet Dent. 2007;97:S119–25.
11. Crespi R, Capparè P, Gherlone E. Radiographic evaluation of marginal bone levels around platform-switched and non-platform-switched implants used in an immediate loading protocol. Int J Oral Maxillofac Implants. 2009;24(5):920–6.
12. Fickl S, Zuhr O, Stein JM, Hürzeler MB. Peri-implant bone level around implants with platform-switched abutments. Int J Oral Maxillofac Implants. 2010;25(3):577.
13. Hürzeler M, Fickl S, Zuhr O, Wachtel HC. Peri-implant bone level around implants with platform-switched abutments: preliminary data from a prospective study. J Oral Maxillofac Surg. 2007;65(7):33–9.
14. Lazzara RJ, Porter SS. Platform switching: a new concept in implant dentistry for controlling postrestorative crestal bone levels. Int J Periodontics Restorative Dent. 2006;26(1):9–17.
15. Pieri F, Aldini NN, Marchetti C, Corinaldesi G. Influence of implant-abutment interface design on bone and soft tissue levels around immediately placed and restored single-tooth implants: a randomized controlled clinical trial. Int J Oral Maxillofac Implants. 2011;26(1):169–78.
16. Trammell K, Geurs NC, O'Neal SJ, Liu PR, Haigh SJ, McNeal S, Kenealy JN, Reddy MS. A prospective, randomized, controlled comparison of platform-switched and matched-abutment implants in short-span partial denture situations. Int J Periodontics Restorative Dent. 2009;29(6):599–605.
17. Canullo L, Penarrocha-Oltra D, Soldini C, Mazzocco F, Penarrocha M, Covani U. Microbiological assessment of the implant-abutment interface in different connections: cross-sectional study after 5 years of functional loading. Clin Oral Implants Res. 2015;26(4):426–34.
18. Cássio do Nascimento DM, Paola Kirsten Miani DM, Pedrazzi V, Gonçalves RB, Ribeiro RF, Faria AC. Leakage of saliva through the implant-abutment interface: in vitro evaluation of three different implant connections under unloaded and loaded conditions. Int J Oral Maxillofac Implants. 2012;27(3):551–60.

19. Peñarrocha-Diago MA, Flichy-Fernández AJ, Alonso-González R, Peñarrocha-Oltra D, Balaguer-Martínez J, Peñarrocha-Diago M. Influence of implant neck design and implant–abutment connection type on peri-implant health. Radiological study. Clin Oral Implants Res. 2013;24(11):1192–200.
20. Linkevicius T, Vindasiute E, Puisys A, Linkeviciene L, Maslova N, Puriene A. The influence of the cementation margin position on the amount of undetected cement. A prospective clinical study. Clin Oral Implants Res. 2013;24(1):71–6.
21. Linkevicius T, Vindasiute E, Puisys A, Peciuliene V. The influence of margin location on the amount of undetected cement excess after delivery of cement-retained implant restorations. Clin Oral Implants Res. 2011;22(12):1379–84.
22. Lops D, Chiapasco M, Rossi A, Bressan E, Romeo E. Incidence of inter-proximal papilla between a tooth and an adjacent immediate implant placed into a fresh extraction socket: 1-year prospective study. Clin Oral Implants Res. 2008;19:1135–40.
23. Tarnow DP, Magner AW, Fletcher P. The effect of the distance from the contact point to the crest of bone on the presence or absence of the interproximal dental papilla. J Periodontol. 1992;63(12):995–6.
24. Tarnow DP, Elian N, Fletcher P, Froum S, Magner A, Cho SC, Salama M, Salama H, Garber DA. Vertical distance from the crest of bone to the height of the interproximal papilla between adjacent implants. J Periodontol. 2003;74(12):1785–8.

Cemented Implant Restorations in the Aesthetic Zone: Biological, Functional, and Aesthetic Considerations

12

Alireza Moshaverinia and Todd R. Schoenbaum

Abstract

Implant treatment in the aesthetic zone can be a challenging clinical situation, which requires high level of communication between the surgeon, the technician, and the restoring dentist. In this chapter, different abutment materials available in the market will be discussed, and the rationale for their applications, advantages, and disadvantages will be reviewed. Additionally, screw-retained and cement-retained implant-supported restorations will be briefly compared, and related clinical considerations will be discussed. Furthermore, abutment design parameters and technician factors will be reviewed. Finally, clinical guidelines will be provided to avoid complications and failures.

12.1 Rationale and Success Rates

Implant treatment in the aesthetic zone requires high levels of collaboration between the surgeon, the technician, and the restoring dentist. Selection and design of the definitive restoration/abutment is the final stage of the process. There is often much discussion about which restoration type (screw or cement retained) is better. Fortunately, many reviews have been performed on this topic looking at thousands of crowns from hundreds of dentists. Looking at the data, it becomes quite clear that either screw-retained or cement-retained single-unit crowns can be done with

A. Moshaverinia (✉)
Division of Advanced Prosthodontics, School of Dentistry, University of California, Los Angeles, Los Angeles, CA, USA
e-mail: amoshaverinia@dentistry.ucla.edu

T. R. Schoenbaum
Division of Constitutive and Regenerative Sciences, University of California, Los Angeles, CA, USA

Todd R. Schoenbaum (ed.), *Implants in the Aesthetic Zone*,
https://doi.org/10.1007/978-3-319-72601-4_12

equivalent success rates for both biologic and technical standpoints [1–5]. Technician-related factors (e.g., design), as well as abutment design parameters, set by the clinician certainly affect outcomes.

There are of course certain protocols that must be followed to minimize the risk of failure; with cemented restorations, we are particularly concerned about cement-induced peri-implantitis (Fig. 12.1) [6–8]. Complications will be discussed at the end of this chapter.

There are a few scenarios where a cemented restoration will be the superior choice (as there are also scenarios where a screw-retained option is better). With ideal implant placement, either option can generally be viable. The most obvious case in the aesthetic zone is when the implants are angled out through the facial (Fig. 12.2). This scenario is a relative contraindication to screw-retained restorations due to the screw access location on the incisal edge or on the facial surface. Some manufacturers have overcome this challenge by designing screws and drivers that can work up to 25° off axis.

A cemented option is also indicated when adjacent crowns or veneers are being placed. The rationale is that the technician cannot usually match a screw-retained PFM or PFZ restoration to the materials used for crowns/veneers in the aesthetic zone (Fig. 12.3a, b). For single-unit implant treatment in the aesthetic zone, most technicians can better replicate natural tooth aesthetics with a cemented restoration.

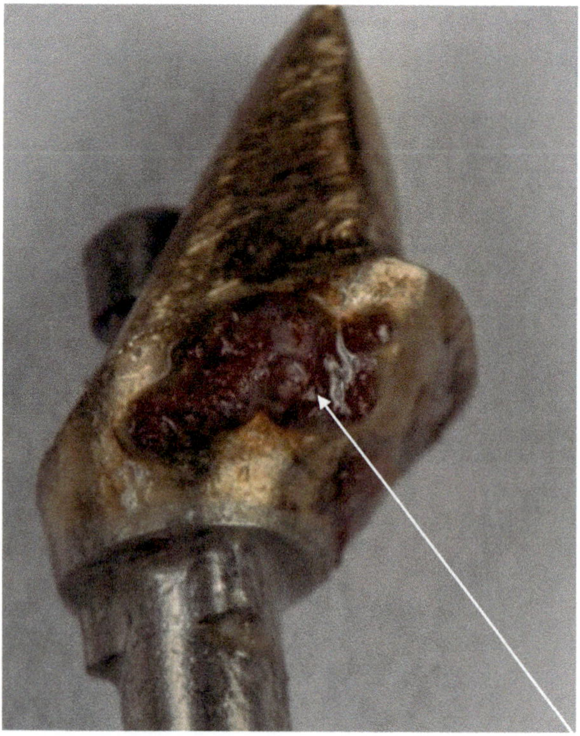

Fig. 12.1 Peri-implantitis has multiple possible etiologies, the most notorious of which is cement retained on the subgingival surface of the abutment. This problem is primarily caused by abutment margins that are too deep subgingivally

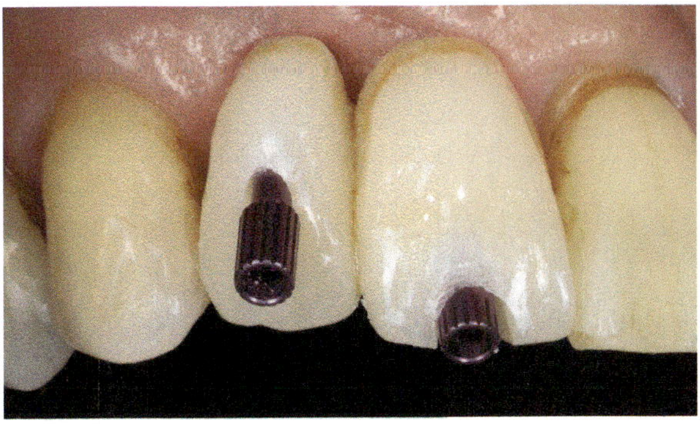

Fig. 12.2 For the partially edentulous patient, cemented restorations are particularly useful when implants have been placed with a facial angulation. There are some esoteric ways around the use of a cemented crown (i.e., angled screw channels, lingual set screws) in such scenarios, but they are proprietary or rarely employed. It is inevitable that restoring implants in the aesthetic zone will require the use of cemented restorations, and it is imperative that the clinician be able to perform this with a high level of success

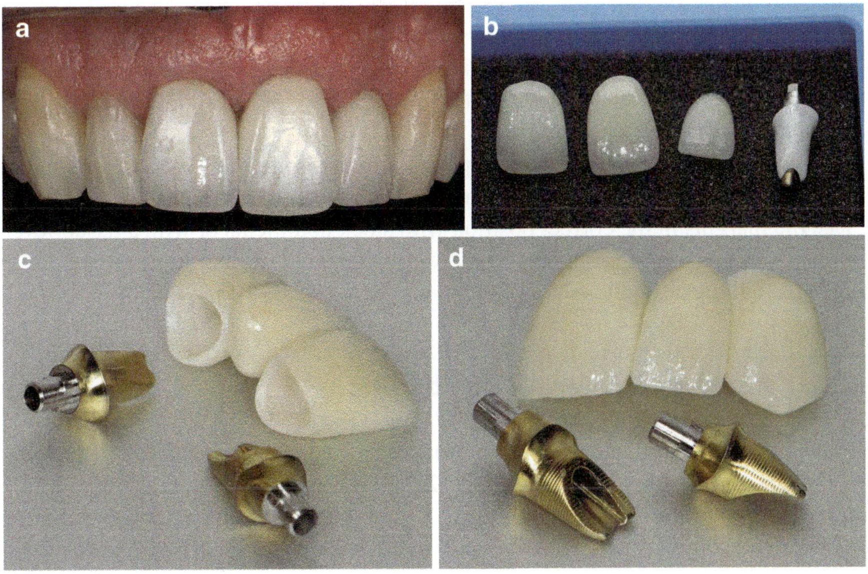

Fig. 12.3 (**a**) Cemented restorations are particularly useful for mixed treatment cases. (**b**) Here a crown, implant crown and a veneer have all been fabricated out of the same material (layered lithium disilicate) to ensure aesthetic harmony. Such results would be extremely difficult and unpredictable with a screw-retained implant PFM restoration. A three-unit-layered zirconia FDP with custom-milled titanium abutments (**c**, **d**). The margins prescribed at −0.5 mm

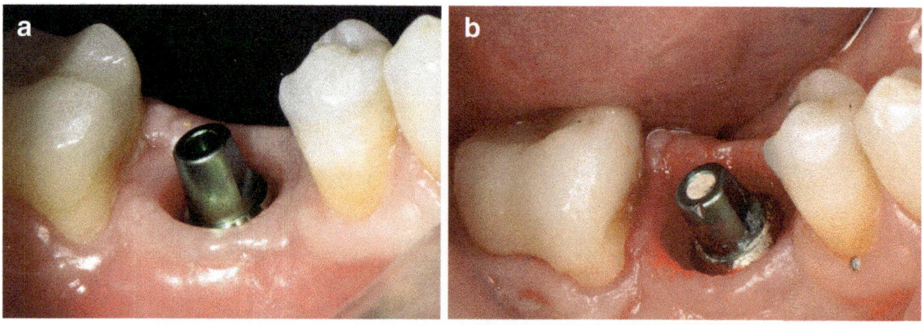

Fig. 12.4 Tissue-level implants should primarily be restored with screw-retained restoration. This implant design is poorly suited to use with cemented restorations or anywhere in the aesthetic zone. The margins of the crown or prosthesis are dictated by the position of the implant, and as such the mesial and distal margins are almost always too deep subgingival to properly manage cement. (**a**, **b**) A tissue-level implant demonstrating the challenge of margin position and subsequent peri-implant mucositis resulting from the deep margins at the mesial and distal

But aesthetics is only one of the concerns and means little if biological and functional risks are too great. To mitigate these concerns, the abutment selection and design are critical. Peri-implantitis has various etiologies, one of which is cement retained in contact with the bone or tissues. This issue has been thoroughly explored later in this chapter. Overall, risk of retained cement decreases significantly when the margins are placed appropriately (i.e., <1 mm deep) [2, 9, 10].

To achieve the above goal, it is imperative to use an implant system which has custom-milled abutments as an option (Fig. 12.3c, d). It is virtually impossible to place the margins in the correct position with stock abutments or with a tissue-level implant designs (Fig. 12.4a, b). There are reasonable scenarios for tissue-level implants, but the aesthetic zone is not among them.

12.2 Abutment Material Considerations

Contemporary abutment material options for the partially edentulous patient include cast gold alloy, titanium (Fig. 12.5a), full-contour zirconia (Fig. 12.5b), and zirconia with a titanium base (Fig. 12.5c). Other options exist (i.e., lithium disilicate, chrome cobalt, alumina) but will not be discussed here due to their limited use. Overall, we will see that zirconia abutments tend to give a better gingival color, though they are more prone to failure under excessive loads [11, 12]. The biocompatibility of the various materials and their effect on the peri-implant tissues is unclear, as good data exists for both Zr and Ti. For functional strength, we will see that titanium (or cast gold alloys) are superior but tend to discolor the tissues more [13]. Zirconia abutments have recently been designed with a titanium base to mitigate many of the issues associated with the full-contour zirconia abutments.

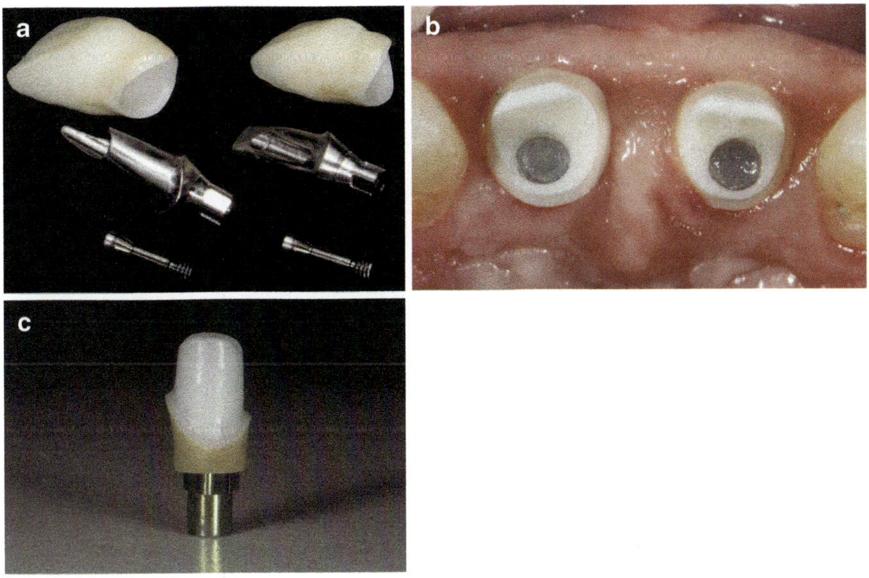

Fig. 12.5 (**a**) Custom-milled titanium abutments with margins prescribed at −0.5 mm. (**b**) Full-contour zirconia abutments with margins prescribed at −0.5 mm. Note that when seated, all margins are clearly visible circumferentially. (**c**) Zirconia abutment mated to a titanium base. This design is ideal (though not available for all implant manufacturers) because it brings the aesthetics of zirconia but removes the risk for zirconia breakage *inside* the implant

When selecting the abutment material, there are three key considerations:

- Biology (Is one material more biocompatible than the others?)
- Function (Is the abutment strong enough?)
- Aesthetics (Will the abutment gray the tissues?)

Titanium is the most biocompatible metal available. The unique property of the titanium abutments (either commercially pure titanium (CP Ti) or titanium alloy (Ti-6Al-4 V)) is due to the possibility of the formation of TiO_2 protective film on the surface of titanium. Therefore, it is the oxide layer, which is in contact with the tissue, and not the metal itself. Titanium has a lower density than base metal casting alloys and possesses much lower density than noble metal casting alloys. In addition, titanium as an abutment material shows desirable mechanical properties. The other desirable characteristics of Ti abutments are their anticorrosive properties. Based on the presence of different elements such as iron (Fe) and oxygen (O), titanium can have four grades (I–IV), where grade IV is the strongest one and has the highest levels of Fe and O. Strengthening of grades I–IV CP titanium is provided by interstitial impurity atoms (C, H, O, and N), where O is the most important [14, 15].

Titanium alloy (Ti-6Al-4 V) or grade V titanium contains 6% aluminum, 4% vanadium, 0.25% (maximum) iron, 0.2% (maximum) oxygen, and the remainder

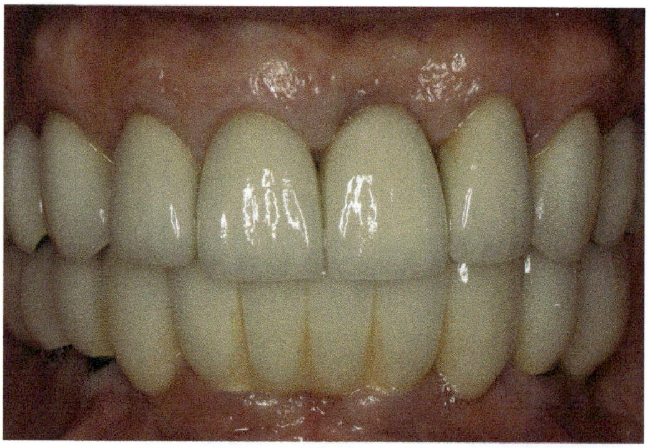

Fig. 12.6 Titanium abutments have the negative effect of graying the color of the soft tissue. This intensity of this effect is dependent on the implant position and tissue thickness. Here, the effect is pronounced in the anterior implant supported metal ceramic restoration

titanium. It is well known that properly manufactured Ti-6Al-4 V has much higher strength and higher fatigue limit than CP titanium. Initially, when these alloys were introduced, concerns were raised about biocompatibility of aluminum (implicated by some for Alzheimer's disease). Additionally, there is not enough body of literature about biocompatibility of vanadium. However, the clinical success of implants suggests that these concerns caused no problems [14, 15].

Due to its grayish color, titanium, and its alloy, is not the material of choice for the aesthetic zone (Fig. 12.6). The grayish discoloration of the peri-implant mucosa by titanium implant impairs the aesthetic result of implant reconstructions in the aesthetic zone [16, 17]. In order to resolve this issue, the surface of the titanium abutment has been plasma coated with titanium nitride (TiN) where titanium and nitrogen ions are combined on the surface and bonded with the titanium substrate of the abutment (thinness of coating 5 μm). Studies have shown that, like Ti, TiN is biocompatible and does not cause any adverse tissue reaction. Additionally, it has been confirmed that TiN behaves like a strong ceramic material with gold hue, which makes it a promising choice to achieve a warm, aesthetic tone under the gingiva. The surface coating in TiN abutments covers the entire abutment excluding the contact area between the abutment/implant and screw/abutment. The indication for this abutment is the clinical satiations when we are treating aesthetically challenging cases for patients with thin biotype and high functional loads [18].

Titanium abutments can have a polished or machined surface. The main difference between these two surfaces is their surface roughness. It is well known that for peri-implant seal, glycoproteins and biofilm are more likely to attach to a rough surface compared to a smooth one. However, several clinical studies have demonstrated no clinically significant difference in the inflammatory response between rough and polished abutment surfaces [19]. Abrahamsson and colleagues showed no significant differences between the soft tissue attachments near the rough and smooth abutments, after 3 months of implantation [20]. Other studies have confirmed a favorable soft tissue response in forming and maintaining peri-implant seal around titanium abutments [21]. Furthermore, Zitzmann et al. explored the reactions of the peri-implant soft tissue to plaque accumulation on titanium implant abutments designed with either a rough or a smooth external surface. The authors concluded that the different surface characteristics of abutments made of commercially pure titanium failed to influence plaque formation and the establishment of inflammatory cell lesions in the peri-implant mucosa [22].

Zirconium dioxide (ZrO_2) has a unique place among other materials in implant dentistry due to its excellent mechanical properties and desirable color. Zirconia can have three crystallographic forms depending on the temperature. At room temperature zirconia possesses a monoclinic structure, which will be remained upon heating up to 1170 °C. After increasing the temperature above 1170 °C and up to 2370 °C, the monolithic (*m*) structure will be transformed to tetragonal (*t*) structure. At temperatures above 2370 °C up to the melting point, zirconia will assume a cubic (c) structure. It is well known that the transformation from the tetragonal (*t*) to the monoclinic (*m*) structure upon cooling is accompanied by a substantial volumetric expansion (~4.5%), adequate to cause a catastrophic failure. In order to stabilize tetragonal workable zirconia at room temperature, stabilizing oxides such as CaO, Y_2O_3, or CeO_2 have been added to the composition of zirconia [23–26].

Due to zirconia's unique mechanical properties, it has gained a wide variety of biomedical applications including in dentistry. In modern dentistry, zirconia is the material of choice for high stress-bearing areas and aesthetic zone. Studies have confirmed that this material exhibits very high fracture toughness and a Young's modulus comparable to that of steel. One of the main distinguishing characteristics of zirconia in comparison with other ceramic is the capability to actively resist crack propagation which leads to very high fracture toughness for the material [23–26].

Several in vivo studies have shown excellent tissue integration properties for zirconia in comparison with other restorative materials. Several other studies have shown enhanced soft tissue and marginal bone around the zirconia abutments in comparison with cast gold alloy abutments. In addition, zirconia has shown excellent biocompatibility showing outstanding tissue response while showing significant reduction of plaque and bacterial adhesion on its surface in comparison with other ceramics and dental materials [27]. Poortinga et al. in their studies showed that bacterial resistance of zirconia abutments might be due to electron conductivity of this material [28].

Other studies have shown lower bacterial load and inflammatory infiltrate around zirconia abutments in comparison with titanium ones. This material can be considered the most hygienic abutment on the market, improving the long-term maintenance of the peri-implant seal and aesthetic soft tissue and preserving the crestal bone [29]. Rimondini et al., Scarano et al., and Hobkirk et al. in their consensus reported high survival rates for ceramic (99.1%) and metal (97.4%) abutments after a mean estimated observation of 5 years.

A systematic review evaluating zirconia abutments concludes that it is as suitable a material for dental implant abutments as titanium [30].

Linkevicius and Vaitelis in their studies found no differences in soft tissue health in peri-implant mucosa adjacent to zirconia and titanium abutments. However, they reported that soft tissue around zirconia abutments heals faster than tissues in contact with titanium ones. They concluded that zirconia has a lower tendency for surface-bound bacterial plaque in early stages in comparison with titanium [12]. In another study, Welander et al. analyzed the soft tissue barrier formed around different implant abutment materials. They reported that soft tissue dimensions at titanium and zirconia abutments remained stable after 5 months of healing. However, gold/palladium alloy abutments caused an apical shift of the barrier epithelium and marginal bone after 5 months of healing [31]. In addition, Linkevicius and Apse in another study analyzed the difference in the stability of peri-implant tissues between titanium abutments, gold alloy, zirconium oxide, and aluminum oxide abutments. They reported titanium abutments did not maintain a higher bone level in comparison with gold alloy, aluminum oxide, or zirconium oxide abutments [32]. Other investigations mentioned no obvious advantage of titanium or zirconia abutments over each other. However, studies consistently conclude that zirconia abutments evoke better color response of peri-implant mucosa and superior aesthetic outcome in comparison with titanium or cast gold abutments.

However, there are disadvantages associated with the application of zirconia ceramics as the abutment material. There are many reports of fracture of zirconia abutment. The other potential issue with the application of zirconia abutments is the greater wear resistance (abrasiveness) of zirconia in comparison with titanium abutments inside the Ti implant. In order to solve these issues, hybrid zirconia abutments or two-piece zirconia abutments have been introduced [33].

In this design, zirconia custom abutments are cemented or compressed to a titanium connection/base. This process is usually done in the lab using a short titanium connection. This design provides a titanium-to-titanium interface with the implant platform. Studies have confirmed that implant–titanium abutment connection has better fit than all implant–zirconia abutment configurations [34]. Truninger et al. [13] studied the fracture load of zirconia abutments with different types of implant–abutment connections after chewing simulation. Four different designs of zirconia abutment were tested: zirconia abutments with one-piece internal implant–abutment connection, zirconia abutments with two-piece internal implant–abutment connection, zirconia abutments with external implant–abutment connection, and zirconia abutments with two-piece internal implant–abutment connection which compared to titanium abutments with one-piece internal implant–abutment connection as the control group. They found that the failure type and bending moments of zirconia abutments vary with respect to their implant–abutment connection after aging and chewing simulation. They concluded that zirconia abutments with internal one- and two-piece implant–abutment connections will perform similarly or even better in a clinical situation than externally connected zirconia abutments [13].

Another study by Sailer and colleagues described that the type of implant–abutment connection has a critical influence on the technical outcome of zirconia abutments [17, 35]. The authors reported significantly higher fracture values for zirconia abutments with internal connection in comparison with the ones with external connection.

Additionally, in their prospective cohort study, Canullo and colleagues did not found any significant difference in marginal gap values and periodontal indices between all zirconia abutments and Ti base zirconia abutments. They concluded that titanium–zirconia abutments might be comparable with currently available aesthetic implant abutments.

Alternatively, other studies (Degidi et al.) have shown higher expression of inflammatory markers around titanium healing caps in comparison with zirconia healing caps showing that zirconia provokes a superior biological response due to reduced bacterial accumulation [29]. Other studies confirmed these findings showing better healing response, less inflammatory infiltrate, and reduced plaque adhesion around zirconia abutment material in comparison with titanium. Furthermore, Scarano et al. [36] in their studies reported significant reduction in bacterial adhesion for zirconia when compared to titanium. Moreover, in vivo human studies have showed greater amounts of inflammatory infiltrate around titanium abutment materials compared to that of zirconia.

Rimondini and colleagues found fewer accumulated bacteria around zirconia abutments in comparison with titanium ones [37]. On the other hand, other studies (Lima et al. and Al-Ahmad et al.) reported no difference in protein adsorption, biofilm composition, and bacterial adherence between zirconia and titanium abutments [38, 39].

In summary, zirconia is a unique ceramic material for application as an abutment in implant dentistry. It is the most hygienic abutment in the market, which maintains the mucosal seal better than titanium. It can be considered as the material of choice for anterior aesthetic zone and for patients with thin biotype, and they are especially reliable in the anterior region from both biologic and mechanical points of view.

Cast gold abutments are widely utilized to fabricate implant-level, custom-cast restorations that provided subgingival margins for aesthetics, reduced height for vertical occlusal clearance, and/or custom angles (Fig. 12.7). With the introduction of more sophisticated ceramic and CAD/CAM-milled abutments, cast gold abutments are not as widely used as they once were. Studies have confirmed that cast gold is strong enough even in thin sections [40]. Moreover, studies have demonstrated a favorable soft tissue response around cast gold abutments leading to formation and maintenance of a desirable peri-implant seal. Generally, high palladium or high noble alloys (type II or IV) are used [41]. However, more recently due to the higher gold prices, base metals are being used as an alternative [42].

Abrahamsson and colleagues compared the soft tissue reaction to gold and titanium abutments. They reported after 6 months titanium and aluminum oxide abutments had formed a 2 mm junctional epithelium and a connective tissue portion of 1–1.5 mm in height. In contrast, gold and porcelain abutments had no attachment formed at the abutment level with signs of soft tissue recession and bone loss. They concluded that titanium abutments present better soft tissue

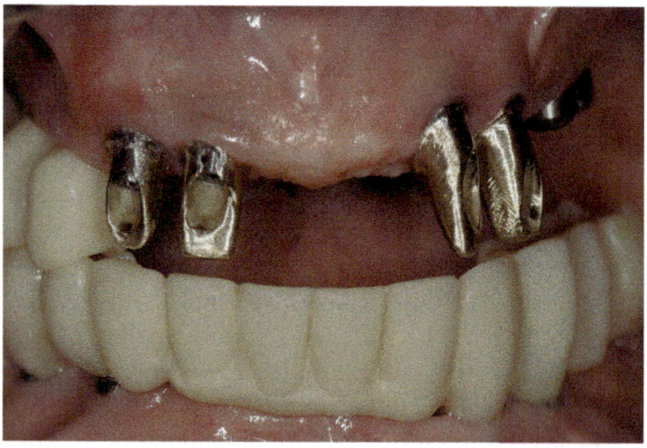

Fig. 12.7 Though largely replaced by the invention of custom-milled titanium and zirconia, custom gold abutments as seen here can also be used for cemented prostheses. Note the equigingival margin position

response compared to gold ones [43]. In another study, Rompen et al. reported that titanium and zirconia abutments exhibit more favorable long-term soft tissue reaction in comparison with gold and porcelain abutments [44].

In a more recent study, Vigolo and colleagues found no significant difference in radiographic peri-implant marginal bone and soft tissue response between titanium and gold alloy abutments [45]. Taylor and colleagues, in an in vitro study, examined the effect of titanium dental implants attached to dissimilar materials on the capacity of osteogenic differentiation of preosteoblasts. They concluded that the presence of commonly used implant abutment biomaterials, attached to titanium dental implants, had no adverse effects on the in vitro osteo-differentiation capacity of preosteoblasts. Furthermore, later studies by Abrahamsson found no significant differences in the transmucosal soft tissue level between titanium and gold abutments [46]. Apart from the high price of gold, the other main disadvantage of cast gold abutments in comparison with titanium and zirconia abutment is the inability to utilize CAD/CAM technology requiring a time-consuming laboratory procedure by lab technician. Other concerns with a cast gold alloy are aesthetic concerns regarding the screw access for screw-retained restorations, the increasing cost of alloy, and the labor required in their fabrication.

Studies have shown that the type and design of the implant abutment material and its design could impact the fracture resistance of implant/abutment/restoration assemblies. Titanium has been widely used as an implant abutment material with high fatigue strength and favorable biological response from surrounding soft tissue [47]. It is well known that titanium abutments are associated with the highest fracture resistance, as previously reported. However, application of titanium abutments for aesthetic zone might be disadvantageous, especially in cases where patient has a high smile line, labially placed implants, or thin biotype. In these clinical scenarios, the grayish hue of titanium abutment can lead to unfavorable aesthetic outcomes. As an alternative treatment modality, ceramic abutment materials have been developed and used in implant dentistry. Ceramic abutments have major advantages over the metal abutments, for instance, superior aesthetics, fit, translucency, and ease of fabrication compared to titanium abutments. Due to their low fracture resistance, alumina abutments have generally been replaced in clinical use by stronger zirconia options. Several in vitro and in vivo studies have reported that the application of alumina abutments can result in numerous abutment fractures [27, 48–50].

Subsequently, the one-piece zirconia abutment was introduced and utilized in implant clinics. However, one-piece zirconia abutments are not immune to fracture either. Several studies have shown that one-piece zirconia abutments exhibit lower fracture resistance in comparison with titanium abutments [51, 52]. Formation of high internal stresses and fractures has been reported during tightening of these abutment screws prior to abutment seating [53]. Additionally, it has been shown that zirconia can cause wear on the internal connection of the titanium implant [54]. Foong et al. in their stepped fatigue study reported that there are significantly lower fracture resistance values for one-piece zirconia abutment in comparison with titanium ones [55].

To overcome these concerns associated with one-piece zirconia abutment, a zirconia abutment with a titanium interface (hybrid zirconia abutment) was introduced which provides a titanium-to-titanium implant–abutment interface. The titanium interface may be in the form of a sleeve or a ring that can be either cemented or friction fitted. Studies have shown that these abutments have exhibited significantly higher fracture resistance in comparison with the one-piece ones.

Another important factor to take into account is the type and design of the implant–abutment connection that can influence the fracture resistance of implant/abutment complex. Some studies have shown that two-piece internal connection designs exhibit significantly higher fracture resistance than one-piece internal connection. Therefore, it can be suggested that failure mode of zirconia abutments might be dependent on the design and geometry of the connection and abutment itself. While titanium abutment fracture has been reported less frequently than zirconia abutments, potential contribution factors could be improper abutment design, manufacturing defects, and non-passive fit of the framework or biomechanical overload. Manufacturing flaws or imperfections in zirconia abutments can weaken zirconia abutments leading to compromised mechanical strength of the material due to formation of cracks or voids in the structure of zirconia and ultimately clinical failure. The presence of cracks when combined with high biomechanical loads leads to crack propagation and failures. Additionally, the design of the zirconia abutment can also be another important factor in mechanical breakdown of zirconia abutments. Due to the brittle nature of the material, unsupported material or uncontrolled biomechanical stress can lead to catastrophic failures. Unfavorable designs such as sharp angles and thin segments need to be avoided.

Therefore, in order to choose the most durable restoration, it is necessary to choose the right abutment material. A proper biomechanical and patient biological assessment seems to be necessary prior to material selection. In aesthetic cases (single unit) in which very low biomechanical load is expected, a zirconia/TiBase abutment can be the material of choice in patients with high smile line or thin biotype. Exercise extreme caution in utilizing one piece Zirconia abutments (those without a TiBase).

12.3 Margin and Cement Considerations

The two key factors for predictable success with cemented implant restorations are proper margin placement and the presence of robust keratinized tissue (Fig. 12.8). Linkevicius et al. have done the most substantial work looking at margin placement and the effect it has on the amount of retained cement [9, 10]. They have examined this both in vitro and in vivo. In Chap. 16, the histology of the peri-implant tissues is examined and clearly shows why implants are more vulnerable to cement-induced problems than natural teeth [56].

Not only are natural teeth and their surrounding tissues more resistant to cement-induced problems, but so too is the clinician limited by the depth of the margin on the natural teeth. When a tooth is prepped for a crown, the tissues must be retracted to obtain the impression. Deep margins are increasingly difficult to obtain an impression and so limit the depth to which the clinician can prep. The cementum on the root is also notoriously difficult to get any dental material to bond to. Lastly and perhaps most importantly, the periodontal fibers insert into the cementum providing a strong barrier to cement penetration subgingivally.

Conversely, with implants, the impression copings allow impressions at virtually any depth. So an accurate impression can be made 4+ mm subgingival and the restoration fabricated. The problem hinges on the fact that the cement cannot be reliably removed any deeper than 1 mm subgingival. In addition, the lack of periodontal fibers inserting into the implant, and that many cements (especially resins) have a high bond strength to titanium, and the problem becomes obvious [57]. As a clinical guideline, all margins on implant abutments should be as close to the gingival margin as aesthetically

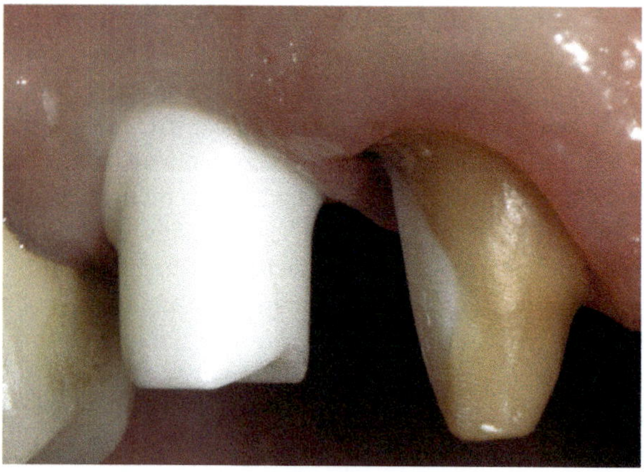

Fig. 12.8 For cemented implant crowns, margin placement is *critical* to mitigating the risk of retained cement and subsequent peri-implantitis. In the aesthetic zone, clinicians and patients are concerned with the possibility of gingival recession and/or visibility of the abutment. The solution to this problem is not to sink the margins deep, but to change to a zirconia abutment with margins placed very near the gingival margin

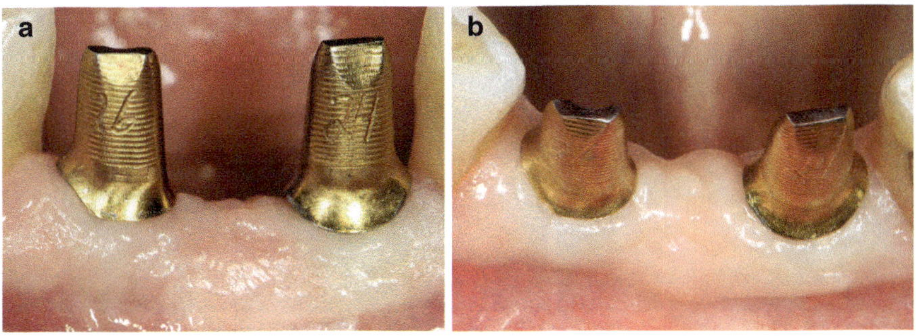

Fig. 12.9 (**a**, **b**) In this lower anterior scenario, custom titanium abutments with a titanium nitride (TiN) coating have been prescribed. The TiN coating is of gold color which helps mitigate graying of the tissues and the overlying prosthesis. Margins are always to be placed in a cleansable position. Here, equigingival margins have been selected

tolerable. In non-aesthetic zones, the margins should be placed equigingival or supragingival (Fig. 12.9a, b). In the aesthetic zone, there is the concern of tissue recession and the abutment material becoming visible. This problem is mitigated, not by placing margins deeper but rather by changing the abutment material to zirconia. The surface of the zirconia can also be stained to resemble the cervical area of the crown or the natural root surface (Fig. 12.10a, b). This material selection is key to allowing the clinician the confidence to prescribe the margins to be placed *no deeper than 1 mm* subgingival.

Cement selection for implant restorations is highly varied. Some clinicians opt for cements with poor bond strengths with the idea that the crown is then retrievable should *something* go wrong. While others opt for cements that better retain and strengthen the prosthesis. In a survey by Tarica et al. [58], they asked all directors of the prosthodontic residencies in the United States what cement they used for implant restorations. The results were widely varied, with the most popular being RMGI, ZOE, and resin cements. These choices represent the entire spectrum of cement choices, with the ZOE cement having low bond strengths and resins having very high bond strengths. Other factors to consider include radiopacity, antibacterial activity, viscosity, solubility, compatibility with Ti, and color.

While it would be advantageous if the implant cement were radiopaque, this does not in any way assure the clinician that a radiograph can prove that no excess cement exists. Low-viscosity cements will only leave a thin film along the abutment surface that would be very difficult to detect on a radiograph and only helpful for large amounts of cement left on the mesial and distal.

The idea of needing a cement that is "retrievable" is common. However, most problems for implant crowns that require removal (peri-implantitis, porcelain failure, shade mismatch, or poor fit) will all require complete replacement of the crown (Fig. 12.11a, b). As for prosthetics on natural teeth, the solution for a failing or problematic implant restoration is removal and replacement, rendering the idea of "retrieval" moot. The additional downside to the use of a weak retrievable cement (i.e., ZOE) is poor long-term retention.

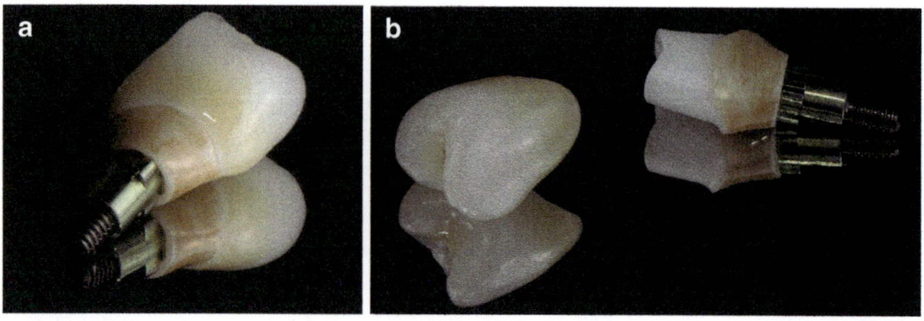

Fig. 12.10 (a, b) In areas of thin gingival biotype or high aesthetic concerns, the emergence area of the zirconia should be stained to resemble the natural root surface. Note the use of a titanium base within the zirconia abutment to minimize risk of zirconia failure and complications

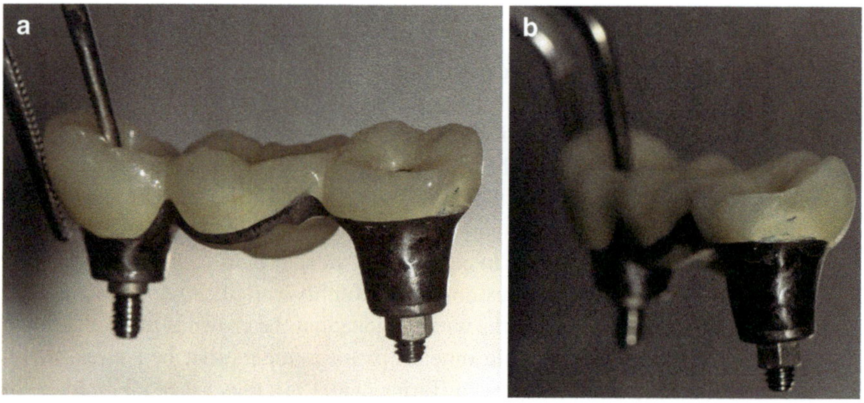

Fig. 12.11 (a, b) A screw-retained PFM FDP demonstrating premature failure of the porcelain at the interproximal contact. This is the most common mode of failure for this type of restoration. The etiology of this failure is usually due to insufficient framework design or poor technique in stacking the feldspathic porcelain. Unfortunately, neither problem is clearly evident to the clinician until after the failure occurs. Such failures are best resolved by complete redesign and replacement of the prosthesis

As the cementum on a natural tooth is resistant to cement adhesion, we can alter the surface of the abutment prior to placement in an attempt to prevent cement adhesion (Fig. 12.12). Petroleum jelly should be applied to the tissue-contacting surfaces of the abutment prior to placement. This should help prevent and cement from sticking to the abutment surface (Table 12.1).

12.4 Complication Avoidance

Rightly so, the primary concern with cemented implant crowns is the potential for cement-induced peri-implant mucositis or peri-implantitis. Published rates for the incidence of peri-implantitis range from 2 to 44% [6]. There are likely many reasons

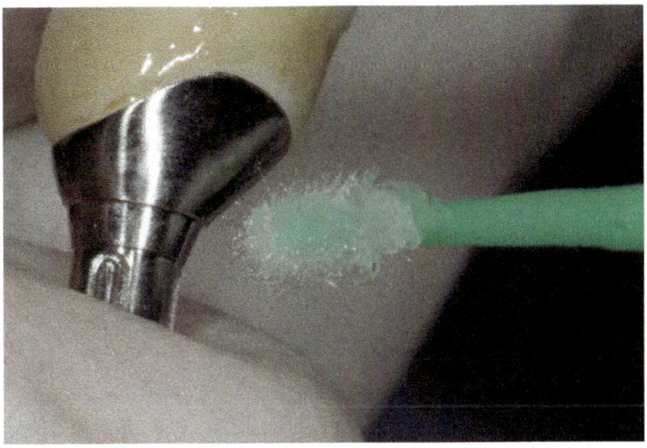

Fig. 12.12 In an effort to further reduce the likelihood of cement retention on the abutment, the emergence area is thoroughly coated with petroleum jelly prior to insertion

Table 12.1 Strategies for success with cemented implant restorations

1. Margins no deeper than 1 mm subgingival
2. Cemented implant crowns should only be used when robust, mature, keratinized tissue is present
3. Use of zirconia abutments should be limited to the "aesthetic zone" or patients with limited occlusal forces
4. Zirconia abutments should have a titanium interface with the implant [59]
5. Use original manufacturer parts whenever possible
6. Use a minimum amount of cement
7. Apply petroleum jelly to the emergence surface of the abutment prior to placement
8. Choose a cement appropriate for the specific conditions of the restoration

for this wide discrepancy in incidence rate. The two most obvious factors are a lack of agreement in the research community on what the requirements for a diagnosis of peri-implantitis actually are, and wide variability in the implants and protocols used in practice. Regardless, whatever definition is used, atypical bone loss, inflammation, bleeding, and infections around implants need to be prevented.

The first decision in implants that may affect the rate of peri-implantitis is the implant body itself. As stated above, if the long axis of the implant exits through the facial, a cemented restoration becomes the appropriate choice. But if a tissue-level implant has been used, then the margin position has to be preset by the surgeon. Due to the natural scalloping of the gingiva in the aesthetic zone, placement of the facial margin slightly subgingival will place the mesial and distal margins several millimeters subgingival (Fig. 12.13a, b). This is an untenable scenario and will undoubtedly leave residual cement subgingival. Cement cannot be predictably removed more than 1 mm subgingival [2, 9, 10]. As such, the tissue-level implant design is strongly contraindicated for the aesthetic zone and any site with scalloped gingival.

Abutment selection is the next most crucial aspect in the prevention of peri-implantitis. Most manufacturers offer a wide variety of stock abutment designs. Most have margins at an equal height all around the abutment, thus creating the same problem as with the tissue-level implants. Most stock abutments also have far too short of an emergence area to sufficiently bring the margins within a range that

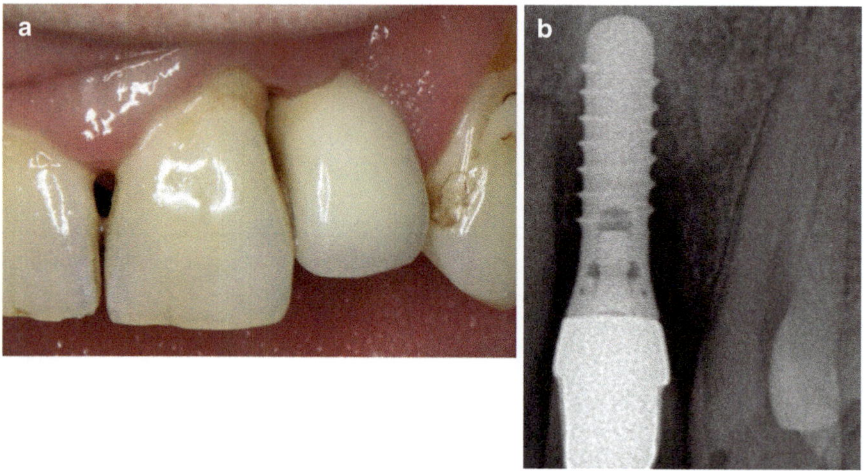

Fig. 12.13 (**a**, **b**) Tissue-level implant designs are poor choices in the aesthetic zone, due to the fact that the margin position is not correctable with the abutment. At placement, the surgeon will generally place the midfacial margin of this implant type about 1 mm subgingival. Subsequently, the mesial and distal margin positions will be located >4 mm subgingival, virtually guaranteeing that cement removal will be impossible. Here a tissue-level implant has been placed for the lateral maxillary incisor. Margin positions at the mesial and distal are 5 mm subgingival, and retained cement has induced aggressive peri-implantitis

can be cleaned at cementation. Some manufacturers offer scalloped or "aesthetic" stock abutments. These attempt to match the scalloped tissue of the aesthetic zone. Far too often, they present the same problems as the other stock abutments as there are only a few choices to match an infinite variation of clinical presentation. While better than the standard stock abutments, the scalloped abutments generally result in margins that are either exposed (aesthetic failure) or too deep (leading to cement-induced peri-implantitis).

The solution to the above scenarios in the aesthetic zone is to use a bone-level implant that allows the creation of a custom-designed abutment. This will allow the team to place the margins at an *exact* appropriate position for each clinical case (Fig. 12.14a, b). The custom abutments can be cast with gold alloy or milled from titanium or zirconia. The cast gold alloy abutments have fallen out of favor due to the increased cost of gold, higher rates of porcelain failure, and higher incidences of screw loosening [3, 4]. Custom-milled titanium abutments are highly durable and biocompatible but may discolor the gingival tissues (even when anodized gold or pink). Custom-milled zirconia abutments change the tissue color less than any other option but have been prone to fracture under excessive loads [11–13]. With earlier designs, the entirety of the abutment was zirconia, and the failure usually happened *inside* the implant connection [59]. Retrieval of the broken zirconia fragments is usually challenging. Contemporary designs utilize a titanium base that is bonded or compressed to the zirconia abutment (Fig. 12.15). This mitigates the tissue and crown coloration concerns, as well as moving the zirconia *outside* the implant.

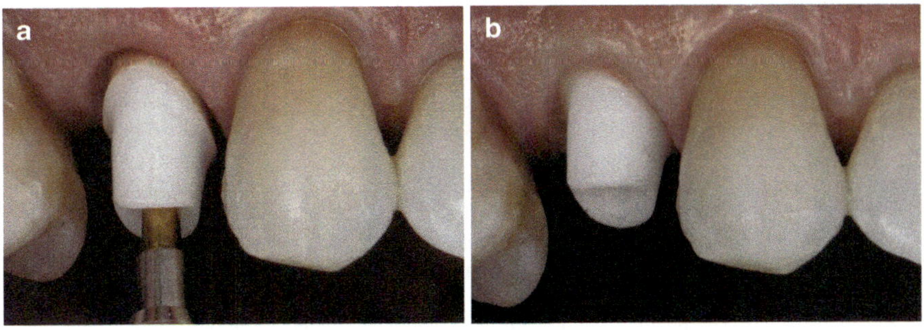

Fig. 12.14 (**a**, **b**) The use of a custom zirconia abutment in the aesthetic zone allows for placement of the margins within 0.5 mm of the gingival margin. This creates a result that is biologically predictable and highly aesthetic and has minimal chance of cement-induced peri-implantitis

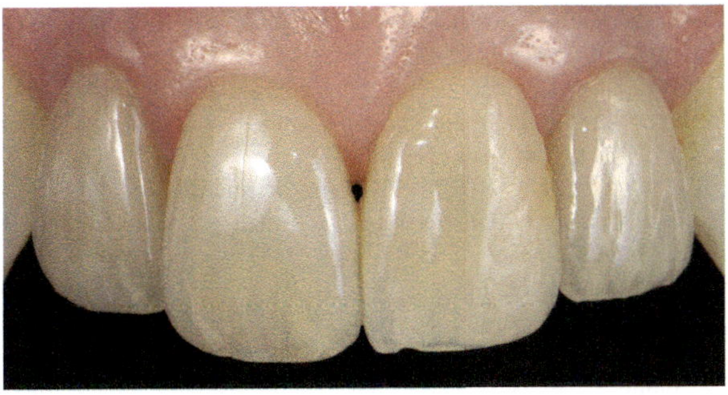

Fig. 12.15 The maxillary left lateral incisor has been replaced with a bone-level implant, a zirconia abutment with a titanium base, margins within 0.5 mm of the gingival margin, and a cemented, layered zirconia crown. This treatment modality allows for aesthetic results and minimal risks of biologic or technical complications

Thus, should the zirconia fail, its removal and replacement are quite simple. It is important to understand that these Ti/Zr abutments appear to be working well [60, 61], but further long-term testing is still ongoing. The primary problem with this abutment design is likely to be debonding of the zirconia from the Ti base. Though incovienient, this is a relatively easy to fix.

References

1. Chaar MS, Att W, Strub JR. Prosthetic outcome of cement-retained implant-supported fixed dental restorations: a systematic review. J Oral Rehabil. 2011;38(9):697–711.
2. Kotsakis G, Zhang L, Gaillard P, Raedel M, Walter MH, Konstantinidis IK. Investigation of the association between cement-retention and prevalent peri-implant diseases: a cross-sectional study. J Periodontol. 2015;5:1–4.
3. Millen C, Brägger U, Wittneben JG. Influence of prosthesis type and retention mechanism on complications with fixed implant-supported prostheses: a systematic review applying multivariate analyses. Int J Oral Maxillofac Implants. 2015;30(1):110–24.

4. Sailer I, Mühlemann S, Zwahlen M, Hämmerle CH, Schneider D. Cemented and screw-retained implant reconstructions: a systematic review of the survival and complication rates. Clin Oral Implants Res. 2012;23(s6):163–201.
5. Wittneben JG, Millen C, Brägger U. Clinical performance of screw-versus cement-retained fixed implant-supported reconstructions-a systematic review. Int J Oral Maxillofac Implants. 2014;29:84–98.
6. Huynh-Ba G. THEMATIC ABSTRACT REVIEW: peri-implantitis: "tsunami" or marginal problem? Int J Oral Maxillofac Implants. 2013;28(2):333–7.
7. Korsch M, Robra BP, Walther W. Cement-associated signs of inflammation: retrospective analysis of the effect of excess cement on peri-implant tissue. Int J Prosthodont. 2015;28(1):11–8.
8. Wilson TG Jr. The positive relationship between excess cement and peri-implant disease: a prospective clinical endoscopic study. J Periodontol. 2009;80(9):1388–92.
9. Linkevicius T, Vindasiute E, Puisys A, Linkeviciene L, Maslova N, Puriene A. The influence of the cementation margin position on the amount of undetected cement. A prospective clinical study. Clin Oral Implants Res. 2013;24(1):71–6.
10. Linkevicius T, Vindasiute E, Puisys A, Peciuliene V. The influence of margin location on the amount of undetected cement excess after delivery of cement-retained implant restorations. Clin Oral Implants Res. 2011;22(12):1379–84.
11. Bressan E, Paniz G, Lops D, Corazza B, Romeo E, Favero G. Influence of abutment material on the gingival color of implant-supported all-ceramic restorations: a prospective multicenter study. Clin Oral Implants Res. 2011;22(6):631–7.
12. Linkevicius T, Vaitelis J. The effect of zirconia or titanium as abutment material on soft peri-implant tissues: a systematic review and meta-analysis. Clin Oral Implants Res. 2015;26(Suppl 11):139–47.
13. Truninger TC, Stawarczyk B, Leutert CR, Sailer TR, Hämmerle CH, Sailer I. Bending moments of zirconia and titanium abutments with internal and external implant-abutment connections after aging and chewing simulation. Clin Oral Implants Res. 2012;23:12–8.
14. Lekholm U, Gunne J, Henry P, et al. Survival of the Brånemark implants in partially edentulous jaws: a 10-year prospective multicenter study. Int J Oral Maxillofac Implants. 1999;14:639–45.
15. Osman RB, Swain MW. A critical review of dental implant materials with an emphasis on titanium versus zirconia. Materials. 2015;8:932–58.
16. Martínez-Rus F, Prieto M, Salido MP, Madrigal C, Özcan M, Pradíes G. A clinical study assessing the influence of anodized titanium and zirconium dioxide abutments and peri-implant soft tissue thickness on the optical outcome of implant-supported lithium disilicate single crowns. Int J Oral Maxillofac Implants. 2017;32:156–63.
17. Sailer I, Philipp A, Zembic A, Pjetursson BE, Hämmerle CH, Zwahlen M. A systematic review of the performance of ceramic and metal implant abutments supporting fixed implant reconstructions. Clin Oral Implants Res. 2009;20(Suppl 4):4–31.
18. Scarano A, Piattelli M, Vrespa G, Petrone G, Iezzi G, Piattelli A. Bone healing around titanium and titanium nitride-coated dental implants with three surfaces: an experimental study in rats. Clin Implant Dent Relat Res. 2003;5:103–11.
19. Wu-Yuan CD, Eganhouse KJ, Keller JC, Walters KS. Oral bacterial attachment to titanium surfaces: a scanning electron microscopy study. J Oral Implantol. 1995;21(3):207–13.
20. Abrahamsson I, Zitzmann NU, Berglundh T, Linder E, Wennerberg A, Lindhe J. The mucosal attachment to titanium implants with different surface characteristics: an experimental study in dogs. J Clin Periodontol. 2002;29:448–55.
21. Nakamura T, Saito O, Mizuno M, Kinuta S, Ishigaki S. Influence of abutment substrates on the colour of metal-free polymer crowns. J Oral Rehabil. 2003;30(2):184–8.
22. Zitzmann NU, Marinello CP. A review of clinical and technical considerations for fixed and removable implant prostheses in the edentulous mandible. Int J Prosthodont. 2002;15:65–72.
23. Denry I, Kelly JR. State of the art of zirconia for dental applications. Dent Mater. 2008;24(3):299–307.

24. Glauser R, Sailer I, Wohlwend A, Studer S, Schibli M, Schärer P. Experimental zirconia abutments for implant-supported single-tooth restorations in esthetically demanding regions: 4-year results of a prospective clinical study. Int J Prosthodont. 2004;17(3):285–90.
25. Piconi C, Maccauro G. Zirconia as a ceramic biomaterial. Biomaterials. 1999;20(1):1–25.
26. Sadan A, Blatz MB, Lang B. Clinical considerations for densely sintered alumina and zirconia restorations: part 2. Int J Periodontics Restorative Dent. 2005;25(4):343–9.
27. Sghaireen MG. Fracture resistance and mode of failure of ceramic versus titanium implant abutments and single implant-supported restorations. Clin Implant Dent Relat Res. 2013;17:1–8.
28. Poortinga AT, Bos R, Busscher HJ. Measurement of charge transfer during bacterial adhesion to an indium tin oxide surface in a parallel plate flow chamber. J Microbiol Methods. 1999;38:183–9.
29. Degidi M, Artese L, Scarano A, Perrotti V, Gehrke P, Piattelli A. Inflammatory infiltrate, microvessel density, nitric oxide synthase expression, vascular endothelial growth factor expression, and proliferative activity in peri-implant soft tissues around titanium and zirconium oxide healing caps. J Periodontol. 2006;77:73–80.
30. Jung RE, Zembic A, Pjetursson BE, Zwahlen M, Thoma DS. Systematic review of the survival rate and the incidence of biological, technical, and aesthetic complications of single crowns on implants reported in longitudinal studies with a mean follow-up of 5 years. Clin Oral Implants Res. 2012;23(Suppl. 6):2–21.
31. Welander M, Abrahamsson I, Berglundh T. The mucosal barrier at implant abutments of different materials. Clin Oral Implants Res. 2008;19:635–41.
32. Linkevicius T, Apse P. Influence of abutment material on stability of peri-implant tissues: a systematic review. Int J Oral Maxillofac Implants. 2008;23(3):449–56.
33. Joda T, Brägger U. Management of a complication with a fractured zirconia implant abutment in the esthetic zone. Int J Oral Maxillofac Implants. 2015;30:21–3.
34. Mitsias ME, Silva NR, Pines M, Stappert C, Thompson VP. Reliability and fatigue damage modes of zirconia and titanium abutments. Int J Prosthodont. 2010;23:56–9.
35. Sailer I, Sailer T, Stawarczyk B, Jung RE, Hammerle CH. In vitro study of the influence of the type of connection on the fracture load of zirconia abutments with internal and external implant-abutment connections. Int J Oral Maxillofac Implants. 2009;24:850–8.
36. Scarano A, Piattelli M, Caputi S, Favero GA, Piattelli A. Bacterial adhesion on commercially pure titanium and zirconium oxide disks: an in vivo human study. J Periodontol. 2004;75:292–6.
37. Rimondini L, Cerroni L, Carrassi A, Torricelli P. Bacterial colonization of zirconia ceramic surfaces: an in vitro and in vivo study. Int J Oral Maxillofac Implants. 2002;17(6):793–8.
38. Al-Ahmad A, Wiedmann-Al-Ahmad M, Faust J, Bächle M, Follo M, Wolkewitz M, Hannig C, Hellwig E, Carvalho C, Kohal R. Biofilm formation and composition on different implant materials in vivo. J Biomed Mater Res B Appl Biomater. 2010;95B:101–9.
39. Lima EMCX, Koo H, Vacca-Smith AM, Rosalen PL, Del Bel Cury AA. Adsorption of salivary and serum proteins, and bacterial adherence on titanium and zirconia ceramic surfaces. Clin Oral Implants Res. 2008;19:780–5.
40. Knosp H, Holliday RJ, Corti CW. Gold in dentistry: alloys, uses and performance. Gold Bull. 2003;3:93–102.
41. Jivraj S, Chee W. Treatment planning of implants in the aesthetic zone. Br Dent J. 2006;201(2):77–89.
42. Abichandani SJ, Nadiger R, Kavlekar AS. Abutment selection, designing, and its influence on the emergence profile: a comprehensive review. Eur J Prosthodont. 2013;1(1):10.
43. Abrahamsson I, Berglundh T, Glantz P-O, Lindhe J. The mucosal attachment at different abutments. An experimental study in dogs. J Clin Periodontol. 1998;25:721–7.
44. Rompen E, Domken O, Degidi M, Pontes AEF, Piattelli A. The effect of material characteristics, of surface topography and of implant components and connections on soft tissue integration: a literature review. Clin Oral Implants Res. 2006;17(suppl 2):55–67.

45. Vigolo P, Givani A, Majzoub Z, Cordioli G. A 4-year prospective study to assess peri-implant hard and soft tissues adjacent to titanium versus gold-alloy abutments in cemented single implant crowns. J Prosthodont. 2006;15(4):250–6.
46. Abrahamsson I, Linder E, Larsson L, Berglundh T. Deposition of nanometer scaled calcium-phosphate crystals to implants with a dual acid-etched surface does not improve early tissue integration. Clin Oral Implants Res. 2013;24:57–62.
47. Ribeiro CG, Maia ML, Scherrer SS, Cardoso AC, Wiskott HW. Resistance of three implant-abutment interfaces to fatigue testing. J Appl Oral Sci. 2011;19:413–20.
48. Prestipino V, Ingeber A. All-ceramic implant abutments: esthetic indications. J Esthet Restor Dent. 1996;8(1):255–62.
49. Prestipino V, Ingeber A. Esthetic high-strength implant abutments. Part I. J Esthet Restor Dent. 1993;5(1):29–36.
50. Prestipino V, Ingeber A. Esthetic high-strength implant abutments. Part II. J Esthet Restor Dent. 1993;5(2):63–8.
51. Saponaro PC, Lee DJ, McGlumphy EA. Managing a fractured one-piece zirconia abutment with a modified plastic periodontal probe: a clinical report. J Prosthet Dent. 2016;117(5):587–91.
52. Stimmelmayr M, Sagerer S, Erdelt K, Beuer F. In vitro fatigue and fracture strength testing of one-piece zirconia implant abutments and zirconia implant abutments connected to titanium cores. Int J Oral Maxillofac Implants. 2013;28:488–93.
53. Aboushelib MN, Salameh Z. Zirconia implant abutment fracture: clinical case reports and precautions for use. Int J Prosthodont. 2009;22(6):616–9.
54. Cavusoglu Y, Akca K, Gurbuz R, Cehreli MC. A pilot study of joint stability at the zirconium or titanium abutment/titanium implant Interface. Int J Oral Maxillofac Implant. 2014;29(2):338–43.
55. Foong JKW, Judge RB, Palamara JE, Swain MV. Fracture resistance of titanium and zirconia abutments: an in vitro study. J Prosthet Dent. 2013;109(5):304–12.
56. Rodríguez X, Navajas A, Vela X, Fortuño A, Jimenez J, Nevins M. Arrangement of peri-implant connective tissue fibers around platform-switching implants with conical abutments and its relationship to the underlying bone: a human histologic study. Int J Periodontics Restorative Dent. 2016;36(4):533.
57. Agar JR, Cameron SM, Hughbanks JC, Parker MH. Cement removal from restorations luted to titanium abutments with simulated subgingival margins. J Prosthet Dent. 1997;78(1):43–7.
58. Wadhwani CP, Schwedhelm ER, Tarica DY, Chung KH. Implant luting cements. In: Cementation in dental implantology. Berlin: Springer; 2015. p. 47–82.
59. Kelly JR, Rungruanganunt P. Fatigue behavior of computer-aided design/computer-assisted manufacture ceramic abutments as a function of design and ceramics processing. Int J Oral Maxillofac Implants. 2016;31(3):601–9.
60. Zembic A, Bösch A, Jung RE, Hämmerle CH, Sailer I. Five-year results of a randomized controlled clinical trial comparing zirconia and titanium abutments supporting single-implant crowns in canine and posterior regions. Clin Oral Implants Res. 2013;24(4):384–90.
61. Zembic A, Philipp AO, Hämmerle CH, Wohlwend A, Sailer I. Eleven-year follow-up of a prospective study of zirconia implant abutments supporting single all-ceramic crowns in anterior and premolar regions. Clin Implant Dent Relat Res. 2015;17(S2):e417–26.

Screw-Retained Implant Restorations in the Aesthetic Zone

13

Tomas Linkevicius and Algirdas Puisys

Abstract

One of the choices to rehabilitate dental implant in aesthetic zone can be cement-screw-retained restoration, usually referred as hybrid prosthesis. It combines some features from cemented and screwed way of restoring implants. The system consists of the crown with palatinal opening, which is cemented to special retentive metal base on the working model. The cement excess is cleaned and restoration is screwed to the implant in the mouth. Retrievability is also a very important factor for success in implant restorations.

In addition this approach is good for peri-implant tissues, as it combines titanium as material for retentive base, which is good for connective tissue part of peri-implant tissues. Highly polished zirconia is appropriate material for epithelial adhesion of more coronal peri-implant tissues.

It is obvious that traditionally clinician can select between cemented or screw-retained restorations, when the time to restore implant in aesthetic zone occurs. Choosing between these constructions is mostly dependent on clinical situation and clinician's preference because there is no definite superiority of either of these means of retention. Some clinicians have better outcome with screw-retained, while others enjoy success with cemented implant-supported restorations (Fig. 13.1).

There are myriad factors to discuss in order to make an informed choice. The factors that are affected by different methods of retention of the prostheses to the implants include ease of fabrication, cost, aesthetics, access, occlusion, retention,

T. Linkevicius (✉)
Faculty of Medicine, Institute of Odontology, Vilnius University, Vilnius, Lithuania

A. Puisys
Vilnius Implantology Center, Vilnius, Lithuania

Todd R. Schoenbaum (ed.), *Implants in the Aesthetic Zone*,
https://doi.org/10.1007/978-3-319-72601-4_13

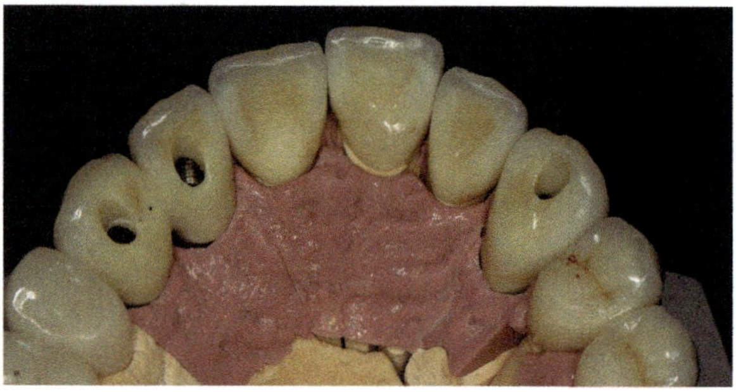

Fig. 13.1 Screw-retained restorations on anterior segment

incidence of loss of retention, retrievability, passivity of fit, restriction of implant position, effect on peri-implant tissue health, provisionalization, immediate loading, impression procedures, porcelain fracture, and clinical performance [1]. Although the purpose of this chapter is not to show the inferiority or superiority of each module, it is a must to say that current systematic reviews show significantly more bone loss around cemented restorations compared to screw-retained solution [2]. That being said, of course, might be due to different reasons; however, the main disadvantage of cemented restorations is of course possible cement extrusion into peri-implant tissues and difficulties to remove the remnants [3]. Recent clinical study by Wasyliuk et al. has shown that even 1 mm below gingival margin on individual abutments was not possible to remove all cement remnants [4]. Additional problem is created, if cemented crown becomes mobile due to abutment screw loosening, as then occlusal perforation must be made to reach the screw and tighten it back [5]. According to Wittneben et al.'s systematic review in 2014, total rate of biological and technical complications of cemented restorations was greater compared to screw-retained prosthesis [6]. On the other hand, rate of ceramic fracture and chipping appeared to be higher in screw-retained metal-ceramic restorations.

This brings us to the other choice—to use screw-retained restorations, a cement-free solution, free from residual cement risk, and offering long-term predictable outcome.

13.1 Indications and Advantages/Contraindications and Disadvantages

Generally, strict indications for screw-retained restorations are not that numerous. Generally, a lack of interocclusal space is strong indication to have one-piece screw-retained restoration while other being rather choice of the clinician, not strict indications. It is considered that if interocclusal clearance is less than 4 mm, screw-retained solution should be considered. Also, if the peri-implant tissue is poorly keratinized or irregular, screw-retained restorations are preferred.

Two major advantages of this approach can be listed: (1) screw-retained design of implant-based restorations allows for easy and nondestructive retrievability of the restoration for maintenance or repair procedures and (2) no risk of residual

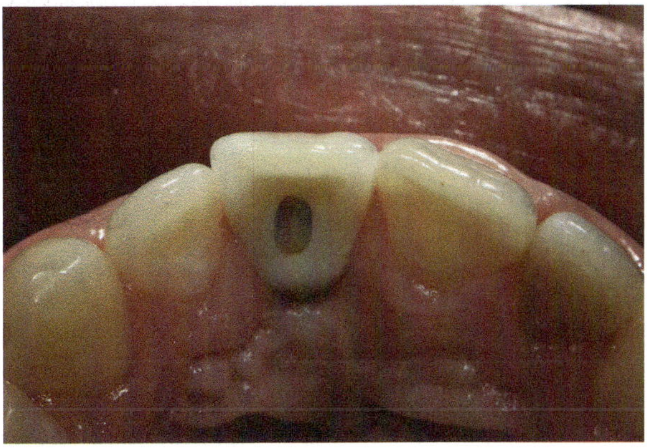

Fig. 13.2 Palatinal screw access channel after 5 years of delivery. Discoloration and microleakage of the composite are obvious

subgingival cement excess. A screw-retained design is a contribution toward healthy peri-implant tissues.

Occlusal or, in case of anterior teeth, palatal access to the screw opening is usually considered as the biggest disadvantage, which sometimes can compromise the treatment (Fig. 13.2). If the implant is angled to the facial, the screw access presents an aesthetic contraindication for traditional screw retention.

Screw-retained prosthesis on implants is impossible without the screw access channel, which must be sealed after delivery. Usually a screw access channel is closed with direct restoration that may affect aesthetics; however there is a quick and convenient way to finish the treatment with better control of aesthetics and occlusion. This alternative to a screw hole closure with composite restorations is the implant crown adhesive plug (ICAP), proposed by Wadhawi et al. [7]. The plug is made of custom-pressed porcelain that matches the same shape of the hole and same shade of the crown. The procedure is similar to inlay cementation: porcelain plug is etched, silanized, and bonded with composite resin luting cement into the crown. This type of restoration can eliminate the poor aesthetics of the screw channel and provide better control of the occlusal contacts. On the other hand, not all clinical situations warrant such sophisticated treatment.

13.2 Fabrication of Screw-Retained Restorations

Fabrication of the screw-retained restoration can be achieved in several ways: (1) casted with the use of plastic sleeves (gold alloy or Cr-Co) and (2) milled one-piece (titanium, zirconium, Cr-Co) and (3) milled two-piece hybrid (milled zirconium coping connected to titanium base).

Casting, as a method, already belongs to the past; poor qualities of gold or Cr-Co in terms of biocompatibility, casting irregularities, and increasing and fluctuating costs make this method less applicable than it once was.

One-piece screw-retained frameworks can be milled, thus eliminating inner tension problems inherent in the investment and casting process [8]. However it is not advisable to use titanium in aesthetic area, as the major drawback of these abutments is that their dark color shines through soft peri-implant tissues (Fig. 13.3), creating a grayish appearance of the peri-implant mucosa, which is aesthetically unacceptable [9].

In contrast zirconia frameworks offer a much better aesthetic outcome, especially in thinner peri-implant mucosa cases [10]. Nevertheless, its brittleness might be considered as one of the shortcomings of zirconium framework. Fractures of one-piece zirconia abutments with internal connection were reported in short-term studies [11] and in longer follow-up observations [12]. In addition, it was reported that zirconia hexagon could damage the implant, as it is stiffer than titanium alloy.

Therefore, it is clear that there should be a more convenient and contemporary way to produce screw-retained restoration. The use of a two-piece system, where the restoration superstructure is produced separately and later by means of cement or mechanical adaptation is connected to a titanium base, is the way to restore in aesthetic area. We can distinguish two most commonly used systems to connect the titanium base to the restoration: (1) cementation and (2) mechanical adaptation.

The most currently used and predictable is cement-screw-retained restoration of hybrid solution, where the zirconia-based restoration is fabricated and glazed, cemented on an appropriate titanium base in the laboratory, and then screw-retained to the implant intraorally. This construction eliminates the cement remnants, as crown is cemented to abutment on the model and technician can easily remove cement excess. Biomechanically this kind of restoration is cement-retained; thus, passive fit is achieved due to the layer of the cement between abutment and the crown.

This method has its roots from modification of Rajan and Gunaseelan. They described very similar technique of cement-screw-retained restoration [13]. They also proposed to use standard abutments (predecessor of titanium base) and metal ceramic restoration with occlusal opening; however, their cementation

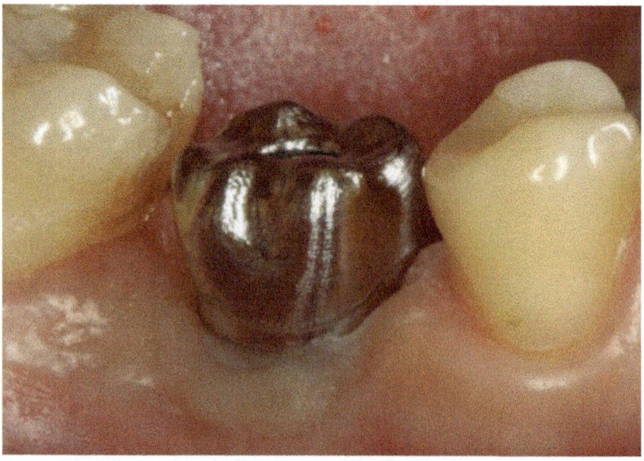

Fig. 13.3 Grayish appearance of soft peri-implant tissues when metal framework is used

procedure was to be performed intraorally. After that, abutment-restoration complex was retrieved, cement remnants cleaned, and restoration returned to the mouth. Currently proposed technique has several advantages. First, the cementation procedure is more controlled on the model, than on the mouth, especially if the implant is placed deeply. In the latter case, it is difficult to fully seat the crown on the implant in the mouth, due to resistance of the peri-implant tissues. Secondly, less clinical time is spent, as cementation and excess cleaning procedures are done in the laboratory. Despite these clear advantages, there are some clinicians who still prefer to cement crowns of cement-screw-retained restorations in the mouth.

The sequence of fabrication can be seen in (Figs. 13.4 and 13.5).

The question arises: what is the success and long-term data of this approach of screw-retained restorations? Indeed, long-term in vivo evidence is still being gathered; however, we can extrapolate from the data of individual prosthetic abutments for cemented restorations. These reports in increased loading situations showed 100% success [14, 15]. It is interesting to note that these excellent-outcome studies used zirconium abutment with external connection or internal hexagon two-piece construction, where zirconium abutment-like coping is cemented on a titanium base. Finally, Zembic et al. showed no fractures of zirconium abutment glued to titanium substructures in an 11-year prospective clinical trial [16].

The other way to connect zirconia to titanium base is via metallic adapter. This is a more unique way, when zirconia is connected to titanium base during the process of tightening. This eliminates the cement line, and connection relies on mechanical precision and adaptation. This system is unique to a few manufacturers. And we do not yet know if the unfilled micro-gap between the titanium base and the zirconia superstructure will prove to be a problematic reservoir of pathogenic bacteria.

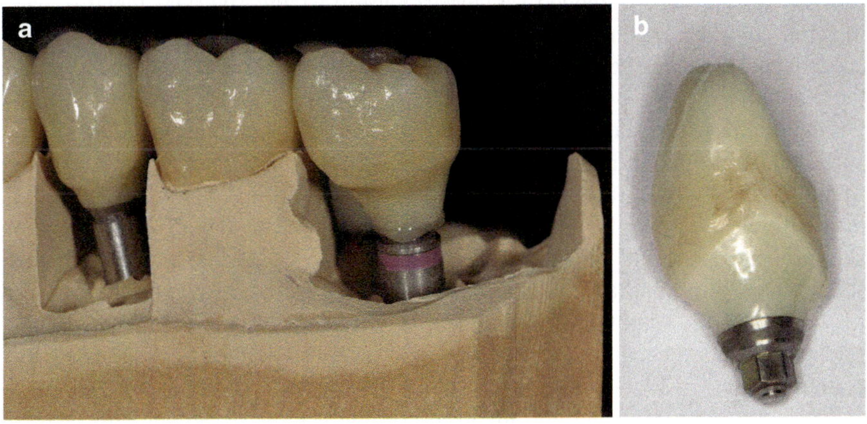

Fig. 13.4 (**a**) Luting of finished restoration to titanium base on the model. This allows to completely clean cement remnants. (**b**) Completely finished hybrid restoration free of residual cement

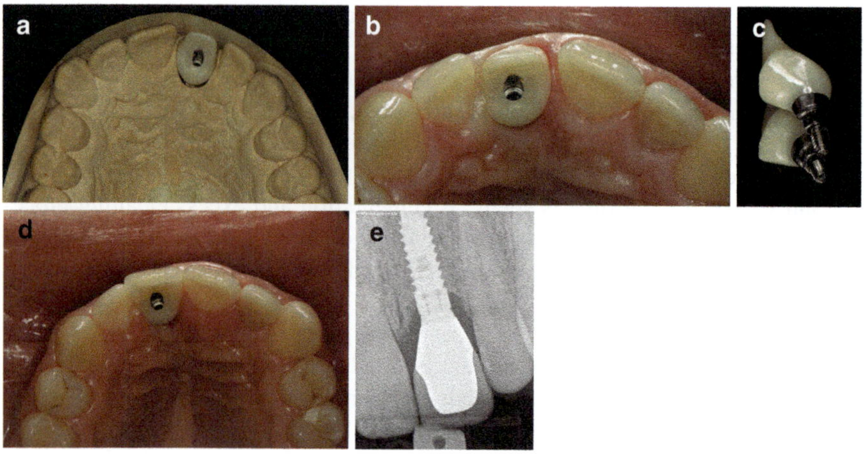

Fig. 13.5 (**a**) Zirconia framework temporary glued to titanium base. (**b**) Clinical verification of the framework. (**c**) Zirconia framework within Ti base without ceramic layering. (**d**) Finished restoration screw-retained to the implant. (**e**) Radiological image of finalized treatment

13.3 Material Selection

The very important factor for the screw-retained restorations is selection of material because part of the restoration ends up subgingivally and plays a direct role in establishment and maintenance of biologic width around implants. Thus, material selection has direct influence on soft tissue stability and functioning of the implant. It is in closest contact with the peri-implant tissues, which is the first and only barrier from oral bacteria—a threat to osseointegration.

Before going into details, we need to distinguish three main parts of the screw-retained restoration—framework material, veneering material, and metallic base material. If we are using cement-screw-retained restoration, we have the fourth component—adhesive resin cement, which is used to connect the superstructure to the titanium base.

Metallic base is usually titanium alloy, which is a biocompatible material with sufficient strength to withstand loading. Recently, manufacturers started to offer titanium bases with different height not only for retention of suprastructure but also with different heights for subgingival part (Fig. 13.6). The base with higher subgingival part might be used in case we want to move the cementation line further from the bone and also in case we are using metal-ceramic crown for restoration of the implant. This reduces the exposure of peri-implant tissues to feldspathic ceramics, gold alloys, and Cr-Co, as more titanium surface is gained from the base.

Currently, various materials are used for fabrication of individually screw-retained restorations, like metals, ceramics, and composites. For many years, cast gold alloy was considered as the state of the art in customized prosthetic solutions;

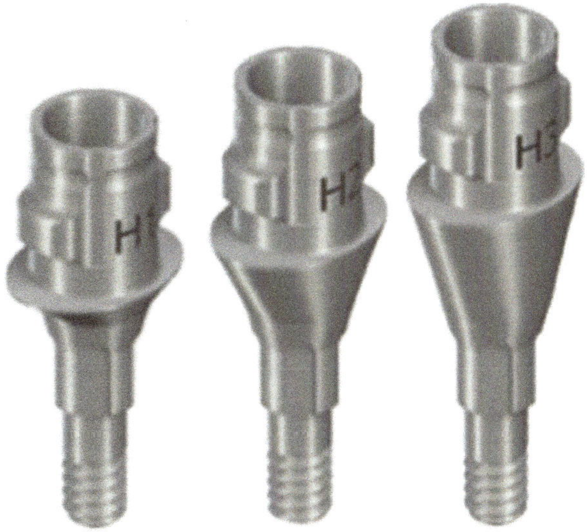

Fig. 13.6 Titanium bases with different height of the gingival part

however, their use recently is rapidly decreasing due to lack of biocompatibility and higher pricing. It was shown in animal studies that peri-implant soft tissues do not form sufficient seal with gold abutments; as such, significant soft tissue recession and crestal bone loss can be expected. Similarly, dental porcelain appeared not to be a proper material for establishment of reliable soft tissue adherence. In fact the outcome with feldspathic ceramics was least favorable, as soft tissue recession and bone loss were highest among the tested materials [17].

Properties of zirconium allow achieving good and stable clinical results. One of the major justifications for zirconia as prosthetic material for implants restorations is biocompatibility. This reason for zirconium oxide's high biocompatibility is its ability to evoke positive reaction of the host tissues. It has been suggested that the biocompatibility is influenced by the following features of zirconia—chemical composition, polishing properties, adhesion of fibroblasts, and bacteria. Zirconia is an inert material, structurally stable, with almost no corrosion, producing side products, thus no threat to the host tissues.

Polishing properties are also very important to the maintenance of the peri-implant tissues. It has been shown that it is possible to polish zirconia to a mirror-like finish (Fig. 13.7). Many studies show that fibroblasts and epithelial cells have better proliferation and retention to a polished zirconium surface when compared to a rough one. Additionally, it has been shown that fibroblasts have better proliferation and adhesion to polished zirconia, while bacteria seem to be least attracted to smooth zirconia. It has been shown clinically that zirconia-healing abutments evoked less inflammation when compared to titanium. This leads to the conclusion that this material is best material currently available for framework fabrication. Although a systematic review did not confirm the superiority of zirconium abutments for crestal bone preservation over titanium abutments, reaction of soft tissues seem to be more favorable clinically.

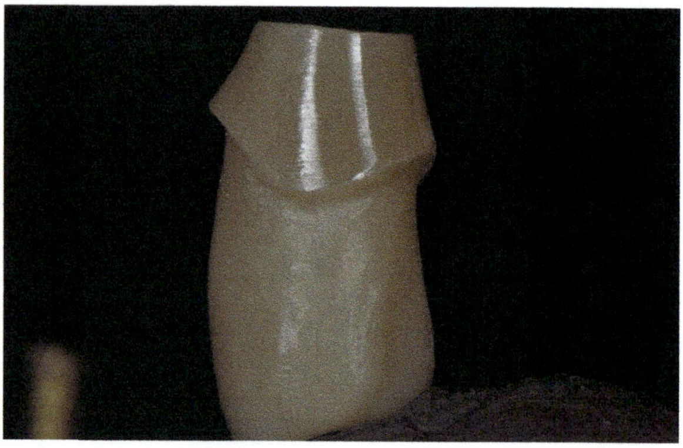

Fig. 13.7 Surface of polished zirconia, achieved with hand polishing

To completely understand the role of framework and veneering materials on peri-implant tissues, we need to look at the schematic picture of a screw-retained restoration.

It is well known that vertical biologic width consists of connective tissue portion (CT) and the epithelial attachment (JE). An overwhelming number of studies show that the connective tissue is approximately 1 mm in length, despite the design of an implant, depth of the placement, and roughness of the abutment. Therefore, it is rather constant figure. In contrast, the epithelial portion varies from 2–3 mm and is formed of a small layer of epithelial cells. It has been shown that the apical part of the epithelium is very thin and attaches to implant surface with hemidesmosome-like structures. Thus, if we are using titanium bases, which are 1 mm in height, we have fibroblasts in contact with titanium, while there is no direct interaction between zirconia and fibroblasts, as connective tissue is lined with epithelial cells that adhere to zirconia surface via hemidesmosomes. This is very important to understand, as majority of in vitro studies study interaction of Zr with fibroblasts, as in fact this interaction usually does not occur intraorally. The zirconia in this design is only in contact with epithelial cells (Fig. 13.8).

Additionally, we must address the interaction between the framework and the veneering materials. One of the common protocols is to completely cover the framework with feldspathic porcelain. Screw retaining of the finished restoration on the implant results in placement of the feldspathic veneering porcelain under the peri-implant mucosa. If this protocol is followed, the zirconia framework is blocked from the tissues by the veneering porcelain, and the reconstruction becomes so called $Zr0_2$ without ZrO_2, where no direct or only minimal contact between ZrO_2 and soft tissues is achieved (Fig. 13.9).

Finally, patients do not receive the benefits of zirconia, as the major part of peri-implant tissues has contact with dental porcelain, which is much less biocompatible. The rational for masking zirconia with feldspathic ceramics may be based on the notion that ZrO_2 can age and subsequently become weaker when confronted by oral environment [10]. Therefore, veneering porcelain protects ZrO_2 from contact with

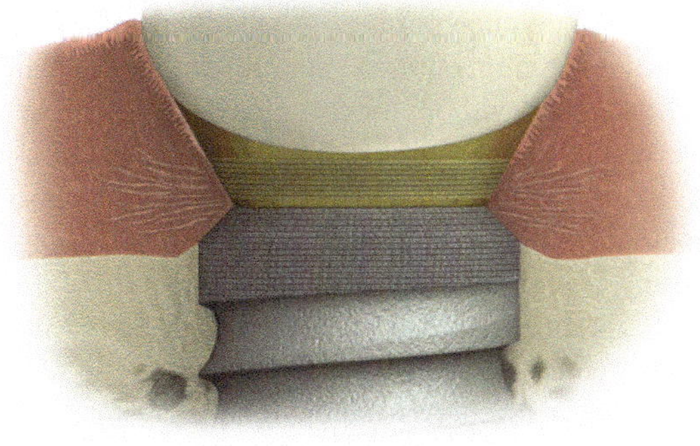

Fig. 13.8 Schematic drawing of peri-implant tissues. It can be seen that connective tissue direct contact is with titanium base, while moving coronal connective tissues are lined with epithelium, which contacts zirconia

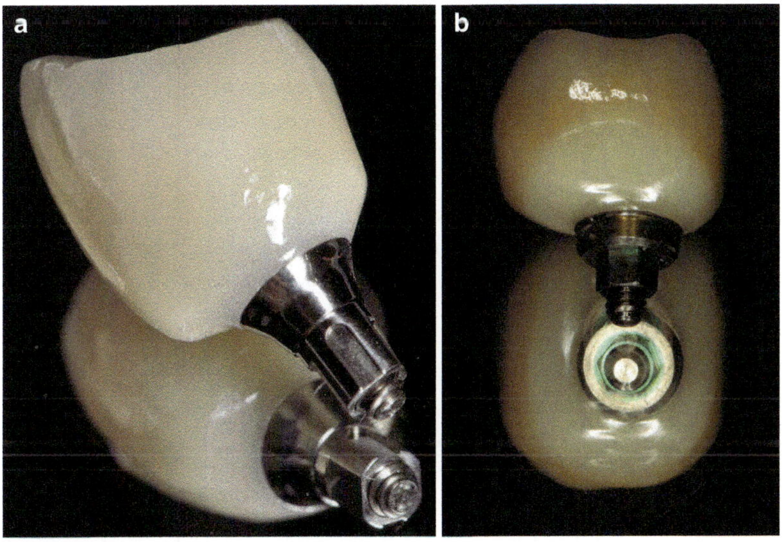

Fig. 13.9 (**a**) "Zirconia without zirconia" restorations. Zirconia framework is covered with veneering porcelain and hidden from peri-implant tissues. (**b**) Restoration with zirconia not covered with feldspathic porcelain

saliva and precludes weakening of the material. However, recent studies do not confirm the idea that saliva can make ZrO_2 weaker with time [11]. Therefore it can be speculated that if Zr_2O screw-retained restoration is designed in the traditional way, no difference in peri-implant soft tissue response will occur, compared to metal-ceramic restorations, since biological properties of veneering porcelain for zirconia and metal are the same.

The scaffold of such restorations can be divided into two areas: (1) peri-implant tissue area with pure ZrO_2 and (2) ceramic area, where only porcelain is applied

(Fig. 13.5). It is designed in such a manner that the veneering ceramics would start only from emergence point of the restoration from peri-implant tissues and do not go into the subgingival area. Subsequently feldspathic porcelain is layered on the ZrO_2 framework without touching the soft tissue area.

It could be suggested that this novel Zr_2O screw-retained restoration, when zirconia is maximally exposed to peri-implant tissues, offers significant advantages, compared to implant-supported crowns, which subgingival parts are covered with veneering porcelain. The benefits of biocompatibility can be obtained only if soft tissues have direct contact with zirconia. This is why we have less soft tissue recession due to integration of the implant.

One of the restrictions to screw-retained restorations has been incorrect 3D implant position because that usually results in an access hole through the facial surface of the crown, which leaves aesthetically unacceptable results. Using custom-milled abutments and cemented restorations solves this problem. However, recent advances have made it possible to have screw-retained restoration with angulated access, thus avoiding cemented solution. Angulated screw channel systems (Fig. 13.10) with a gimbaled screw/screwdriver construction, allowing an angulation of the screw channel and screwdriver axis of up to 25°. This solution is not available for all implant systems (Fig. 13.11).

In conclusion it can be stated that screw-retained restoration is viable solution for prosthetic rehabilitation of implants in aesthetic region, if a cementless solution is desired.

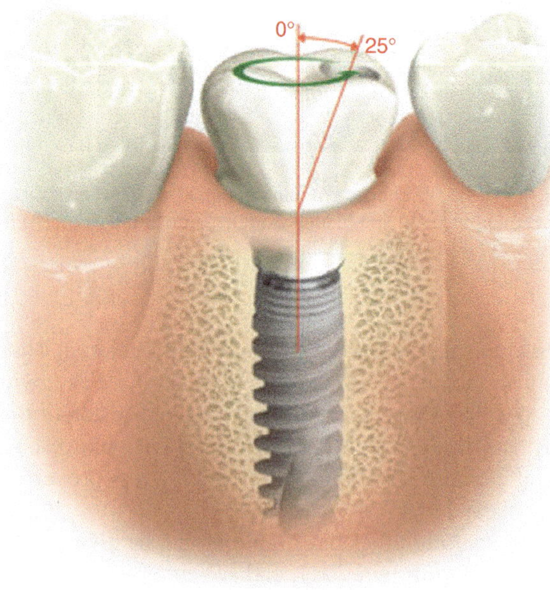

Fig. 13.10 Schematic visualization of angulated screw access possibilities up to 25°

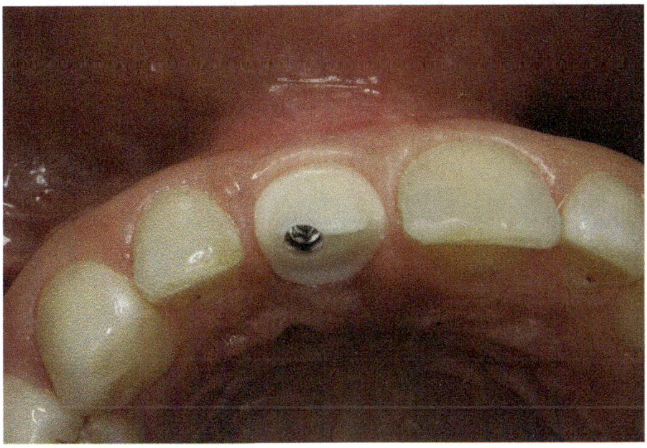

Fig. 13.11 The case, there screw angulation could be used—individual abutment and screw hole is on incisal; therefore, regular screw-retained restoration would compromise aesthetics

References

1. Hebel KS, Gajjar RC. Cement-retained versus screw-retained implant restorations: achieving optimal occlusion and esthetics in implant dentistry. J Prosthet Dent. 1997;77:28–35.
2. Sailer I, Muhlemann S, Zwahlen M, Hammerle CHF, Schneider D. Cemented and screw-retained implant reconstructions: a systematic review of the survival and complication rates. Clin Oral Implants Res. 2012;23(Suppl 6):163–201.
3. Linkevicius T, Vindasiute E, Puisys A, Peciuliene V. The influence of margin location on the amount of undetected cement excess after delivery of cement-retained implant restorations. Clin Oral Implants Res. 2011;22:1379–84.
4. Wasiluk G, Chomik E, Gerhrke P, Pietruska M, Skurska A, Pietruski J. Incidence of undetected cement on CAD/CAM monolithic zirconia crowns and customized CAD/CAM implant abutments. A prospective case series. Clin Oral Implants Res. 2016;28(7):1–5.
5. Michalakis KX, Hirayama H, Garefis PD. Cement-retained versus screw-retained implant restorations: a critical review. Int J Oral Maxillofac Implants. 2003;18:719–28.
6. Wittneben JG, Millen C, Brägger U. Clinical performance of screw- versus cement-retained fixed implant-supported reconstructions-a systematic review. Int J Oral Maxillofac Implants. 2014;29:84–98.
7. Wadhwani CH, Piñeyro A, Avots J. An esthetic solution to the screw-retained implant restoration: introduction to the implant crown adhesive plug: clinical report. J Esthet Restor Dent. 2011;23:138–45.
8. Kano SC, Bonfante G, Binon PP, et al. Effect of casting procedures on screw loosening in UCLA-type abutments. J Prosthodont. 2006;15:1–5.
9. Park SE, Da Silva JD, Weber HP, Ishikawa-Nagai S. Optical phenomenon of peri-implant soft tissue. Part I. Spectrophotometric assessment of natural tooth gingiva and peri-implant mucosa. Clin Oral Implants Res. 2007;18:569–74.
10. Jung RE, Holderegger C, Sailer I, Khraisat A, Suter A, Hammerle CH. The effect of all-ceramic and porcelain-fused-to-metal restorations on marginal peri-implant soft tissue color: a randomized controlled clinical trial. Int J Periodontics Restorative Dent. 2008;28:357–65.
11. Carrillo de AA, Vignoletti F, Ferrantino L, Cardenas E, De SM, Sanz M. A randomized trial on the aesthetic outcomes of implant-supported restorations with zirconia or titanium abutments. J Clin Periodontol. 2014;41:1161–9.
12. Passos SP, Linke B, Larjava H, French D. Performance of zirconia abutments for implant-supported single-tooth crowns in esthetic areas: a retrospective study up to 12-year follow-up. Clin Oral Implants Res. 2014;27(1):47–54. https://doi.org/10.1111/clr.12504.

13. Rajan M, Gunaseelan R. Fabrication of a cement- and screw-retained implant prosthesis. J Prosthet Dent. 2004;92:578–80.
14. Zembic A, Bosch A, Jung RE, Hammerle CH, Sailer I. Five-year results of a randomized controlled clinical trial comparing zirconia and titanium abutments supporting single-implant crowns in canine and posterior regions. Clin Oral Implants Res. 2013;24:384–90.
15. Glauser R, Sailer I, Wohlwend A, Studer S, Schibli M, Scharer P. Experimental zirconia abutments for implant-supported single-tooth restorations in esthetically demanding regions: 4-year results of a prospective clinical study. Int J Prosthodont. 2004;17:285–90.
16. Zembic A, Philipp AO, Hammerle CH, Wohlwend A, Sailer I. Eleven-year follow-up of a prospective study of zirconia implant abutments supporting single all-ceramic crowns in anterior and premolar regions. Clin Implant Dent Relat Res. 2014;17(Suppl 2):e417–26.
17. Abrahamsson I, Berglundh T, Glantz PO, Lindhe J. The mucosal attachment at different abutments. An experimental study in dogs. J Clin Periodontol. 1998;25:721–7.

Delivery of the Definitive Abutment/ Prosthesis: Biologics, Aesthetics, and Mechanical Considerations

14

Chandur P. K. Wadhwani, Luigi Canullo, and Todd R. Schoenbaum

Abstract

The aim of implant therapy is integration, not only host tissue integration but also in the form of biology, esthetics, and mechanics, whereby the implant works as a system in harmony with the human body. Research inspired, this chapter will evaluate the fundamentals of soft tissue integration, the seal that protects the bone and acts as a barrier to the oral environment. Written by practicing clinicians, the goal is to provide information on how to optimize health through understanding handling, cleaning, aesthetics, and mechanics of the restorative componentry.

Traditional dentistry has relied on the adjacent teeth or the mobile soft tissues when providing prostheses that substitute for and replace the missing dentition. This has led to the necessary destruction of healthy sites with the potential for future compromise of the patient's oral health. Dental implants have provided a solution to these issues and can be used as individual or multiunit medical devices to support the missing teeth or tooth. However, the invention and use of the dental implant have also led to some new issues not encountered by dentistry in the past, especially with respect to biologics, aesthetics, and mechanics. This chapter will deal with some of the issues when delivering the implant restoration with clinical guidance on how

C. P. K. Wadhwani (✉)
Department of Restorative Dentistry, University of Washington, Seattle, WA, USA

Loma Linda University School of Dentistry, Loma Linda, CA, USA

L. Canullo
University of Valencia, Valencia, Spain

T. R. Schoenbaum
Division of Constitutive and Regenerative Sciences, University of California, Los Angeles, CA, USA

Todd R. Schoenbaum (ed.), *Implants in the Aesthetic Zone*,
https://doi.org/10.1007/978-3-319-72601-4_14

these problems can be circumvented. Modification of the thought processes and a need to adapt to the new challenges that dental implants have brought are essential if the implant restoration is to be of value and provide good service to our patients.

14.1 Biologics: Delivering Abutments Without Introducing Potentially Harmful Foreign Materials

One of the prerequisites when delivering any prosthesis is that it should not introduce potentially harmful foreign materials. Considering dental implants, there is the potential for such material to inadvertently contaminate the peri-implant tissues. Examples of this are when the components are not adequately cleaned, impression material remnants, retraction cord, and luting cements. All of these events have been proven to cause insult to the soft tissues. The most common causes, contaminated components (Fig. 14.1) and residual excess cement (Fig. 14.2a, b), will be discussed in this section.

14.2 Component Contaminants

Much has been written on material selection for implant components and how this has the potential to affect long-term health of the peri-implant soft tissues.

One study reported on the biological contaminants that have been detected on previously used, cleaned, and sterilized healing abutments, thus indicating that only new abutment components are to be used on the implant and should be considered the standard of care. However, even with new components, microscopic impurities on the surface of the abutment due to the industrial processes have been detected after prepackaging industrial procedures. Additional metallic microparticles mixed

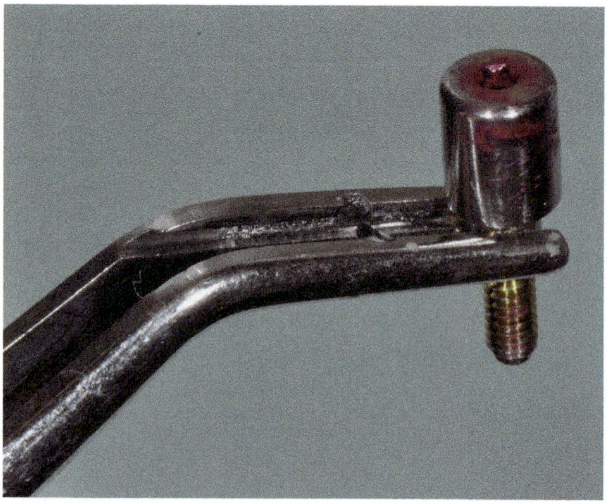

Fig. 14.1 A used Cleaned and sterilized healing abutment, red stain indicates protein contamination after use. Abutments cannot be reused if tissue integration is to occur

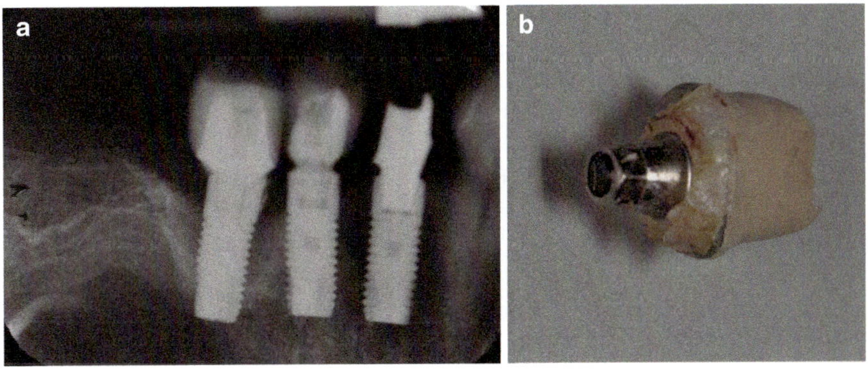

Fig. 14.2 (**a**) Radiograph, highlighting the excess cement associated with a failing implant. (**b**) Abutment retrieved from implant seen in radiograph. The excess residual cement is clearly visible, indicating poor clinical use of cement

with lubricant and oxide layers can be produced during the laboratory work flow, and adsorbed contaminants can be accumulated during the delivery.

Abutment cleaning procedures such as cleansing with decontaminates such as alcohol, soaps, or steam vapor at the end of the laboratory phases should be routinely carried out. The effectiveness of such methods has been questioned as impurities may still be detected on the abutment surface. It is considered that under certain circumstances, this exogenous material can trigger soft and hard tissue inflammatory responses.

To date, no clear cleaning protocols exist, and as such the introduction in the clinical practice of cleaning technologies able to maintain or even positively affect host cell response constitutes a very important area of research. In this context, cold plasma technology represents an efficient clinical option. Plasma is defined as a partially or wholly ionized gas with a roughly equal number of positively and negatively charged particles. Two types of plasma exist: high and low temperature. Only the last one (ionized gases generated at pressures between 13 and 266 Pa and temperature below 60 °C) could be considered for clinical purpose such as surface modification and organic cleaning.

With appropriate plasma parameters, argon plasma removes all chemical traces from former treatments, in effect producing cleaner and more well-controlled surfaces than with conventional preparation methods.

As mentioned, plasma cleaning produces two notable effects:

1. Cleaning and corrosion protection
2. Increasing the surface energy

It has been demonstrated that this procedure can produce a cleaning effect on customized abutments after 12 min comparable with the one after 45 min in an ultrasonic bath. At the same time, it was demonstrated to increase the surface energy (wettability), showing in vitro cell adhesion both to the abutment and implant surfaces.

Advantages of plasma cleaning were demonstrated in vivo to enhance the soft tissue response during prosthetic implant phases. Such a modified surface, unlike traditional machined-polluted surface abutment, might provide improved opportunities for a direct fibro-collagenous attachment, preventing soft tissue downgrowth. From a clinical point of view, these favorable events may result in a long-term hard and soft tissue stability. Early data suggest significantly improved preservation of the bone at 5 years with the use of argon plasma to clean abutments prior to placement.

14.3 Cements

Work by Wilson and others has demonstrated a positive relationship between excess cement and peri-implant disease. This foreign material may cause serious implant heath issues with an etiology, though not fully understood, considered to be multifactorial. Cement type, abutment design, cement application amount, and margin position have all been studied, illustrating that each may have a positive or negative effect on the implant.

The excess cement issues related to cement materials are likely derived from the bacterial interaction, chemical effects, host response, and sensitization producing negative tissue responses.

Few cements have ever been tested for their antibacterial effects as they relate to the microbes implicated in peri-implant disease. Many claims are made about antibacterial properties simply because the cement may contain chemicals such as triclosan. Without proper bacterial tests being made, these claims should be ignored, and the manufacturers held to a higher standard whereby they truly understand the products they sell. Dental cements for teeth are frequently tested for their antimicrobial activity against caries-producing bacteria; surely implant cements and the bacteria associated with diseases specific to implants need to be considered.

The first study to evaluate the response of peri-implant-related, Gram-negative microbes was conducted by Raval in 2012. His work suggested that Temp-Bond (Kerr) with eugenol inhibited both planktonic and biofilm growth of *A. actinomycetemcomitans*, *P. gingivalis*, and *F. nucleatum*. Although a rudimentary study design, it gave some indication of the need for such studies. The results of this study indicated that zinc oxide with eugenol appeared to be a very effective antibacterial material especially against the "specially formulated" implant cements.

Further negative effects of cements used with implant restorations have been reported. Cement particles have been found in soft tissue biopsies of failed removed implants, initially reported by Ramer and then by Burbano. The cement may be a result of the cementation process itself or be a result of fragments breaking off after the cement has fully set. In the authors' opinion, it is possible that the cement is being implanted within the soft tissues during the final cementation process. The sulcular tissue around the implant is very different compared to that around the tooth. The attachment is easily stripped away; it also shows high permeability and has a poor blood supply, which reduces the ability to repair. Some cements also

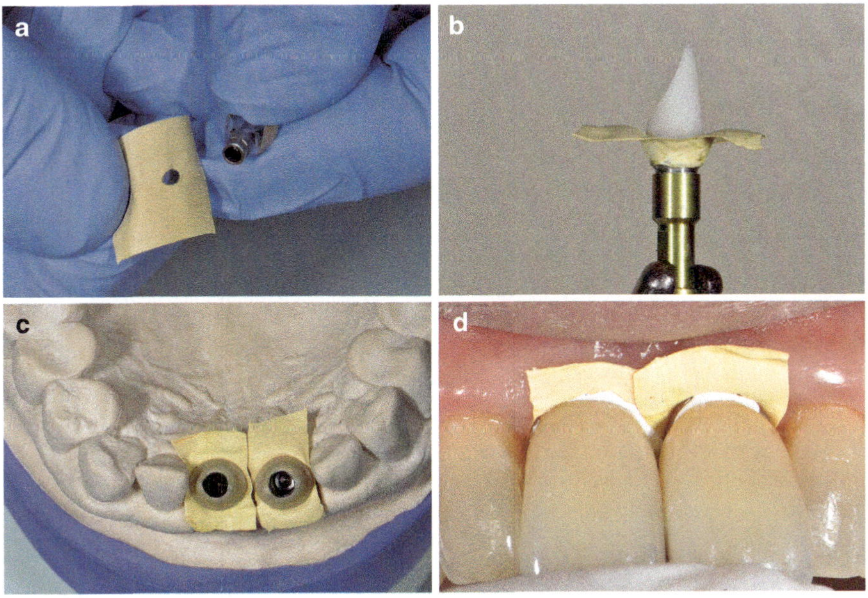

Fig. 14.3 (**a**) A square piece of PTFE yellow tape, cut and a hole punched in the center using a rubber dam punch. (**b**) The PTFE piece placed over the abutment, checking that it will not be caught in the connection of the implant site (by seating an analog over the connection allows this to be confirmed). (**c**) Model showing how the barrier PTFE works, again it must not encroach onto the margin area, or it will be trapped during cementation. (**d**) PTFE barrier in place as the crowns are being seated with finger pressure first. The barrier protects the vulnerable soft tissues from cement insult

have very thin film thickness which allows them to be pushed directly into the tissues. Although it does not seem logical that materials can penetrate soft tissues, any clinician that has ever encountered an amalgam tattoo will understand that this occurs commonly. Allergic response to the chemicals used by cement manufactures is also a cause for concern. Most, if not all, material substance data sheets (MSDS) warn that the cements must be handled with care, often recommending gloves to protect the skin. The skin tissue has been shown to be multiple times less permeable than mucosa, and protection of the peri-implant soft tissues is almost never considered. This can be readily achieved by using rudimentary dams made with polytetrafluoroethylene (PTFE) tape (Fig. 14.3a–d). Finally, some cements contain fluoride, which can become associated with hydrogen to produce hydrofluoric (HF) acid. This particular acid can result in corrosion of titanium and titanium alloys. Not only does it roughen the surface allowing more bacteria to adhere, reactive oxidative species can be produced by the body that leads to host tissue destruction.

To date almost all cements are developed for natural teeth which have very different requirements compared to implant restorations. Currently, there is no ideal implant cement, but selection should be based on sound clinical criteria, with the

Table 14.1 Outlines some of the differences in cement selection criteria for implant restorations and cement properties for the natural tooth

	Implant restoration	Natural tooth
Substructure	Metal, ceramic, acrylic	Dentine, enamel
Biological tissue association	Peri-implant tissues	Periodontal tissues, pulp
Primary disease issue	Peri-implant disease	Caries, pulpal, periodontal
Restorations finish line		½–1 mm below anterior aesthetic sites, often above the free gingival margins
Cement margin	May or may not follow scallop of the tissues	Preparation follow gingival tissues
Need for cement seal	Questionable	Absolute (prevent caries)
Anti-caries agents	May be detrimental	Desirable
Corrosion	Corrosion of titanium possible	Not applicable
Radiopacity	Highly radiopaque	Similar to dentine (relatively low)
Microbial challenge	Bacteria found in peri-implant sites	Caries-producing bacteria

clinician understanding desirable and undesirable qualities of the selection made. Wadhwani and Schwedhelm summarized in detail the different considerations for material selection specific to teeth and implant-cemented restorations (Table 14.1).

Abutment design has evaluated the cement margin location, indicating this is most critical. Linkevicius has shown that a cement margin site as minimal as 1 mm below the soft tissues can result in excess cement extrusion into the soft tissue sulcus and recommends the margin be placed equi-gingival. Abutment modifications that control cement flow have also been described, as have techniques to limit cement volume and control application site. All these measures should be taken into account when considering cementation of the implant restoration.

Cement application techniques with implants have been poorly studied. Most clinicians have never been taught how to optimize cement flow within the crown abutment system, and the authors believe that many of the problems related to residual excess cement come from a lack of knowledge on cement materials and how they are used. In a survey of over 400 clinicians as to where and how cement is applied, three distinct patterns were noted. Cement was either grossly applied, applied at the margin of the crown, or painted on the intaglio walls of the crown. Apart from the application technique, most clinicians were unaware of how much cement was required for the finite lute space between the crown and the abutment, with most applying far in excess of what is ideally required. Cement knowledge must not be limited to chemistry or setting characteristics; understanding the mechanics of flow is required. Wadhwani studied this using a super computer and specialized fluid dynamic software. It was determined that the optimum site for most cements was an application near to the cervical margin of the in the form of a circumferntial hoop. Also, speed of seating was determined to be optimal when around 14 mm per second. Too fast and the cement due to its inherent non-Newtonian character shear thinned and was pushed past the margin. Too slow and the occlusal aspect was not fully filled, again resulting in an excess of cement extrusion through the margin. Currently, all implant-abutment components have little if any science behind their shape. Most are simply machined to conform to the shape dentists have been preparing teeth for over 50 years. There is no understanding of the shape, which today defies all reasoning. With the expense of implant abutments, we should demand their shape be made to follow their function. With metal and ceramic abutments, there is no need to have them conform to a tooth form—they may have vents, spiral cement spill ways, conical inserts, and many other designs that will help the clinician prevent cement excess extrusion—all we need is to drive the science behind implant component design.

14.4 Aesthetics and Simple Implant-Abutment Modifications

Aesthetics has always been of great concern in the dental industry, with color, contour, and soft tissue emergence profiles high on our list to help satisfy both the patient and the clinician. When implants are employed as replacements for the teeth, there are multiple issues in trying to emulate the natural tooth. One such example is how aesthetics and biologics may interact. For instance, the current gold standard for implantable materials used in the dental implant industry is titanium. This silver gray metal with excellent biocompatibility, strength, and ability to withstand the challenges of the oral environment is used widely for the implant body, abutments, and prosthetic components.

However, the color of titanium has become an aesthetic issue, especially when it reflects through the gingival tissues and produces a blue/gray discoloration. Such aesthetic demands have resulted in newly developed and measured tests for color as well as form of the peri-implant tissues. Fürhauser was the first to describe the so-called pink esthetic score. This index compared the shape, color, and form of the implant and restoration on the peri-implant tissues. Others added and modified the index to measure the restoration related to the existing dentition and surrounding environment.

One method of overcoming the blue/gray hue of titanium was the introduction of zirconia-based abutments. They also provided an improved foundation base color for all ceramic restorations used in highly aesthetic cases. However, zirconia is not as strong as titanium, and the literature report abutment fracture issues (Fig. 14.4a, b). Also, if the restoration requires cementation to the zirconia abutment, this is not always predictable due to zirconia's low adhesive properties. Finally, the interface of zirconia with titanium implants may promote titanium particle discoloration within the tissues as a result of dissimilar wear rates.

To overcome these issues and help with abutment aesthetics, some manufacturers of titanium abutments use a titanium nitride (TiN) coating method, producing a yellow/gold-colored surface effect. This places a surface coating layer of dissimilar material onto the surface of the titanium. However, case reports have suggested patients may be allergic to this surface, and the biocompatibility of TiN does not appear to be as sound as the titanium dioxide that spontaneously forms on titanium metal in an oxygen environment. Some orthopedic studies have reported that the TiN layer can crack off the surface of the titanium.

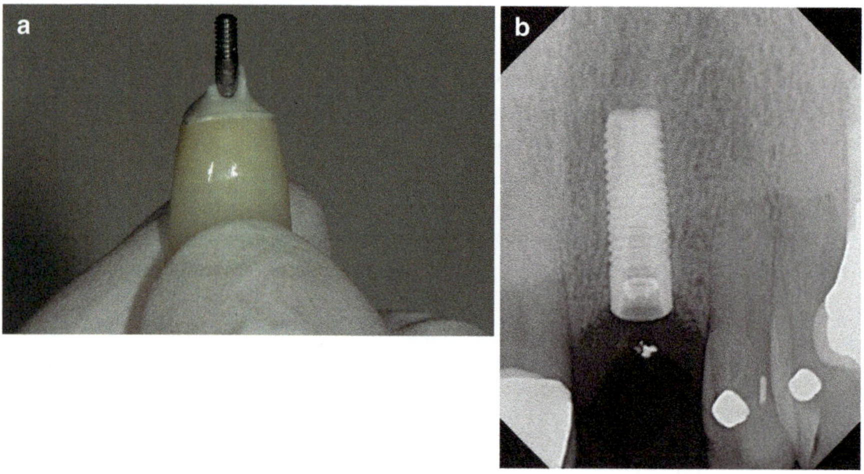

Fig. 14.4 (**a**) Zirconia abutment fracture at the implant-abutment connection, considered a weak site. (**b**) This fracture has left some of the zirconia still within the implant itself, which can be challenging to remove

Fig. 14.5 Abutments have been anodized using batteries and diet soda. By varying the voltage applied, yellow/gold colors can be used for the core abutment color. Pink hues can be produced for the abutment beneath the tissues. Both pink and yellow can also be produced by selective anodization

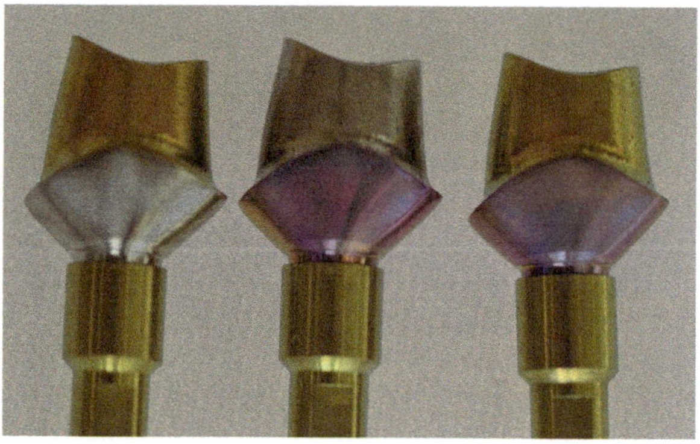

An improved way of coloring titanium has been described in the literature, which uses a very different technique to provide aesthetic-colored abutments (Fig. 14.5). Anodization is a physicochemical controlled method of thickening the titanium dioxide surface layer. This is the same layer that naturally and sponaneously evolves if the titanium is left in air and is the basis of the biocompatibility of titanium itself. This is a simple, fast, and inexpensive technique for coloring the titanium that has been described in the dental literature and can be done by anyone, using common materials. When the titanium dioxide layer is thickened, a physical phenomenon occurs, whereby natural white light is absorbed and reflected back as a thin film

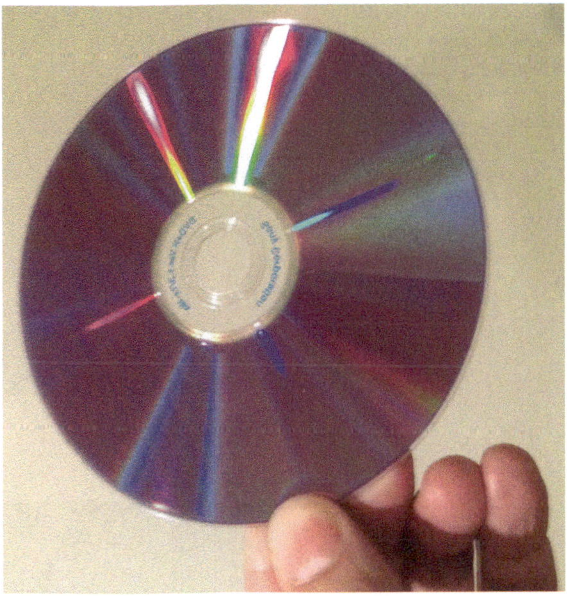

Fig. 14.6 Anodization uses the properties of reflected light passing through a clear film—the same effect is seen when a CD-ROM is rotated. It has no intrinsic color, but colors are seen through this effect

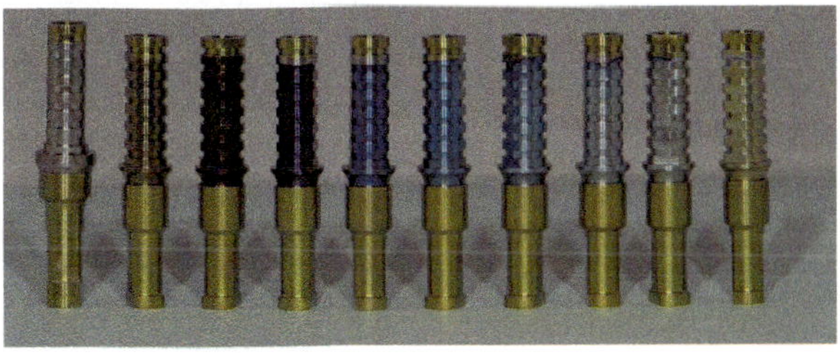

Fig. 14.7 Some of the many colors that can be produced by anodization of titanium and titanium alloy, simply by using different voltages

interference pattern, similar to what is commonly seen with oil films on water or when a CD-ROM reflects colors (Fig. 14.6). A series of colors can be produced, each of which is dependent upon the thickness of the titanium dioxide layer. Some of the colors are very useful for improving abutment aesthetics, either relative to the soft tissues, the restoration, or both. The anodization can easily produce many different colors including clinically useful yellows, golds, and pinks (Fig. 14.7) all of which are dependent upon the applied electrical direct current voltage. This natural phenomenon is easily achieved using common electrolytes—usually acids, including products such as diet cola (Fig. 14.8).

The process involves placing a positive electrical charge on the titanium to be anodized and placing it in an electrolyte which has a negative electrode immersed

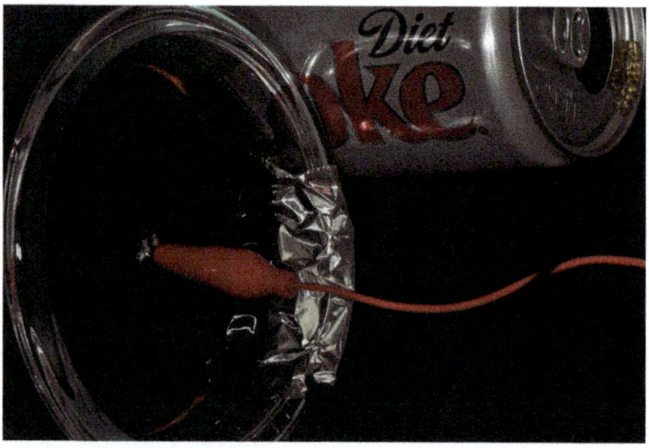

Fig. 14.8 Using weak acids, including diet soda which contains food-grade phosphoric acid, as an electrolyte for anodization. Note the aluminum cooking foil provides the negative terminal for the solution

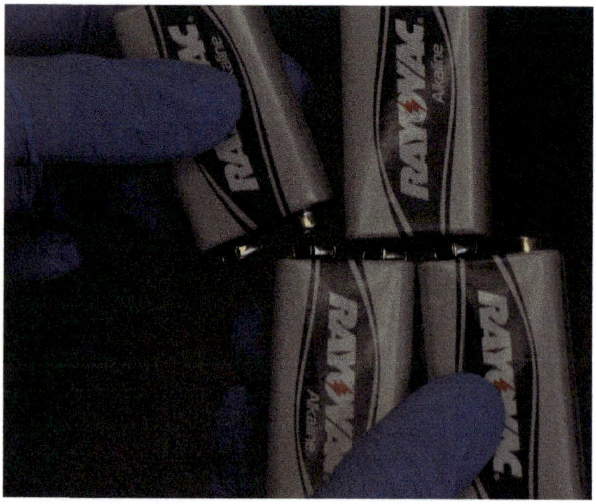

Fig. 14.9 Flat, 9 V household batteries are ideal to use for the electrical power with anodization. Generally, linking them in series by "connecting them" allows the voltages to be increased in increments of 9 V. Nine of these batteries produce a "pink" hue, and seven linked gives a "yellow" hue

in it. The negative electrode can pass electrical current through the electrolyte if attached to aluminum cooking foil (Fig. 14.8). The electrical supply can be a dedicated direct current generator or simply common household batteries (Fig. 14.9). Because electric current must flow onto the surface of the titanium, it must be clean and free of oils. Similarly, at the conclusion of the anodization process, the abutment must be thoroughly washed with deionized water to remove any residue left by the electrolyte used. At 63 V (seven 9 V batteries connected in series), a gold color is produced. At 81 V (nine 9 V batteries connected in series), a pink hue results (Fig. 14.5). This technique is highly effective, does not change the biocompatibility of the titanium, and is fast (taking less than 10 s). However, care must be

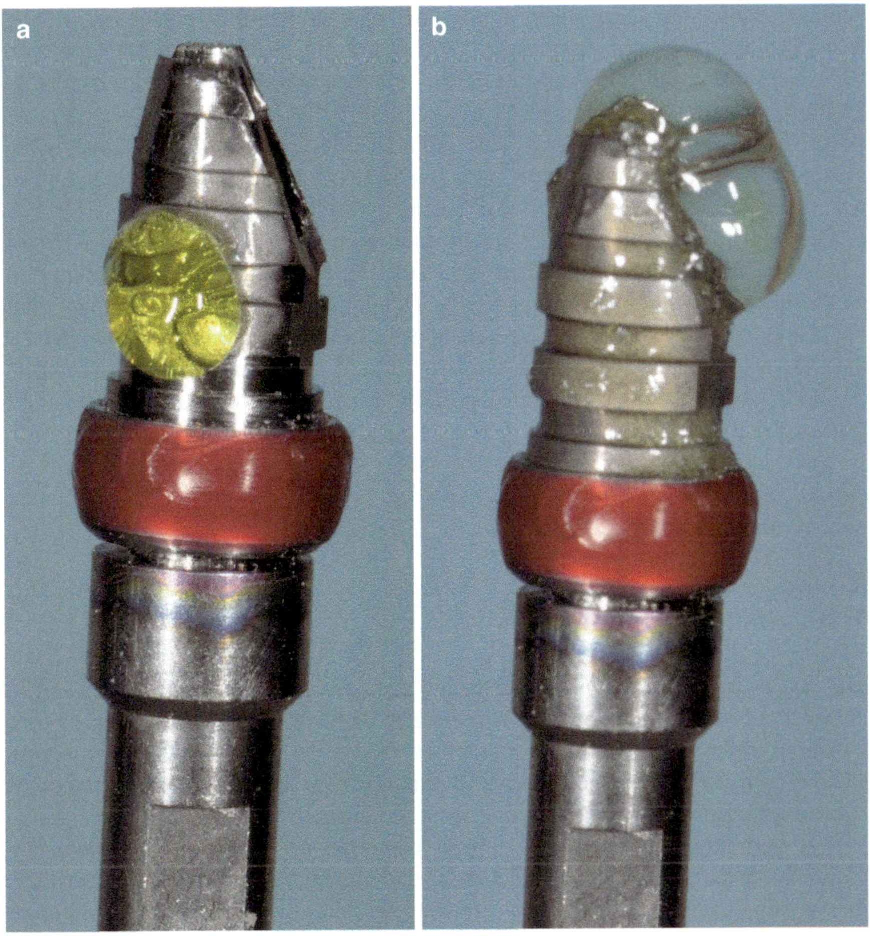

Fig. 14.10 (**a**) This abutment has HF (hydrofluoric acid 9.5%) applied. Within seconds the titanium surface starts to bubble (**b**). This is hydrogen being liberated. It can be used to etch the abutment; red wax is applied as a protective barrier at sites where etching is undesirable

exercised whenever electrical currents are employed, even household batteries can induce an electric shock if incorrectly handled.

Titanium has other very useful properties also, for example, in contrast to zirconia, titanium can be acid etched with 9.5% hydrofluoric acid for 30 s (Fig. 14.10a, b). This results in an increase in surface area which improves micromechanical bonding.

14.5 Delivery of the Restoration

Many implant restorations provided by the laboratory have residual contamination present. This may result from machining processes as described by Kelly or from simply handling the components in a contaminated environment. Because these items come into close proximity with the tissues, and in an ideal situation have some cellular attachment, these materials should be biocompatible, clean, and sterile. Many offices do not possess plasma equipment to pretreat components. However, some chemical cleansing is possible. Citric acid, a natural food substance, is readily available from many grocery stores. Made into a 40% solution, it has been used to effectively decontaminate implant surfaces affected by peri-implantitis. Placing the abutment in an ultrasonic bath for 5 min and then rinsing thoroughly with deionized water provide a cheap and effective decontaminant.

During the final stages of the implant restoration being delivered, irrespective of the type (cement- or screw-retained), the contact points with the adjacent dentition should always be carefully evaluated. They should allow floss to pass through, but not be too light especially at the mesial contact site where natural teeth exist. Recent data suggest that these will often present issues in the future with open contacts developing as a result of the natural anterior mesial drifting that occurs with natural teeth, but not with implants.

Also, routinely radiographs must be made, to confirm component fit, and no excess cement remains (Fig. 14.2b) as well as providing a baseline for evaluating bone changes that may occur.

14.6 Implant Restorations

The vast majority of implant abutments are held onto the implant body via a screw, although a few manufacturers use friction grip connections, but these can be problematic if the componentry must be removed. Restoring the implant superstructure, such as a crown or a bridge, is generally undertaken either by a screw-retained or cement-retained restoration.

Although there are proponents of each technique, neither is ideal, and both systems involve the use of a screw attaching to the implant body. The cemented restoration is separated to an abutment screwed onto the implant. It introduces more variables into the system, with two attachment sites, the abutment and the crown, as well as introduce another material into the system, namely, the cement which is known to cause biological issues in some cases. The screw-retained option has only one attachment as the abutment and restoration are an integral component. It may have aesthetic issues associated with the screw access channel and has an access hole with the potential to compromise the structure of the restoration.

With either of the systems discussed, the screw and how it works has been reported on. Early implants tended to have screw loosening issues, predominantly related to the poor tightening techniques involved. The screws were usually tightened to finger tight, which produces a very inefficient use of the screw mechanics. Eventually, engineering principles were employed with the introduction of dedicated torque wrenches. These are used to deliver a specific torque, known as preload, which is dictated by the screw manufacturer. What this essentially does is cause a mechanical stretch within the screw itself, turning the screw into a "spring"-type device that pulls the components tightly together and makes the most effective joint. However, there is still a lack of understanding on how best to provide the preload with some authorities suggesting waiting up to 10 min between repeated torque application. When one evaluates how other industries approach screw loosening of critical components, it appears waiting between torque applications is not needed. A prime example is the motor racing industry, where formula one tires are replaced within seconds, using torque devices and a single screw. They never wait 10 min! The authors consider tightening torque should be repeated but within a second or so during the development of the preload and always to the manufacturers specifications.

14.7 Mechanics of the Implant-Abutment Connection: Delivery of Componentry

The screw connection must be very carefully considered, as it is a potential site of implant failure, with screw loosening or breakage occasionally occurring.

Factors that can negatively affect this joint include how the components match or fit together. Manufacturers design their joints to fit perfectly with predefined machining tolerance, using specific metal alloys. If the tolerance or the alloy used differs from the prescribed dimensions, then the joint may not work as intended. Enlarged discrepancies at the implant-abutment junction will compromise the seal and lead to premature screw loosening and larger microgaps which may harbor pathogenic bacteria. For these reasons, prosthetic components should be made by the implant manufacturer; predictable joints are essential to implant success.

Even with original componentry, errors can occur in the mechanics of the joint, if, for example, a damaged screw is used or an incorrect torque delivered or the joint is not fully seated. Care must be taken with all these aspects, and where a joint cannot be physically inspected by tactile probing, or visualized well made, radiographs are essential.

Once the screw has been tightened, the screw head should be covered to maintain the ability to use a screw driver in the event that the screw needs to be re-torqued. Several materials have been proposed to do this, ranging from cotton wool, wax, impression material, gutta-percha, and zinc oxide/eugenol; however, the authors consider polytetrafluorethylene (PFTE)—also known as plumbers tape—to be a good alternative. It is readily available, is inexpensive, can be autoclaved, and has been shown not to support bacteria in an in vitro experiment when used as an access hole spacer for endodontics.

14.8 Summary

Delivery of the final abutment/prosthesis is at the control of the clinician; he or she may improve the biologics, esthetics, and mechanics by the choices made. Understanding the value of the physical properties of the materials such as titanium, as well as knowing how to make simple modifications, can vastly improve these factors, usually in a simple, inexpensive, and clinically useful way.

Planning is always essential; knowing where to place margins, how to control cement flow, and choice of materials in situations where cementation is necessary will help reduce the incidence of cement issues. A correct understanding of how the joint works will also improve the long-term stability and outcome of the implant restoration.

Bibliography

1. Canullo L, Micarelli C, Iannello G. Microscopical and chemical surface characterization of the gingival portion and connection of an internal hexagon abutment before and after different technical stages of preparation. Clin Oral Implants Res. 2013;24(6):606–11.
2. Canullo L, Gotz W, Cassinelli C, Tarnow D. Cell growth on titanium disks treated by plasma of argon. Int J Oral Maxillofac Implants. 2013;28:957–62.
3. Canullo L, Micarelli C, Iannello G. Microscopical and chemical surface characterization of the gingival portion and connection of an internal hexagon abutment before and after different technical stages of preparation. Clin Oral Implants Res. 2013;24(6):606–11.
4. Canullo L, Tallarico M, Peñarrocha-Oltra D, Monje A, Wang HL, Peñarrocha-Diago M. Implant abutment cleaning by plasma of argon: 5-year follow-up of a randomized controlled trial. J Periodontol. 2016;87(4):434–42.
5. Da Silva JD, Kazimiroff J, Papas A, Curro FA, Thompson VP, Vena DA, Wu H, Collie D, Craig RG, Practitioners Engaged in Applied Research and Learning (Pearl) Network Group. Outcomes of implants and restorations placed in general dental practices: a retrospective study by the practitioners engaged in applied research and learning (PEARL) network. J Am Dent Assoc. 2014;145(7):704–13.
6. Dawson DV, Drake DR, Hill JR, Brogden KA, Fischer CL, Wertz PW. Organization, barrier function and antimicrobial lipids of the oral mucosa. Int J Cosmet Sci. 2013;35(3):220–3.
7. Fürhauser R, Florescu D, Benesch T, Haas R, Mailath G, Watzek G. Evaluation of soft tissue around single-tooth implant crowns: the pink esthetic score. Clin Oral Implants Res. 2005;16(6):639–44.
8. Garcia B, Camacho F, Peñarrocha D, Tallarico M, Perez S, Canullo L. Influence of plasma cleaning procedure on the interaction between soft tissue and abutments: a randomized controlled histologic study. Clin Oral Implants Res. 2017;28(10):1269–77.
9. Hebel KS, Gajjar RC. Cement-retained versus screw-retained implant restorations: achieving optimal occlusion and esthetics in implant dentistry. J Prosthet Dent. 1997;77(1):28–35.
10. Kasemo B, Lausmaaa J. Material-tissue interfaces: the role of surface properties and processes. Environ Health Perspect. 1994;102(Suppl 5):41–5.
11. Kelly JR, Rungruanganunt P. Fatigue behavior of computer-aided design/computer-assisted manufacture ceramic abutments as a function of design and ceramics processing. Int J Oral Maxillofac Implants. 2016;31(3):601–9.
12. Lim HP, Lee KM, Koh YI, Park SW. Allergic contact stomatitis caused by a titanium nitride-coated implant abutment: a clinical report. J Prosthet Dent. 2012;108(4):209–13.
13. Liu CM, Huang FM, Yang LC, Chou LS, Chou MY, Chang YC. Cytotoxic effects of gingival retraction cords on human gingival fibroblasts in vitro. J Oral Rehabil. 2004;31(4):368–72.
14. Mansour A, Ercoli C, Graser G, Tallents R, Moss M. Comparative evaluation of casting retention using the ITI solid abutment with six cements. Clin Oral Implants Res. 2002;13(4):343–8.
15. Millen C, Brägger U, Wittneben JG. Influence of prosthesis type and retention mechanism on complications with fixed implant-supported prostheses: a systematic review applying multivariate analyses. Int J Oral Maxillofac Implants. 2015;30(1):110–24.
16. Mishra PK, Wu W, Rozo C, Hallab NJ, Benevenia J, Gause WC. Micrometer-sized titanium particles can induce potent Th2-type responses through TLR4-independent pathways. J Immunol. 2011;187(12):6491–8.

17. Moisan M, Barbeau J, Crevier MC, Pelletier J, Philip N, Saoudi N. Plasma sterilization. Methods and mechanisms. Pure Appl Chem. 2002;74:349–58.
18. Moráguez OD, Belser UC. The use of polytetrafluoroethylene tape for the management of screw access channels in implant-supported prostheses. J Prosthet Dent. 2010;103(3):189–91.
19. Sailer I, Mühlemann S, Zwahlen M, Hämmerle CH, Schneider D. Cemented and screw-retained implant reconstructions: a systematic review of the survival and complication rates. Clin Oral Implants Res. 2012;23(Suppl 6):163–201.
20. Ntrouka VI, Slot DE, Louropoulou A, Van der Weijden F. The effect of chemotherapeutic agents on contaminated titanium surfaces: a systematic review. Clin Oral Implants Res. 2011;22(7):681–90.
21. Sheets JL, Wilcox C, Wilwerding T. Cement selection for cement-retained crown technique with dental implants. J Prosthodont. 2008;17(2):92–6.
22. Squier RS, Agar JR, Duncan JP, Taylor TD. Retentiveness of dental cements used with metallic implant components. Int J Oral Maxillofac Implants. 2001;16(6):793–8.
23. Sawase T, Wennerberg A, Hallgren C, Albrektsson T, Baba K. Chemical and topographical surface analysis of five different implant abutments. Clin Oral Implants Res. 2000;11(1):44–50.
24. Tarica DY, Alvarado VM, Truong ST. Survey of United States dental schools on cementation protocols for implant crown restorations. J Prosthet Dent. 2010;103(2):68–79.
25. Taylor TD, Agar JR. Twenty years of progress in implant prosthodontics. J Prosthet Dent. 2002;88(1):89–95.
26. van Hove RP, Sierevelt IN, van Royen BJ, Nolte PA. Titanium-nitride coating of orthopaedic implants: a review of the literature. Biomed Res Int. 2015;2015:485975.
27. Varthis S, Randi A, Tarnow DP. Prevalence of interproximal open contacts between single-implant restorations and adjacent teeth. Int J Oral Maxillofac Implants. 2016;31(5):1089–92.
28. Wadhwani CP, O'Brien R, Kattadiyil MT, Chung KH. Laboratory technique for coloring titanium abutments to improve esthetics. J Prosthet Dent. 2016;115(4):409–11.
29. Wadhwani C, Chung KH. In-office technique for selectively etching titanium abutments to improve bonding for interim implant prostheses. J Prosthet Dent. 2016;115(3):271–3.
30. Wadhwani C, Hess T, Pineyro A, Chung KH. Effects of abutment and screw access channel modification on dislodgement of cement-retained implant-supported restorations. Int J Prosthodont. 2013;26(1):54–6.
31. Wadhwani C, Chung KH. Effect of modifying the screw access channels of zirconia implant abutment on the cement flow pattern and retention of zirconia restorations. J Prosthet Dent. 2014;112(1):45–50.
32. Wadhwani C, Hess T, Piñeyro A, Opler R, Chung KH. Cement application techniques in luting implant-supported crowns: a quantitative and qualitative survey. Int J Oral Maxillofac Implants. 2012;27(4):859–64.
33. Wadhwani C, Goodwin S, Chung KH. Cementing an implant crown: a novel measurement system using computational fluid dynamics approach. Clin Implant Dent Relat Res. 2016;18(1):97–106.
34. Wadhwani C, Piñeyro A, Hess T, Zhang H, Chung KH. Effect of implant abutment modification on the extrusion of excess cement at the crown-abutment margin for cement-retained implant restorations. Int J Oral Maxillofac Implants. 2011;26(6):1241–6.
35. Wadhwani C, Piñeyro A, Avots J. An esthetic solution to the screw-retained implant restoration: introduction to the implant crown adhesive plug: clinical report. J Esthet Restor Dent. 2011;23(3):138–43.
36. Weber HP, Kim DM, Ng MW, Hwang JW, Fiorellini JP. Peri-implant soft-tissue health surrounding cement- and screw-retained implant restorations: a multi-center, 3-year prospective study. Clin Oral Implants Res. 2006;17(4):375–9.
37. Winkler S, Ring K, Ring JD, Boberick KG. Implant screw mechanics and the settling effect: overview. J Oral Implantol. 2003;29(5):242–5.
38. Wittneben JG, Millen C, Brägger U. Clinical performance of screw- versus cement-retained fixed implant-supported reconstructions—a systematic review. Int J Oral Maxillofac Implants. 2014;29 Suppl:84–98.

Implants in the Aesthetic Zone: Occlusal Considerations

15

Richard G. Stevenson III and Anirudha Agnihotry

Abstract

Occlusion is the relationship of the mandibular teeth to those in the maxillary arch, when they are brought together. Knowledge of occlusion is key in developing a successful implant restoration as most technical implant complications are related to biomechanical issues: fractured crowns, chipping, screw loosening, fractured abutments, and also fractured implants are attributed to uncontrolled forces on the implant-restoration complex. Understanding and delivering optimal occlusal schemes for *natural teeth* will serve as a premise for majority of this chapter, as it is important to note that very little evidence exists to support most of the recommendations with respect to implant occlusion. Therefore, the strategy recommended here is to utilize known concepts of occlusion for natural dentition with the added understanding that implants fail by a completely different mechanism. Although little is known, the material outlined here provides a sound, logical, and perhaps growing evidence base for delivery of implant restorations in the aesthetic zone. There is emphasis on certain principles of occlusion which, if ignored, cause early failures of implants and implant restorations. The ultimate goal of this chapter is to describe the clinical techniques required to fabricate implant restorations which are aesthetically appealing with significantly successful longevity—not just survival.

R. G. Stevenson III (✉)
Stevenson Dental Solutions, Inc., San Dimas, CA, USA
e-mail: dr.s@rgsdds.com

A. Agnihotry
Arthur A Dugoni School of Dentistry, San Francisco, CA, USA

Todd R. Schoenbaum (ed.), *Implants in the Aesthetic Zone*,
https://doi.org/10.1007/978-3-319-72601-4_15

15.1 Occlusion and Dental Implants

Occlusion is the relationship of the mandibular teeth to those in the maxillary arch, when they are brought together. Knowledge of occlusion is key in developing a successful implant restoration as most technical implant complications are related to biomechanical issues: fractured crowns, chipping, screw loosening, fractured abutments and also fractured implants are attributed to uncontrolled forces on the implant-restoration complex. Understanding and delivering optimal occlusal schemes for *natural teeth* will serve as a premise for majority of this chapter, as it is important to note that very little evidence exists to support most of the recommendations with respect to implant occlusion. Therefore, the strategy recommended here is to utilize known concepts of occlusion for natural dentition with the added understanding that implants fail by a completely different mechanism. Although little is known, the material outlined here provides a sound, logical, and perhaps growing evidence base for delivery of implant restorations in the aesthetic zone. There is emphasis on certain principles of occlusion which, if ignored, cause early failures of implants and implant restorations. The ultimate goal of this chapter is to describe the clinical techniques required to fabricate implant restorations which are aesthetically appealing with significantly successful longevity—not just survival.

15.1.1 Optimal Occlusion

Knowledge of the fundamentals of accepted occlusal concepts is paramount when approaching the implant restoration occlusal scheme. However, there are few clinical studies that elaborate on a set criteria of occlusal considerations for dental implants. The following are some terms that should be understood well for conceptual understanding of occlusion:

- Maximum intercuspal position (MIP): It is the complete intercuspation of the antagonistic teeth independent of condylar position, sometimes referred to as the best fit of the teeth regardless of the condylar position [it is important to note that the term "centric" has been historically used to describe this position; however, the terms have been updated by the Glossary of Prosthodontic Terms, 8th Ed. [1]].
- Anterior guidance: It is the pattern of the contacting surfaces of anterior teeth on the antagonistic teeth limiting mandibular movements, including right and left laterotrusive and protrusive guidance.
- Balanced articulation (BA)/balanced occlusion: It is the bilateral, simultaneous, anterior, and posterior occlusal contact of teeth in centric and eccentric positions.
- Balancing interference: It is the undesirable contact(s) of antagonistic occlusal surfaces on the nonworking (mediotrusive) side.
- Working interference: It is the undesirable contact(s) of the antagonistic occlusal surfaces on the working (laterotrusive) side.

- Canine protected articulation (canine guidance): It is a form of mutually protected articulation or guidance, in which the horizontal and vertical overlap of the canine teeth on one side disengages the posterior teeth in the excursive movements of the mandible on the same side.
- Condylar guidance: It is the mandibular guidance generated by the condyle and articular disc traversing the contour of the glenoid fossae.
- Group function: It is the multiple contact relations between the upper and lower teeth in lateral movements of working side, whereby simultaneous contact of several teeth acts as a group to distribute occlusal forces.
- Centric relation: It is the most superior, anterior position of the condyles in the glenoid fossa braced against the articular disc. A jaw position and not a tooth position.
- Centric occlusion: It is the first tooth contact recorded when the jaws are rotating into closure from a centric relation position. [It is important to note that this term has been used for various definitions including maximum intercuspal position (MIP); however, this is currently an incorrect use as per the Glossary of Prosthodontic Terms 8th Ed. [1]]
- Mutually protected articulation: The most favorable occlusion scheme for implants is mutually protected occlusion. In this scheme, the anterior teeth and posterior teeth mutually protect each other in MIP and excursive movements of the lower jaw. When in MIP, the posterior teeth bear all the load, and there is minimum load on the anterior teeth, and during lateral and protrusive excursions of the mandible, the cusps of the posterior teeth dis-occlude, guided by the anterior teeth, which helps protect posterior teeth from wear and oblique forces. This scheme describes the movements of the teeth through manipulation of casts on an articulator and through directed jaw movements, but not necessarily in actual function. Patients chew, speak, and swallow often without ever replicating these protected movements [2]. Thus, mutually protected articulation/occlusion is actually a mutually protected "parafunction," as it is usually most helpful to have anterior and canine guidance when patient is not performing normal jaw activities. Mutually protected articulation is definitely a starting point for all dental rehabilitations, because it provides the dentist and laboratory with principals to build the teeth and tooth contacts and interfaces. It must be emphasized, however, that patients may or may not utilize this scheme when functioning. The actual jaw pathways during normal function cannot be reproduced on an articulator, as they happen in the mouth, and must be considered in their dynamic state [2]. CR and MIP are approached during deglutition, which occurs more than 2000 times daily. Maximum intercuspal position (MIP) occurs naturally at CO in only one of the ten adult individuals [3–5]. However, most dentate individuals have an anteriorly positioned MI to CO by a millimeter [6–9], which might develop a mesial drift of posterior teeth when a tooth is missing.
- Simply having a patient bite down and slide side to side and forward and backward is a part of the occlusal adjustment step, but clearly not the sole step required. Refer to the chew test and crossover check further in the chapter.

15.2 Implant vs Tooth: Biomechanics

On a broad note, the differences of occlusal loads between teeth and implants can be explained by an analogy of sitting on a cushioned chair (tooth) versus a non-cushioned chair (implant). The tooth has a cushion of periodontal ligament (PDL), while the implant is embedded in the bone. This has implications on the biomechanics of implants while in function.

There are mechanoreceptors within the periodontal ligaments which deliver impulses of the occlusal load very effectively to the brain, and it is also a shock absorber for the tooth. Implants do not have periodontal ligaments and show relatively lower occlusal sensations as the nervous innervation around an implant is not as profound as natural dentition. Natural teeth have an estimated 8.75 times higher tactile sensation than an implant [10]. This makes implant occlusion prone to trauma more than natural teeth as there is no feedback of pain sensation to kick off any protective reflexes to high occlusal forces. The occlusal neural cognizance is measured as tactile sensitivity, which could be measured by either applying pressure on the occlusal surface of the tooth/implant until the person reports tactile sensation [passive tactile sensitivity; measured in Newtons (N)] or by measuring thickness of the narrowest foreign material that can be detected between two opposing natural teeth/implants/or their combination [active tactile sensitivity; measured in microns (μ)]. It has been found that passive tactile sensitivity of the tooth-tooth combination is 0.3 N, while tooth-implant combination is 15 N [11]. Active tactile sensitivity is also found to be considerably higher for implants than natural teeth (over nine studies have reported 10–70 μ active tactile sensibility for implants) [11]. Moreover, the mobility of a tooth in its socket is more when compared to an implant. The natural tooth can be displaced 25–100 μ in axial compressive forces, while, horizontally, it can move up to 50 μ [12]. In occlusal loading, the forces are dissipated equally in an apical direction [13]. The tooth is more elastic than the implant and can also respond to forces by rotation of the root and other displaced movements, which support shearing stresses of the excursive movements of the teeth in a dynamic fashion. The dental implant is connected directly to the bone, eliminating space for physiologic movement. In contrast to a tooth, implants can only be displaced by 3–5 μ axially and 10–50 μ in horizontal direction while subject to normal occlusal forces [12]. Thus, while a tooth may adapt to movement through intrusion or rotation, the dental implant-bone interface may absorb all of the forces. Although forces are evenly distributed along the natural tooth, the forces are concentrated at the crestal bone level surrounding the implant. The fibers around the implant are oriented circumferentially around the implant body. Conversely, the fibers of the PDL around a natural tooth insert into the root surface and are oriented perpendicularly to oppose axial loads. This is vital for the health of the tooth because vertically directed physiologic occlusal loads do not induce mobility, as lateral occlusal loads can. Without fibers oriented to mitigate axial loads, an implant is more susceptible to lateral forces which create bending moments [12]. The movement phases between the natural teeth and implants differ as well, impacting the response to occlusal loads of the surrounding bone. In a natural tooth, the

Table 15.1 Summary of biological and biomechanical factors influencing the occlusion of dental implants

Biological/ biomechanical factors	Tooth	Implant
Periodontal ligament (PDL)	A vital tissue surrounding the tooth. It attaches the tooth to the bone. It offers cushioning effect and repair to protect the tissue from trauma	There is no such peri-implant specialized tissue present
Nervous innervation	PDL is innervated by nerve endings which are sensitive to pressure, called mechanoreceptors. These act as feedback source for pain sensation due to excessive occlusal force	Peri-implant nerve innervation is present, but it is not as specific and as dense as around a tooth
Compressive forces (axial forces)	Due to resilience of the PDL, a tooth can be compressed to about 25–100 μm in the socket	An implant can be compressed only 3–5 μm
Shearing forces (excursive movements)	Horizontal movements due to shearing forces are 50 μm Elasticity of the tooth makes it invulnerable to subtle bending moments caused by excursive movements	Horizontal movements due to shearing forces are 10–50 μm Rigidity of the implant makes it vulnerable to bending moments caused by excursive movements
Tactile sensitivity	Due to high innervation of nervous tissue, a force as low as 0.3 N can be detected	Due to low innervation of nervous tissue, a force of at least 15 N can be detected

movement is not linear. It begins with an initial phase, where the tooth moves within the boundaries of the PDL [14]. Continued force involves the secondary phase, which involves elastic deformation of the alveolar bone. In contrast, the implant lacks an initial, adaptive phase of movement. The implant moves (<50 μ) in a linear and elastic fashion (Table 15.1).

15.3 Consequences of Overloading

Occlusal overload has been implicated as one of the contributing factors for atypical peri-implant bone loss. Theoretically, this is possible though unproven. As previously mentioned, the stress distribution of an implant occurs at the crestal bone level. The difference in the elasticity modulus of bone compared with that of the titanium implant suggests that forces are directed to the first area of bone-implant contact (BIC), the crestal bone. Microfractures in this area could in turn produce marginal bone loss. Conclusions from the best available literature are varied: ranging from a possible association, a possible relationship including other factors, to no probable association. Proper clinical trials are needed in this area to determine a conclusive link between occlusal overload and atypical peri-implant bone loss.

In a small animal study, Kozlovsky et al. [15] found that dynamic occlusal overload created marginal bone loss; however, the extent of the bone loss was determined by the presence of ligature-induced inflammation. Without inflammation, the bone resorption did not occur below the implant neck with "overloaded" implants. The presence of plaque-induced inflammation led to significantly greater bone loss. Clinicians have theorized that, if occlusal overload is indeed associated with marginal bone loss, the micro-movements could lead to the development of peri-implantitis.

Similar controversy surrounds a possible association between occlusal overload and the loss of osseointegration. There is no high-quality evidence on the relationship between osseointegration and supraoccluded implants in humans, and the available animal studies contradict such association in healthy conditions [16]. However, animal studies have shown that occlusal overload (mimicked by supraocclusal contacts with inflammation) increases the plaque-induced bone resorption quite significantly [16].

Still, there are some cases reported with bone loss attributed to overloading in dental implants [17–20]. These mixed results can be attributed to complicated nature of studying occlusal overload in a clinical setting. In light of the incomplete and inconclusive evidence, let us deal with occlusal overload by a precautionary principle. Because, even if overloading only leads to biomechanical complications (screw loosening, prosthesis failure, and the fracture of screws, veneering material), or failure of the implant, it can be costly and time-consuming to restore them back to optimal form and function.

15.4 Dynamic Occlusion: Function

Although the use of an articulator is indicated for oral rehabilitations and is particularly important for implant restorations, one must come to terms with the fact that the articulator, no matter how sophisticated, is not a reliable device capable of replicating the patients' *actual* function [21]. The properly adjusted articulator is essential to establish the anterior occlusal plane for aesthetics, phonetics, pathways of the planned guidance to decrease forces and protect posterior teeth from untoward lateral forces, posterior cusp heights to enhance chewing efficiency while reducing interferences, anterior lingual anatomy, and inclination angles to coordinate with the condylar guidance and posterior cusp inclines, and it serves to allow the technician the ability to create restorations that may be transferred to the mouth with minimal modifications and adjustments. A properly adjusted articulator is indispensable to be sure; however, the actual occlusal function of the patient, chewing, speaking, swallowing, and respiration, cannot be accurately or precisely predetermined with the use of an articulator.

After following the well-known principles of occlusion on the articulator, it is critical to be able to determine the *dynamic* occlusion of the patient—that is, that actual pathways and patterns exhibited by the patient. We will discuss and describe the practical steps which will provide the clinician with a plan for anterior implant restoration delivery.

15.5 Occlusal Considerations in History, Examination, and Treatment Planning

15.5.1 Acceptable Occluding Surfaces and Relationships

1. Bilaterally stable and uniform posterior occlusal contacts in MIP, with the anterior teeth not making any contact unless the individual squeezes.
2. Absence of occlusal trauma to the dentition, which may be indicated by: pain in the individual tooth; a widened PDL with increased mobility, root resorption, cementum resorption, alveolar bone changes, pulpitis, tooth/restoration fractures, or a combination of these conditions.
3. Absence of tooth structure loss from occluding surfaces. In vivo studies have confirmed that occlusal wear of natural enamel opposing natural enamel is approximately 15–17 μ in the premolar region and twice that (29–35 μ) in the molar region per year (Table 15.2) [22, 23].
4. Wear that exceeds these amounts on the tooth-tooth, tooth-restoration bearing interfaces or is isolated indicates attrition (tooth-tooth) or abrasion (tooth-restoration). However, erosion (corrosion) from intrinsic or extrinsic factors must be ruled out or treated accordingly. Simply diagnosing wear as parafunction is an incorrect and incomplete diagnosis. It lacks a specific diagnosis which will require a specific treatment protocol. Fabricating night guards for any individual with wear is not an appropriate treatment. Anecdotally, the authors have seen patients with obvious erosion from undiagnosed and untreated GERD (possibly associated with sleep disorders) treated with occlusal splints, without any improvement in their progressing condition.
5. Absence of non-axial loading or tooth migration. If diastema is developing, particularly over the recent years, this is an indication that occlusal forces are currently overloading the normal tooth positions which is further exacerbated by the lack of bone support, posterior occlusal support, and mobility due to advanced periodontitis [24, 25]. Placing dental implants in patients with active periodontal disease negatively affects long-term success [26, 27]. Placement of implants in these patients, without stabilizing the posterior dentition and controlling the active disease process, is contraindicated.
6. Absence of anterior and posterior occlusal plane discrepancies. If the anterior and posterior occlusal planes are not symmetrical and uniform in anteroposterior, sagittal, and frontal planes, this is not only an aesthetic issue but an occlusal discrepancy as well. Attention must be given to understand these discrepancies and treat them with orthodontics and/or maxillofacial surgical interventions, if needed for optimal results, as part of an overall treatment strategy.

Table 15.2 Normal occlusal wear with advancing age based on documented evidence

Age	30	40	50	60	70	80
Amount of tooth loss *first molar* (mm)	0.72	1.02	1.32	1.62	1.92	2.22
Amount of tooth loss *premolar* (mm)	0.27	0.42	0.57	0.72	0.87	1. 02

15.5.2 Acceptable Occlusal Vertical Dimension (OVD)

The OVD cannot be corrected in most cases without an impact on the amount of display of the anterior teeth while at rest (repose) and smiling. Although OVD corrections may be indicated due to loss of tooth structure in the posterior teeth, it is incumbent on the clinician to determine what effect this will have on the anterior component of the teeth with respect to aesthetics. There are numerous instances where the OVD simply cannot be corrected without creating unwanted or unnatural display of the anterior teeth. The desire to correct the OVD to improve the occlusal pathways and occlusal planes may need to be considered more carefully prior to initiating a major reconstruction. It may create a more ideal occlusion, however, with undesirable aesthetics. It is important to note that for most patients, they are driven by aesthetics, not occlusion. The clinician must consider a reconstruction focused on facial aesthetics and work from this when considering functional (occlusion), biomechanical (structural), and periodontal treatment planning.

15.5.3 Acceptable MI Position (MIP) and Centric Occlusion (CO)

Very few individuals will have an MIP coincident with the condyles in a fully seated position (centric relation). An occlusal slide from the first point of contact (centric occlusal contact) to MIP of <2 mm with intact proprioception is acceptable for the vast majority of patients. A CR-MIP slide only becomes an issue when it is large or when the patient develops symptoms which make the MIP position unacceptable. In such instances, further diagnostic tests are indicated, including a comprehensive TMJ examination, muscle testing, and centric relation mounting/evaluation of casts.

The use of deprogrammers (anterior bite planes) and monitoring of symptoms are critical to obtain a stable and pain-free position of the joints and teeth. The treatment may include occlusal equilibration/restorations in cases of occlusal dysfunction and orthodontics/surgery/rehabilitations in cases where movements of the anterior teeth are constricted (constricted chewing patterns or constricted envelopes of function) [28].

Preferably centric occlusion and MIP are coincident; in other words, when the jaws are in the superior midmost and anterior braced position (CR), the teeth are able to achieve a comfortable MIP. When altering occlusal vertical dimension (OVD), or treating cases of occlusal dysfunction, this is a primary objective of achieving a stable (and successful) occlusion.

15.5.4 Occlusal Schemes [Acceptable Anterior Guidance (AG) or Group Function (GF)]

Single Tooth Implant

- Incisors: To maintain good contacts and a suitable emergence profile, light contacts on the marginal ridges are acceptable in maximum intercuspation (MIP), with little or no contacts with protrusive movements.

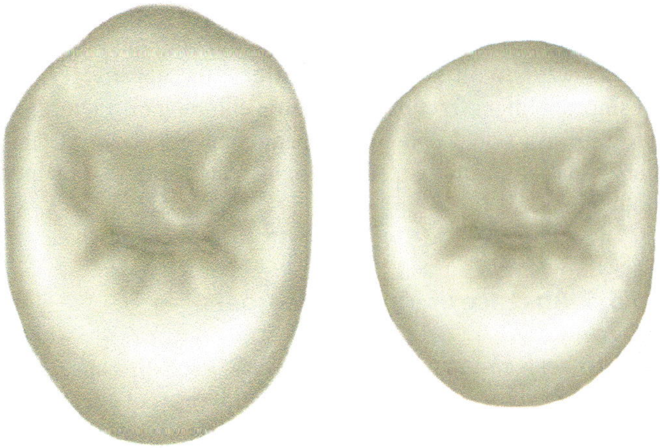

Fig. 15.1 Narrow occlusal table of premolar to reduce shearing forces from excursive (left). An occlusal table of conventional restorative crown compared to implant supported crown (right)

- Canines: The canine should not contact heavily in maximum intercuspation (MIP). The canine should not be used for canine guidance (laterotrusive or protrusive movements), and a group function scheme should be established with premolars, so that no shearing forces act on the implant in unfavorable non-axial directions. On protrusive movement, a light contact is acceptable to maintain the aesthetics, but care should be taken that it is shared with all the anterior teeth, so that there is no undue force on the canine, which could lead to its failure.
- Premolars: For premolars, the cusps ridges involved in contact areas should not be bulky in order to minimize any possibility of contact away from the center of the restoration, to direct forces linearly in the center of the implant. With a narrow occlusal table, and less acute inclines of the cusps, the crown can be kept away from touching opposing cusps in excursive movements. Canine guidance can help here to keep the premolar's dimensions comparable to adjacent posterior teeth for acceptable aesthetics, yet protecting the implant crown from excursive forces (Fig. 15.1).

Multiple Unit Implants in the Aesthetic Zone

- Incisor-Incisor: light contacts on protrusive movements. Canine guidance is favorable.
- Incisor-Canine: light contacts on protrusive movements, group function on laterotrusive movements with little or no contacts on canine.
- Incisor-Canine-Premolar: light contacts on protrusive movements, group function on laterotrusive movements with little or no contacts of restorations on the implants.

15.5.5 Absence of Posterior Balancing Interferences

In cases where patients have posterior interferences, they may develop avoidance patterns which involve moving the mandible forward, thus generating forces outside the pathways of normal function and transferring these unfavorable loads to the anterior teeth. In the natural dentition, we see the negative effects of this by observable and accelerated wear and tooth chipping, tooth mobility, and diastema creation [29]. With implant restorations, the negative effects will include screw loosing, abutment fracture, restoration chipping or fracture, and even implant fracture [30]. As stated above, it is paramount for the posterior dentition to be in a stable and comfortable physiologic state prior to planning anterior implant restorations.

15.5.6 Absence of Muscle Disorders

Muscles get sore and painful, when overworked. Spasms in muscles from continued nonfunctional use are often a sign found in cases of occlusal dysfunction, pathways issues, and, of course, parafunction. For dysfunction and improper pathways of function, the muscles are trying to accommodate the teeth, joints, and nervous system in a trifecta of harmony. Parafunction is different. It is important to note that parafunction is a *brain-mediated* event and cannot be corrected by improving the occlusal contacts of the dentition [31]. Muscle pain from bruxism is reported upon awakening and is not curable perhaps but is entirely amenable to certain treatment strategies. Simply prescribing an occlusal guard without understanding the underlying etiology is unwarranted and contraindicated. Sleep disorders have been reported to correlate highly with the presence of sleep bruxism, and this requires a series of diagnostic tests and evaluations to treat properly [32]. Patients should receive at a very minimum an *Epworth Sleepiness Scale* questionnaire and an airway evaluation prior to embarking on any oral rehabilitation [33]. If a sleep problem is suspected, it is wise to refer to a specialist in this area of dentistry.

15.5.7 Absence of TMJ Disorders

Patients that complain of joint pain or who are incapable of taking loads on the joints (via a joint load test). Temporomandibular issues *must* be resolved or at least mitigated by the appropriate dental experts prior to significant oral rehabilitation.

Criteria for the diagnosis of occlusal dysesthesia (a contraindication of significant restorative treatment) [34]:

1. Complaint of uncomfortable bite sensation.
2. Significant associated emotional distress.
3. TMJ symptoms lasting more than 6 months.
4. History of various bite-altering dental procedure failures.
5. Absence of dental occlusal discrepancies or the occlusal discrepancies present are disproportional to the degree of the complaint.
6. The occlusal discrepancy is not attributed to another disorder (dental pathology, muscle, temporomandibular joint, or neurologic disorder).

15.6 Formulating a Functional Diagnosis

A straight forward approach to determine a functional diagnosis is to perform the following tests:

1. Occlusal questionnaire
2. Joint load test/joint auscultation/joint palpation
3. Muscle palpation
4. Analysis of the dentition (wear, mobility, and excursive movements)

The above tests will allow the clinician to render the following diagnoses: acceptable function, dysfunction, pathway issues, parafunction, or some kind of TMD/neuromuscular issue which will require a dedicated treatment approach outside of the realm of typical restorative procedures.

Acceptable Function: With a diagnosis of acceptable function, the clinician may proceed with treatment of the dentition without occlusal rehabilitation because the system is working within the physiologic boundaries of the patient. Care must be taken not to disrupt the stability of the individual's occlusion in these cases, or serious consequences may arise, which may require additional treatment to resolve. The goals of occlusal therapy should always follow the preception that our restorations will maintain a stable occlusion, and in cases where the occlusion is unstable or destructive, it will correct or improve the stability of the occlusion. With acceptable function, the articulator is used to reproduce the maxillo-mandibular relationships and incisal plane via an accurate face bow [21]. Hand-articulating the casts is generally sufficient to proceed with the case. However, in the event that the OVD will be altered, the casts must be mounted with a centric relation method (like a leaf gauge or deprogrammer) because the MIP position will be altered (Table 15.3) [35].

Occlusal Dysfunction: With patient's whose posterior teeth do not achieve a stable/comfortable MIP, when interference-related posterior wear is noted or accelerated anterior wear exists, it may be possible to confirm the diagnosis with the use of an occlusal deprogrammer. Muscle pain will be a frequent finding in these cases, especially the lateral pterygoids [36]. The deprogrammer will ease the spasms of the offending muscles and allow the mandible to move *posteriorly* on the anterior bite plane. The patient should be completely comfortable while in this position [37]. This usually occurs after 1–4 weeks with 20 h of daily use. Interocclusal records are taken at this new position (CR), and casts are then mounted for analysis. It is often possible to paint the casts with paint (Tempera paint in a contrasting color from the stone color) to track the adjustments made with a trial equilibration made directly on the casts. This approach allows the clinician to evaluate the extent of occlusal grinding necessary to achieve a stable occlusion. During trial equilibration, the anterior teeth should be left unaltered with the end point being that of bilateral posterior contacts on cusps, fossae, and marginal ridges and not on inclines which could produce deflective patterns, non-axial forces, and instability. It can be

Table 15.3 Five possible occlusal diagnoses (Adapted from John Kois, DMD)

Diagnosis	Joint symptoms	Muscle symptoms	Wear patterns	Further tests	Treatment
Acceptable function	None—the joint may be loaded without discomfort	None—the muscle of mastication is pain-free when palpated	Normal wear, or stable wear from previous conditions (accelerated wear not active)	None	Proceed normally, but be aware that new restorations may generate instability if not adjusted properly
Occlusal dysfunction	Joint may be slightly tender when loaded	Muscles usually sore, especially lateral pterygoids	Accelerated anterior wear with flat incisal edges or isolated of unilateral posterior wear	Deprogrammer; jaw finds CR in 1–4 weeks	Equilibration, restorations, or orthodontics
Pathway issues	Joints usually tender, especially when patient closes into MIP	Sore muscles, especially lateral pterygoids	Anterior wear with the lingual of the maxillary anterior teeth and the facials of the mandibular anterior	Deprogrammer; jaw moves forward on bite plane	Orthodontics, replace bulky anterior crowns, or open VDO
Parafunction	Joints may or may not be tender	Muscles may or may not be tender	Wear on all of the teeth, especially posteriors (with bruxism) and isolated wear with habits	Optional deprogrammer to evaluate wear patterns on bite plane	Treat with orthotic and restorations designed for heavy forces and assumed fractures
TMD/neuromuscular disorders	Joints usually painful	Muscles may or may not be tender, but unusual patterns exist, including myofascial pain, etc.	Various	TMJ work-up and definitive diagnosis	Refer to OFP, or treat with extreme caution

further determined which teeth will require restorations due to hypo-occlusion where onlays or crowns may be made to achieve occlusal contact or when extensive adjustments leave the tooth unprotected by enamel. The goal of occlusal equilibration is to spare the anterior teeth from further destruction, and equilibration must be accomplished when indicated, prior to the initiation of aesthetic implant restorations.

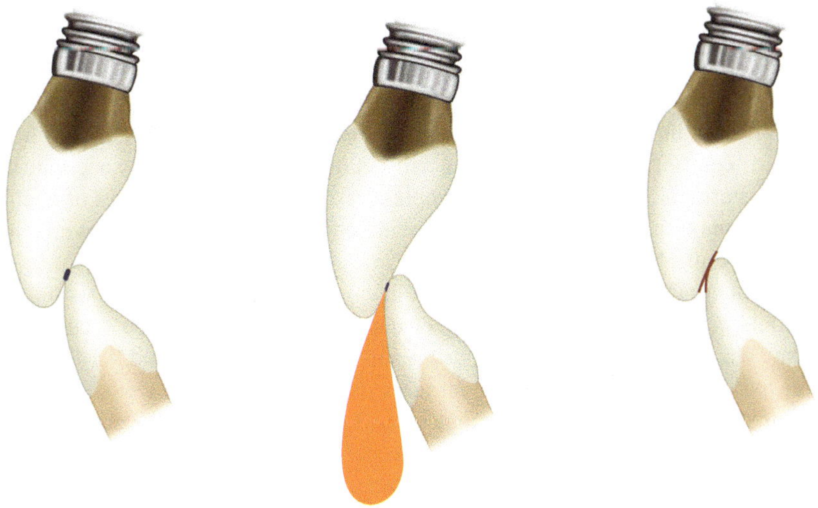

Fig. 15.2 Typical MIP contact area (left), functional pathway (center), and pathway-related wear areas (right)

Pathway Issues (Constricted Envelope of Occlusion, Constructed Chewing Pattern): Perhaps, one of the more poorly understood issues in field of occlusion is the pathways taken by the anterior teeth during normal function. The mandibular movements during chewing mimic a teardrop shape (see Fig. 15.2), where the teeth come close but do not touch until MIP is established. When this natural pathway is altered and the teeth touch during closure, the resultant friction leads to wear of the occlusion tooth surfaces. In a constricted envelope the maxillary anterior teeth are interfering with the normal closing pathway of the mandibular teeth. The facial surfaces of the mandibular incisors and canines are wearing against the lingual surfaces of the maxillary incisors and canines during sleep, phonation, chewing, speaking, or swallowing. This wear pattern seems to occur during normal chewing and often seen clinically when a patient with a class IV composite meeting the requirements of an articulator-based occlusion returns soon after placement with a failure of the restoration. The system is flawed—the patient cannot chew without having the anterior teeth rub against another, which in turn leads to wear, flexing of the teeth, mobility, diastema creation, or distalization of the mandible. Patients with pathway issues may experience the inability to chew hard food; they may be fast eaters (it is uncomfortable to eat) and experience TMJ pain, muscle pain, or frequent problems with anterior restorations as described above. The anterior deprogrammer is an excellent tool to confirm the diagnosis, as the patient will typically move *forward* on the anterior bite plane after treatment. The treatment solution for a pathway issue is to create more space for the anterior teeth to move in and out of MIP without friction. This space may be established via several different approaches: orthodontics (to expand the maxillary teeth or slightly retract the mandibular teeth); orthognathic surgery (to realign the maxilla and mandible to better approximate the dentition), increasing the OVD; or occasionally the placement or replacement of anterior restorations which are either too bulky (maxillary lingual surfaces of crowns are often the culprit), or the repositioning of teeth with crowns (rarely indicated due to pulpal involvement). Pathway issues are not treatable with equilibration. Equilibration will decrease the OVD and exacerbate the issue. It is critical that aesthetic zone implant restorations obey the laws of healthy dynamic function, and NOT interfere with chewing, speech, swallowing, and breathing (Fig. 15.2).

Parafunction: It is the broad definition given to nonfunctional activities that the individual performs either consciously or unconsciously. Often these occur during the day, via clenching, rubbing the surfaces in eccentric patterns and border movements, protruding the mandible and retracting it against the upper teeth, sliding the anterior teeth against each other, and sleep bruxism (associated with breathing issues or not). It is important that adequate guidance be established in order to at least partially protect the teeth from accelerated destruction due to parafunction. Restorations and equilibrations will not cure parafunction, as it is brain mediated, but action should be taken to prevent parafunction activities from destroying restorations and teeth. Parafunction is multifactorial, and it is good to understand the neurological pathways involved and the patterns of jaw movements that occur under different conditions including nocturnal (sleep bruxism and sleep disordered breathing-related wear) and diurnal conditions (clenching, habits with foreign objects, finger nail biting, and other conscious/subconscious habits). Thoughtlessly prescribing a "night guard" is a poor service for the treatment of a disease with a varied but specific etiology. It shows a complete lack of a definitive diagnosis and is potentially dangerous, especially with an untreated sleep disorder. The use of night guards to treat true sleep bruxism (which only occurs in 9.7–15.9% of patients) [38] is appropriate assuming that a sleep breathing disorder is not the primary issue. Using "day guards" to treat habitual clenching is also indicated when this is indeed the issue; however, some individuals cannot tolerate wearing appliance during the day. Nonetheless, after completing a rehabilitation with ceramics (particularly thin or fragile restorations), the use of a night guard (constructed of a soft intaglio and a hard shell) as an insurance policy against an episodic or aberrant nocturnal parafunction is recommended [39]. At the restoration delivery appointment, the clinician should perform a "crossover check," as described in the following section (Table 15.4).

15.7 Clinical Techniques for Occlusal Adjustments During Implant Restoration Delivery

Restoration Cementation/Screw Tightening and Access Closure: These techniques have been covered in Chap. 14 and should be followed precisely, as significant research and much clinical trial and error have gone into the approaches described.

Table 15.4 The five-step occlusal check

Step	1	2	3	4	5
Name of check	MIP	Lateral excursives	Protrusive	Crossover	Chew test
Jaw movement	Close teeth together	Move jaw left and right	Move jaw forward	Position teeth edge to edge, and move side to side	Chew on wax for 30 s, then insert paper, and chew 30 s
Posterior contacts	Even, bilateral *posterior* contacts (cusp tips, marginal ridges, and fossae)	No contacts on *posterior* teeth unless *group function* is designed to lessen load on *canine implant*	No contacts on *posterior* teeth	No contacts on *posterior* teeth	No contacts on *posterior* inclines in group function design
Anterior contacts	*Anterior* teeth touch lightly in MIP	No contacts in *anterior* teeth	Even bilateral *anterior* dis-occlusion	Even, smooth surfaces, no catches, broad contact areas	No contacts on *anterior* teeth with 200 μm paper
Implant restoration contacts	Implant restorations only touch when patient *squeezes* teeth together	No contacts on *anterior* implant restorations if possible	No contacts on *anterior* implant restorations if possible	Light contacts, smooth surfaces, no catches, broad contact areas	No contacts on *anterior* implant restorations with 200 μm paper
Articulating paper used	8–12 μm *BLUE* paper	8–12 μm *RED* paper	8–12 μm *RED* paper	8–12 μm *RED* paper	200 μm paper

The Five-Step Occlusion Check: This system has been developed to respect all aspects of occlusal theory and provides a practical, repeatable, and reliable method of insuring predictable results with implant-retained restorations. It has been shown to provide restorations that are comfortable, more durable, and more successful. During the following steps, the implant restoration is firmly seated and cemented or screwed into place, and in the case of a screw access, the final composite cover has been placed (Table 15.4).

1. MIP Check: With the patient *seated upright*, thin (8 or 12 μm, Arti-Fol (*Bausch*) or Troll Foil (*Troll Dental*)) articulating paper is positioned between the teeth, and the patient is instructed to close several times, tapping on their posterior teeth. Contacts are recorded and analyzed, and the only anterior contact should be the distal of the maxillary canine. The maxillary incisor lingual surfaces should be free of contacts at this stage. Then, shim stock is placed between the anterior teeth and the patient instructed to squeeze. With the teeth held together tightly, the shim stock should be held by the anterior teeth; however, when the patient bites with normal force, the shim stock releases. Contacts are then analyzed for their size. The paper is reinserted, the teeth squeezed together, and the contacts analyzed. The contact sizes

should be "slenderized" to be approximately 0.5 mm in diameter on all anterior teeth, both implant crowns or natural teeth (see Fig. 15.2). It is important that the implant crowns achieve a positive MIP contact at the squeeze step (shim stock barely holds), as this will prevent the over-eruption of the opposing tooth and the lack of occlusal stability. Simply taking the implant crowns "out of occlusion" will destabilize the occlusion. The teeth will eventually erupt into this space, and this uncontrolled event may result in other interferences developing. A "light contact" means that the surfaces do in fact contact, but later and with less force than the adjacent teeth. With anterior teeth, the desired occlusion for natural teeth is lighter than posterior teeth, and the occlusion for implant restorations should be slightly lighter than the natural teeth to allow for the compression of the PDL on the natural teeth, which may be as much as 0.1 mm or more (Figs. 15.3 and 15.4).

2. Lateral Excursive Check: With the patient seated upright, insert thin red articulating paper between the anterior teeth, and instruct the patient to grind in circles, and slide side to side. It may be helpful to demonstrate the movement that is desired with your own jaws. Then insert a thin blue articulating paper, and instruct the patient to tap, and squeeze as in the MIP check step.
   (a) For Canine Guidance: Use when the canine is a natural tooth. Leave the red on the canine; however, adjust the pattern of the mark in a manner which replicates the steepness desired and the width of the pathway taken, as it will provide the proper canine guidance required. When the anterior teeth are not critical to the protection of the implant crown (the canine is a natural tooth), then adjust the red marks away from all of the natural incisors and restored implant surfaces.
   (b) For Anterior Group Function: Use when the canine is an implant, and it is desirable to have the natural anterior teeth assist with the guidance. Analyze and adjust the marks as follows: remove all red contacts from the lingual surface of the canine implant restored tooth, and leave the blue marks. With the anterior teeth, adjust the pattern of the marks in a manner which replicates the steepness desired and the width of the pathway taken, as it will provide the proper anterior group function required.

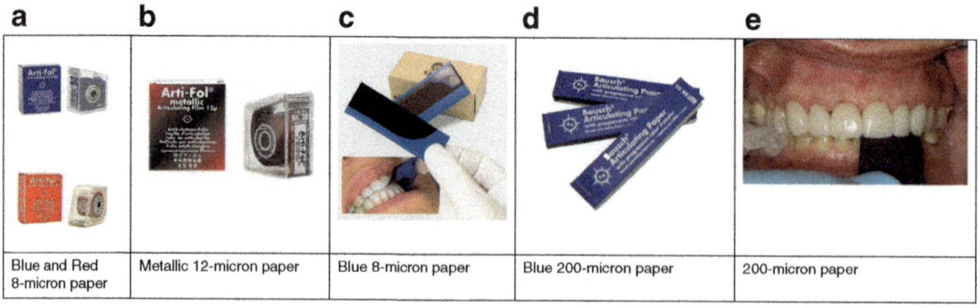

Fig. 15.3 Articulating paper: (**a**) BLUE and RED 8 μm paper (Bausch Arti-Fol, BK23 and BK21). (**b**) Metallic 12 μm paper with shim stock on one surface and ink on the other (Bausch Arti-Fol BK28). (**c**) BLUE 8 μm paper with built-in plastic holder (TrollDental TrollFoil). (**d**) BLUE 200 μm paper for the chew test (Bausch BK05). (**e**) 200 μm paper being used to perform the chew test

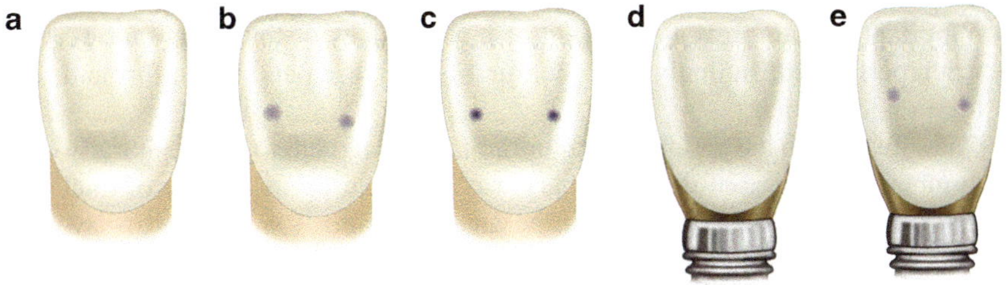

Fig. 15.4 (**a**) Lingual surface of maxillary central incisor tooth. (**b**) Lingual surface of maxillary central incisor tooth with typical MIP contacts (this would barely hold shim stock). (**c**) Lingual surface of maxillary central incisor tooth with typical MIP contacts after patient clenches (this would firmly hold shim stock). (**d**) Lingual surface of maxillary central incisor implant crown in MIP (note: lack of contact marks). (**e**) Lingual surface of maxillary central incisor implant crown in MIP when patient clenches (note: this would barely hold shim stock)

3. Protrusive Check: With the patient seated upright, insert thin red articulating paper between the anterior teeth and instruct the patient to slide forward and back. It may be helpful to demonstrate the movement that is desired with your own jaws. Then use blue thin articulating paper, and instruct the patient to tap and then squeeze as in the MIP check step. Analyze and adjust the marks as follows: remove all RED contacts from the lingual surfaces of the anterior implant restored teeth, and leave the BLUE marks. Reshape the RED marks on the natural anterior teeth to the pattern which replicates the steepness desired and the width of the pathway taken, as it will provide the proper anterior protrusive guidance required. Do not allow implant anterior teeth to perform protrusive guidance, when natural teeth are available to carry the load. When nothing but implant restorations are present in the anterior segment, distribute the forces as evenly as possible among all of the surfaces involved in the guidance.
4. Crossover Check: With the patient sitting upright, insert the thin red paper, and instruct the patient to move into edge-to-edge position, and move their teeth edges against the opposing anterior teeth—side to side and from a protrusive (underbite) position backward. Look to see that the incisal edges are broad and allowing for smooth movements, without catching the corners of the incisal edges. The adjustments may likely require the adjustment of the incisal edges of natural mandibular teeth. This step is best completed in the prototypes, before final impressions are made to avoid the unpleasant situation of explaining the need to fit "their teeth" to "your restorations." This step rarely requires much more than a ceramic polishing abrasive with slow rpm—in lieu of a high-speed carbide or diamond, which may mitigate patient concerns. With anterior aesthetic restorations, this step is necessary on most patients during the prototype phase and met with little resistance from the patient. When it is a preplanned step and is described before treatment is

initiated, it is readily accepted by patients. The crossover check is an extremely important step to prevent chipping of incisal edges of final restorations and, when performed routinely, will measurably enhance patient comfort and restoration longevity.

5. Chew Test: With the patient sitting upright, instruct them to chew naturally on a thimble-sized piece of tray periphery wax, while inserting a piece of thick red 200 μm (*Bausch BK05*) between the anterior teeth. It is helpful to have the patient chew on this piece of "sterile" wax without the clinician watching, which seems to allow the patient to chew more naturally. After 10 s, turn toward them, and instruct them to continue chewing, and insert the paper when access is available, and have them continue chewing, again with your back turned. After another 10 s or so, remove the paper, and then use a blue thin articulating paper, and instruct the patient to tap and then squeeze as in the MIP check step to analyze the marks on the lingual surfaces of the anterior teeth. Remove all red marks on the anterior teeth, as these are the functional pathway interferences which may lead to untoward forces on the teeth and implant restorations. It is best to remove all red marks during this exercise, whether they exist on teeth or implant restorations. Repeat the test until no red marks can be made on the lingual surfaces of the anterior teeth while chewing. The 200 μm paper is thick enough to allow for an adequate space for non-frictional dynamic occlusal functionality (Fig. 15.5).

15.8 Polishing After Adjustments

It is incumbent on the clinician to research the best available polishing systems for achieving a highly polished and comfortable surface after making occlusal adjustments. For all currently available ceramic systems (i.e., zirconia, lithium disilicate, leucite, feldspathic), the correct bur for adjustments is a 30 μm diamond [40]. Carbides are contraindicated on ceramics as they have been shown to cause microcracks. The surface left by the fine diamond must be polished to a high luster to mitigate future crack propagation [40]. Numerous systems exist which provide varying level of smoothness; however, they must be used after the occlusion has been adjusted with the fine diamond bur (Table 15.5).

15.9 Engineering Checks at Follow-Up Appointments

After the final delivery of the aesthetic zone implant restoration, these five checks should be employed at re-care appointments to mitigate forces and fine-tune the occlusion over time, as natural wear and tooth movement occurs over time. True occlusal stability is a dynamic event and hence a moving target that requires our most conscientious attention to detail.

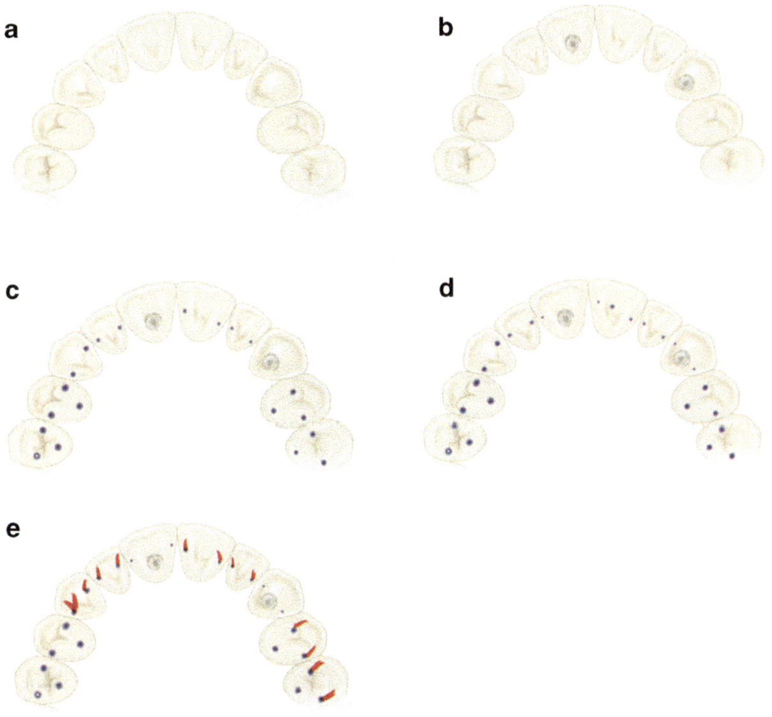

Fig. 15.5 (**a**) Occlusal view of maxillary premolars and anterior teeth. (**b**) Occlusal view of maxillary premolars and anterior teeth with implant restored crowns at the maxillary right central incisor and maxillary left canine positions prior to occlusal analysis with articulating paper. (**c**) Optimal occlusal marking with thin articulating paper of **b** in MIP. (**d**) Optimal occlusal marking with thin articulating paper of **b** in MIP with the patient clenching (note: the lighter occlusion on the implant crowns, which would barely hold shim stock). (**e**) Optimal occlusal marking with thin articulating paper of **b** in eccentric movements with red paper showing canine guidance on the right and optimal protrusive markings (note: no marks exist on the implant crowns in any movement, and group function is established on the left, decreasing the load on the canine)

15.10 Occlusal-Related Failures

When a patient complains that an implant crown "is loose," or "something moved," or "something chipped," it is natural for any conscientious clinician to experience significant concern. Even with best efforts, this is a dynamic situation on a human being and not a static machine. Humans do things with their teeth that cannot be predicted, and their dentistry, however well planned, engineered, integrated, and adjusted into the body, is prone to failure over time. Reentering a fractured screw-retained restoration is relatively simple, but "repairs" nearly always require a

Table 15.5 Occlusal adjustment armamentaria sequence

	Step 1	Step 2	Step 3	Step 4
Abrasive	30 μm diamond	Coarse	Medium	Fine
Purpose	Gross adjustments	Moderate adjustments and finishing	Minor adjustments and surface smoothing	Polishing
Example image	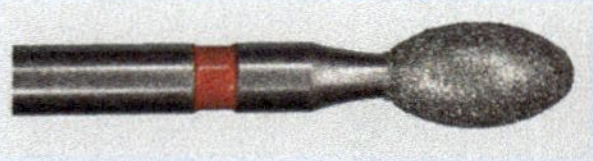	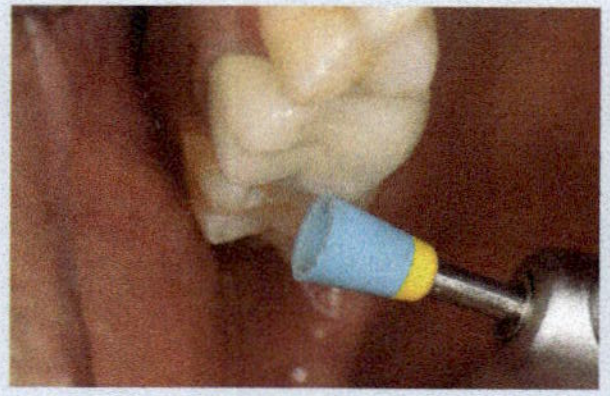	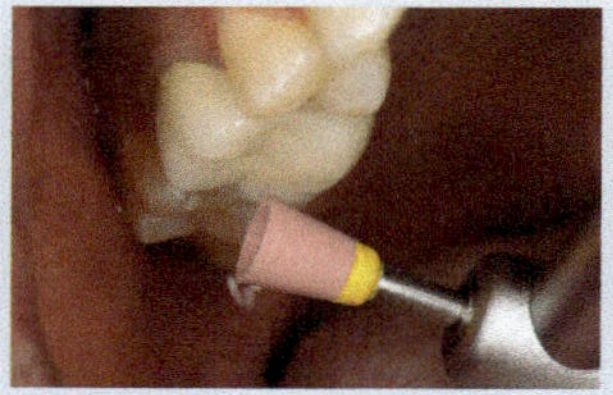	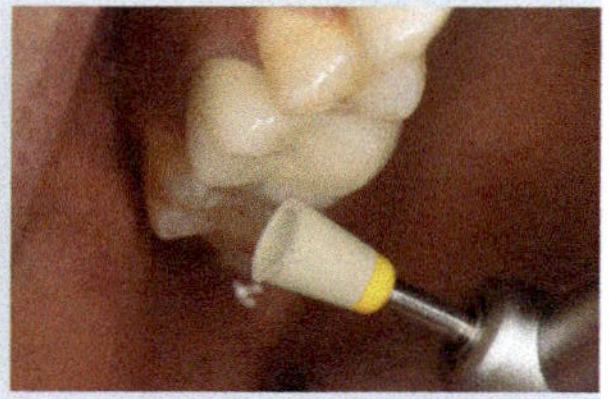
Manufacturer	KS4f (Brasseler USA)	Dialite Blue (Brasseler, USA)	Dialite Pink (Brasseler, USA)	Dialite Pink (Brasseler, USA)

complete remake of the prosthesis. Retrieving a cement-retained restoration may be slightly more complicated but, once removed, also typically requires a complete remake. Failures are not enjoyable, but they are inevitable. The diligent clinician is expected to minimize early failure of restorations by unflinching adherence to best practices and never compromise what is right.

References

1. The glossary of prosthodontic terms. J Prosthet Dent. 2005;94(1):10–92. https://doi.org/10.1016/j.prosdent.2005.03.013.
2. Utz KH, Müller F, Lückerath W, et al. The lateral leeway in the habitual intercuspation: experimental studies and literature review. J Oral Rehabil. 2007;34(6):406–13.
3. Berry HM, Hofmann FA. Cineradiographic observations of temporomandibular joint function. J Prosthet Dent. 1959;9:31–3.
4. Becker CM, Kaiser DA, Schwalm C. Mandibular centricity: centric relation. J Prosthet Dent. 2000;83:158–60.
5. Moss ML. A functional cranial analysis of centric relation. Dent Clin N Am. 1975;19:431–42.
6. Posselt U. Terminal hinge movement of the mandible. J Prosthet Dent. 1957;7:787–97.
7. Posselt U. The physiology of occlusion and rehabilitation. Philadelphia: FA Davis; 1962.
8. Johnston LA. Gnathological assessment of centric slides in postretention orthodontic patients. J Prosthet Dent. 1988;60:712–5.
9. Celenza FV. The centric position: replacement and character. J Prosthet Dent. 1973;30:591–8.
10. Hämmerle CHF, Wagner D, Brägger U, et al. Threshold of tactile sensitivity perceived with dental endosseous implants and natural teeth. Clin Oral Implants Res. 1995;6:83–90.
11. Bhatnagar VM, Karani JT, Khanna A, Badwaik P, Pai A. Osseoperception: an implant mediated sensory motor control- a review. J Clin Diagn Res. 2015;9(9):ZE18–20.
12. Sekine H, Komiyama Y, Hotta H, et al. Mobility characteristics and tactile sensitivity of osseointegrated fixture- supporting systems. In: van Steenberghe D, editor. Tissue integration in oral maxillofacial reconstruction. Amsterdam: Excerpta Medica; 1996. p. 326–32.
13. Hillam DG. Stresses in the periodontal ligament. J Periodontal Res. 1973;8:51–6.
14. Kurashima K. Viscoelastic properties of periodontal tissue. Bull Tokyo Med Dent Univ. 1965;12:240.
15. Kozlovsky A, Tal H, Laufer BZ, et al. Impact of implant overloading on the peri-implant bone in inflamed and non-inflamed peri-implant mucosa. Clin Oral Implants Res. 2007;18(5):601–10.
16. Naert I, Duyck J, Vandamme K. Occlusal overload and bone/implant loss. Clin Oral Implants Res. 2012;23(Suppl 6):95–107.
17. Merin RL. Repair of peri-implant bone loss after occlusal adjustment: a case report. J Am Dent Assoc. 2014;145(10):1058–62.
18. Tawil G. Peri-implant bone loss caused by occlusal overload: repair of the peri-implant defect following correction of the traumatic occlusion. A case report. Int J Oral Maxillofac Implants. 2008;23(1):153–7.
19. Conrad HJ, Schulte JK, Vallee MC. Fractures related to occlusal overload with single posterior implants: a clinical report. J Prosthet Dent. 2008;99(4):251–6.
20. Passanezi E, Sant'ana AC, Damante CA. Occlusal trauma and mucositis or peri-implantitis? J Am Dent Assoc. 2017;148(2):106–12.
21. Quinlan P. Articulators, face bows and interocclusal records. J Ir Dent Assoc. 2016;62(2):102–4.
22. Mundhe K, Jain V, Pruthi G, Shah N. Clinical study to evaluate the wear of natural enamel antagonist to zirconia and metal ceramic crowns. J Prosthet Dent. 2015;114(3):358–63.
23. Lambrechts P, Braem M, Vuylsteke-wauters M, Vanherle G. Quantitative in vivo wear of human enamel. J Dent Res. 1989;68(12):1752–4.
24. Brunsvold MA. Pathologic tooth migration. J Periodontol. 2005;76(6):859–66.

25. Khorshidi H, Moaddeli MR, Golkari A, Heidari H, Raoofi S. The prevalence of pathologic tooth migration with respect to the severity of periodontitis. J Int Soc Prev Community Dent. 2016;6(Suppl 2):S122–5.
26. Wen X, Liu R, Li G, et al. History of periodontitis as a risk factor for long-term survival of dental implants: a meta-analysis. Int J Oral Maxillofac Implants. 2014;29(6):1271–80.
27. Chrcanovic BR, Albrektsson T, Wennerberg A. Periodontally compromised vs. periodontally healthy patients and dental implants: a systematic review and meta-analysis. J Dent. 2014;42(12):1509–27.
28. Seay A. Achieving esthetic and functional objectives with additive equilibration. Compend Contin Educ Dent. 2014;35(9):688–92.
29. Lima AF, Cavalcanti AN, Martins LR, Marchi GM. Occlusal interferences: how can this concept influence the clinical practice? Eur J Dent. 2010;4(4):487–91.
30. Warreth A, Doody K, Al-mohsen M, Morcos O, Al-mohsen M, Ibieyou N. Fundamentals of occlusion and restorative dentistry. Part II: occlusal contacts, interferences and occlusal considerations in implant patients. J Ir Dent Assoc. 2015;61(5):252–9.
31. Reddy SV, Kumar MP, Sravanthi D, Mohsin AH, Anuhya V. Bruxism: a literature review. J Int Oral Health. 2014;6(6):105–9.
32. Huynh NT, Emami E, Helman JI, Chervin RD. Interactions between sleep disorders and oral diseases. Oral Dis. 2014;20(3):236–45.
33. Mungan U, Ozeke O, Mavioglu L, et al. The role of the preoperative screening of sleep apnoea by Berlin Questionnaire and Epworth Sleepiness Scale for postoperative atrial fibrillation. Heart Lung Circ. 2013;22(1):38–42.
34. Melis M, Zawawi KH. Occlusal dysesthesia: a topical narrative review. J Oral Rehabil. 2015;42(10):779–85.
35. Solow RA. Mounted diagnostic casts: the entry into comprehensive care. Gen Dent. 2013;61(5):12–5.
36. Fujii T. Occlusal conditions just after the relief of temporomandibular joint and masticatory muscle pain. J Oral Rehabil. 2002;29(4):323–9.
37. Bynum JH. Clinical case report: testing occlusal management, previewing anterior esthetics, and staging rehabilitation with direct composite and Kois deprogrammer. Compend Contin Educ Dent. 2010;31(4):298–302. 304, 306.
38. Manfredini D, Winocur E, Guarda-nardini L, Paesani D, Lobbezoo F. Epidemiology of bruxism in adults: a systematic review of the literature. J Orofac Pain. 2013;27(2):99–110.
39. Santamato A, Panza F, Di venere D, et al. Effectiveness of botulinum toxin type A treatment of neck pain related to nocturnal bruxism: a case report. J Chiropr Med. 2010;9(3):132–7.
40. Vieira AC, Oliveira MC, Lima EM, Rambob I, Leite M. Evaluation of the surface roughness in dental ceramics submitted to different finishing and polishing methods. J Indian Prosthodont Soc. 2013;13(3):290–5.

The State of the Art of the Implant-Abutment Design to Maximize the Peri-Implant Tissue Potential

16

Xavier Vela and Xavier Rodríguez

Abstract

Nowadays, implant restorations are considered one of the best treatments to replace hopeless teeth. In spite to achieve good aesthetic and functional results several questions about implant restorations remain still unanswered. Can long-term tissue stability be achieved? Can both, the soft tissue recession and early periimplant bone resorption be prevented? Which is the key factor that allows the soft and hard tissue to attain stability? If it exists, how can we do to include it in the implant restoration protocol?

In the past, countless studies about tissue stability focused in the role of the bacterial colonization to explain the loss of tissue stability mainly in the long-term follow up. Nowadays and considering the importance of bacterial colonization too, other factor has become more and more important than the aforementioned bacteria. That is the connective tissue. Currently, not only the connective tissue thickness but also the physiologic mechanisms by which the connective tissue fibres are stabilized on the abutment are recognized as a key factor of tissue stability. Instead of showing the well-known apical soft tissue migration and bone resorption around standard implant restorations while the time goes by, this sort of implant rehabilitations allow the tissues migrate coronally overtime. This chapter reports what and how can it be done to get the long-term tissue stability around implant restorations.

16.1 Introduction

The search of a natural result similar to the teeth and the surrounding tissues is the ultimate goal of implant-supported rehabilitations. The tooth is unique in the human body as it breaks through the epithelium. For this reason, peri-implant tissues must

X. Vela (✉) · X. Rodríguez
Implantology Department, International University of Catalonia (UIC), Barcelona, Spain
e-mail: vela@borgbcn.com; rodriguez@borgbcn.com

Todd R. Schoenbaum (ed.), *Implants in the Aesthetic Zone*,
https://doi.org/10.1007/978-3-319-72601-4_16

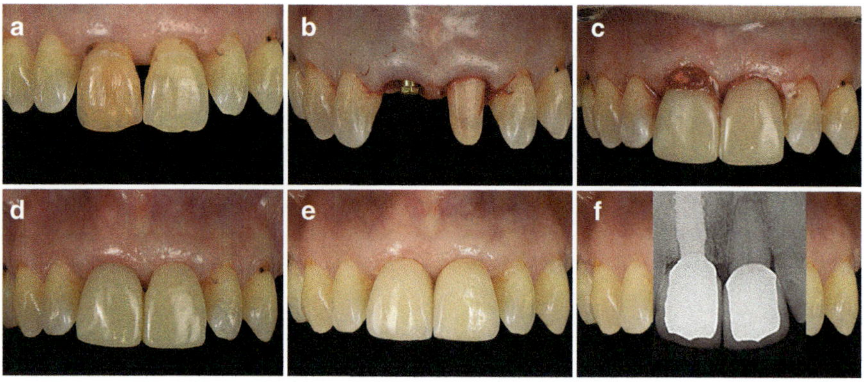

Fig. 16.1 Clinical case. (**a**) Hopeless right central incisor. (**b**) Extraction, immediate implant placement, and restoration with a tapered abutment. (**c**) Postoperative view. (**d**) After 1 year of loading. Provisionals. (**e**) After 1 year of loading. Definitive prostheses. (**f**) Radiograph showing no crestal bone resorption. It must be noted that bone is preserved at the abutment level with the tapered abutment

be organized not only to anchor the implant in the bone but also to form a protective seal around the implant as it emerges into the oral cavity.

When a tooth falls, the implant restoration should mimic both the aesthetics and function of the natural tooth (Fig. 16.1).

One of the most important functions of the natural teeth is their role in providing mechanical soft tissue stabilization. The tooth has the capability to stabilize the connective tissue fibers at the tooth neck level (supracrestally) and allow epithelial adhesion at the tooth crown level, thus preserving crestal bone [1]. The periodontal tissues (connective tissue, epithelium, and cementum) have two functions regarding the protective role. The first one is related to periodontal sealing and adhesion on the tooth which mitigates bacterial contamination. The second role is related to mechanical tissues stability around the tooth.

This chapter will focus on the rehabilitation of the anterior area with improved peri-implant tissues for healthy and aesthetic results. Several aspects of the tissue behavior around teeth and implants will be analyzed here to show the biologic rational of this treatment:

- The biologic function of the tooth.
- The effect of the standard implant rehabilitation on the surrounding tissues: The histomorphogenesis of the peri-implant tissues following the traditional protocol of anatomical (divergent) abutments with several abutment dis/reconnections will be discussed.

16.2 Tooth Function

Understanding the function of the tooth is of crucial importance for the implant restoration success. The tooth will be considered three parts: the root, the neck, and the tooth crown.

- The tooth *crown* is the part of the tooth that drives the “white aesthetics,” while the periodontal soft tissues determine the “pink aesthetics” [2].
  - The function of the tooth crown is shearing or cutting food during mastication. The enamel crown provides a smooth surface where the epithelium adheres and provides a walling-off function. To achieve epithelial attachment to the tooth enamel surface, the connective tissue must first be stabilized. The mechanical connective tissue stabilization on the tooth neck is crucial for allowing the subsequent epithelial attachment [3].
- The periodontal soft tissues at the tooth *neck* level will determine the “pink aesthetics” [2]. The function of this transmucosal portion of the tooth stabilizes the soft tissues by “insertion” of the connective tissue fibers into the cementum [1, 4]. It is important to note also that the stabilized connective tissue on the tooth neck surface provides support and blood supply to the coronally attached epithelium at the level of the enamel crown surface [5]. Both the connective tissue inserted in the cementum and the epithelium adhered to the enamel surface protect the bone from the resorption.
  - The key factor for tissue preservation around the tooth is the connective tissue stabilization on the tooth neck at the supracrestal level. In this way, the connective tissue stops the apical migration of the epithelium during healing and promotes the formation of a short sulcus length. In addition, a shortened sulcus length is related to predictable and aesthetic results [6]. If the connective tissue fibers fail, the soft tissues move apically, and the bone is resorbed.
- In healthy conditions, the *root* is the part of the tooth located in the bone and surrounded by the periodontal ligament. Periodontal ligament fibers go from the tooth root cementum to the alveolar bone. The function of the tooth root is to transmit the load from the crown to the bone [7] (Fig. 16.2)

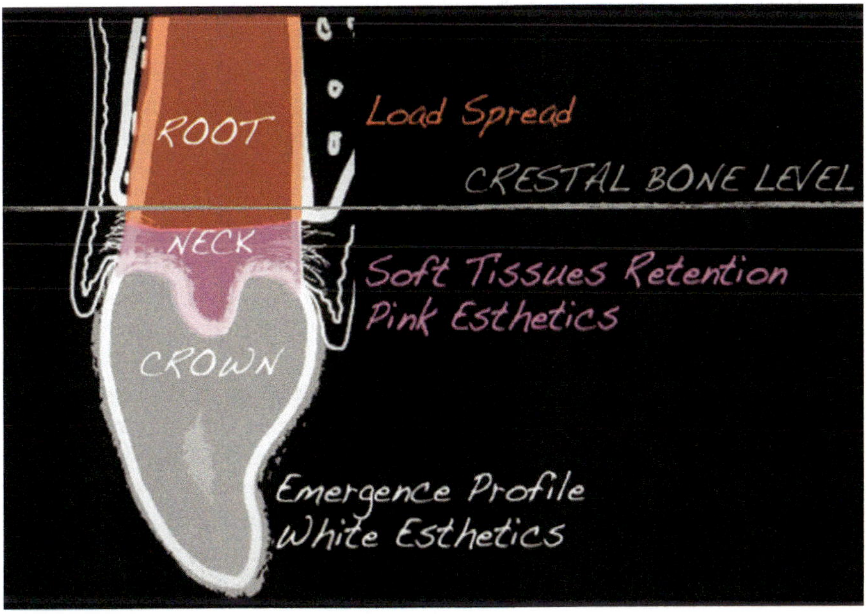

Fig. 16.2 Sketch of the tooth from a functional point of view

The main concern around implant restorations is soft tissue apical migration and subsequent bone resorption. This results in restorations prone to accumulate plaque at the level of the implant platform and potentially result in peri-implantitis. Several features related to the behavior of the peri-implant tissues can be understood from the periodontal tissues around the tooth. Those are palatal position and narrow shape.

- Tooth position: The concept of an alveolar "envelope" has been suggested within which the teeth should be maintained. Severe proinclination appears to be contributory to gingival recession [8]. Buccally placed tooth also contribute to the gingival recession [9, 10].
- Tooth morphology: Convex tooth morphology yields a more apical location of the gingival margin, while a concave shape leads to coronal position of the gingival margin. This is most evident in the gingival zenith position on maxillary anterior teeth [9].

16.3 The Effect of Traditional (Divergent) Implant Rehabilitations on Surrounding Tissues

The use of an implant restoration with an anatomical (divergent) abutment has long been considered an ideal restoration due to its mimicking of the natural tooth shape [11, 12]. The ideal implant restoration and approach must restore not only the aesthetics but also the function of the natural tooth. The implant restoration should also allow the connective tissue fibers to stabilize at a supracrestal level and in turn allow epithelial adhesion at the crown level. Both elements together exert a walling-off function and prevent bone resorption.

The most significant function of the implant restoration is connective tissue stabilization on the restoration at a supracrestal position. This is the key factor in achieving peri-implant bone preservation. In short, the correlation between the function of the three parts of the tooth and the three parts of the implant restoration are as follows:

- The tooth *root* will be replaced by the *implant*, thus the implant function is to transmit the load from the crown to the bone. The implant is firmly anchored to *bone* without any kind of ligament, for this reason the load is transmitted from the implant to the bone interface but in different way than the tooth transmitted the load to the bone interface [13].
- The tooth *neck* (supracrestal area): This part of the restoration is a key factor for maintaining the *connective tissue at supracrestal level* and, in turn, for bone preservation. The *abutment*, in theory, must fulfil this role. Unfortunately, the implant abutment lacks the capability to retain the connective tissue fibers by means of periodontal fiber insertion. This inherent deficiency forces an apical migration of the connective tissue fibers until they are retained at the level of the

first thread of the implant [14]. Therefore the connective tissue will make contact in the area between the implant platform and the first thread. This feature has been found in several studies [14–20]. The area between the implant platform and the first implant thread in traditional anatomical abutments (divergent shape) is the first part of the implant restoration with tapered shape (narrow at the top and wider at the bottom). It is important to understand that this shape is responsible for retaining the circular connective tissue fibers [14, 18, 21]. As it has been found, this feature stops the apical epithelial migration at the level of the implant platform. By using this traditional abutment design, the *implant* itself is responsible for providing the *epithelial attachment*, rather than the abutment (Fig. 16.3).

- The tooth *crown* is replaced by the *prosthetic crown*. Thus, the prosthetic crown will mimic the aesthetics of the tooth and provide a smooth surface where the epithelium can attach as well. Unfortunately, when using traditional abutment designs, the epithelial attachment migrates apically to the level of the implant platform; therefore the prosthetic crown merely provides the aesthetics and chewing function of the teeth and not the sealing capability.

In short, the traditional flared abutment design forces the neck of the implant to provide the function of the root, neck, and crown of the natural tooth. This reality makes it difficult to design the ideal implant restoration regarding its shape and surface characteristics (Fig. 16.4).

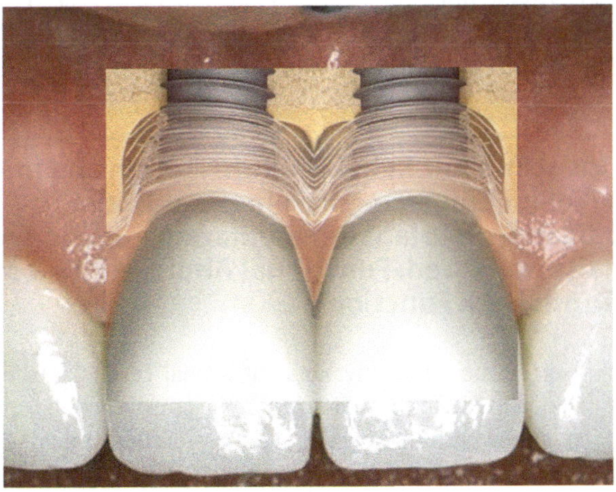

Fig. 16.3 Implant rehabilitation with anatomical abutments is shown. The area where the connective tissue fibers are retained is at the implant level. Circular connective tissue fibers will be stabilized where the diameter of the implant rehabilitation switches from narrow to wider diameter. The compromised area between the implant platform and the first implant thread will be the part of the restoration where the connective tissues are stabilized

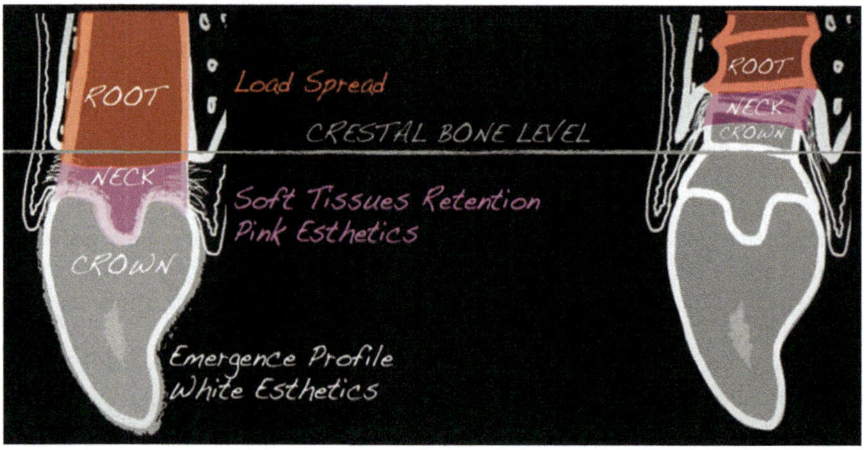

Fig. 16.4 Sketch of the tooth and implant function. Tooth and implant rehabilitation with anatomical abutments are compared. It must be highlighted that the implant surface has three functions (root, neck, and crown tooth)

Regarding the three parts of the implant rehabilitation, implant, abutment, and crown, three general concepts should be considered. In each one, the surface, the shape, and the surgical/prosthetic positioning determine the outcome.

In summary, the main challenge of implant rehabilitation is how to guide and support the soft tissues on the restoration while isolating and protecting the bone without connective tissue fiber insertion into the cementum. The success or failure of the implant restoration is determined by the transmucosal interface area. For improving the clinical results, it is important to look at the early healing events.

16.4 The Ideal Implant Rehabilitation Design and Implant Protocol for Enhancing Peri-Implant Tissue Stabilization: Implant Rehabilitation Function with the Narrowed, Functional Abutment that Mimics the Tooth Neck Function

In order to achieve the most aesthetic and functional result, an accurate implant placement must be achieved. The implant should be considered the apical extension of the restoration, and the preferred design of the restoration should guide the surgical implant placement [11]. Both the implant and the abutment must be placed in the ideal position to produce acceptable results. Consequently, it is mandatory that the surgery be performed with an implant surgical guide.

To achieve good mechanical connective tissue stability, the restoration design is of crucial importance. Whether the abutment is placed at the time of implant placement or at the second stage, once the abutment is connected, it shouldn't be disconnected to ensure the stability of the soft and hard tissues. Several studies have shown that avoiding or diminishing the abutment dis-reconnections also reduced the soft tissue collapse and bone resorption [4, 14, 22]. The challenge with placing the abutment only once is difficulty in achieving an appropriate finish line on the restoration, while the tissues are still healing. This can be solved by means of using a shoulderless abutment. This restoration follows the principles of biologically oriented preparation technique (BOPT) on teeth suggested by Loi [23]. Through this kind of restorations, the tissues adapt to the rehabilitation instead of a margin finish line which adapts to the tissues. For this reason, a protocol with no disconnections of the abutment should be considered. The authors propose the placement of the *definitive shoulderless abutment at the time of implant placement or exposure.*

In both the immediate restoration and second-stage surgery, the biologic interface between the abutment and the soft tissues must be reestablished. This means that the connective tissue must recover its mechanical stability on the rehabilitation surface before achieving the epithelial adhesion [3]. *Due to the presence of the abutment, which prevents healing by primary intention, healing by secondary intention will drive the wound healing.* This will be a key point from which a chain of biologic events will be promoted. Wound healing around the dental implant is a coordinated and sequentially organized repair mechanism. Soft tissue healing progresses in four phases: the hemostasis phase, the inflammatory phase, the proliferative phase, and finally the remodeling phase. All are necessary to repair or regenerate the tissue damage. These phases appear in chronological sequence with some overlap.

16.4.1 Hemostasis (First Minutes): The Phase Responsible for Stopping Hemorrhaging and Preparing the Scaffold for Tissue Regeneration

In the first minute after abutment placement, a blood clot occupies the space between the abutment and the mucosa. The platelets release chemotactic and growth factors. The hemostasis takes place for only a few minutes [24].

What can it do in this short time to improve the peri-implant tissue stability? Two features are important to the clinician during this time: to *provide space* for the blood clot and to promote its *stability*.

16.4.1.1 Providing Space

The abutment should leave as much room as possible to let the clot work. The clot will serve as the three-dimensional scaffold where the tissues will start their regeneration. From the first minute of healing, the role of the provisional prosthesis or healing abutment is to aid in clot formation. The simplest way to make room at the implant platform level is the use of a *platform-switching* (PS) implant and the use of a *tapered (functional) abutment profile* [18, 19, 25–29]. This type of rehabilitation design will better preserve the *fBIC (first bone to implant contact)* [20, 30]. The use of a PS implant and tapered abutment will create more space around the rehabilitation for connective tissue growth [18, 31]. This fact may promote a more coronal and thicker soft tissue stabilization comparing to a standard divergent abutment design [25] (Fig. 16.5).

Thus, both *the use of a platform-switching implant and a tapered abutment* could enhance soft tissue response.

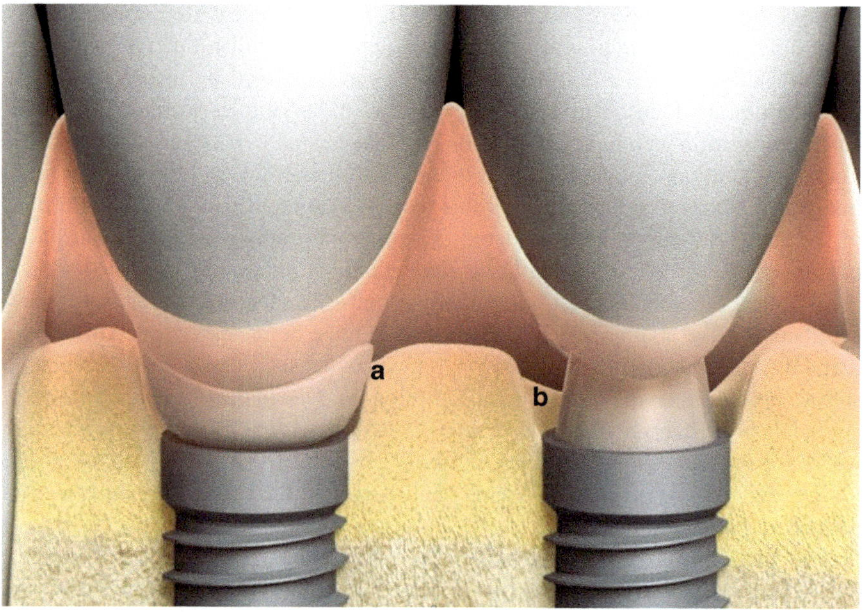

Fig. 16.5 Sketch of a non-platform switching implant (**a**) and platform-switching implant (**b**). (**a**) Matched implant rehabilitation with divergent profile (anatomic abutment). There is no place for the blood clot, the space provided is minimal around this kind of restoration. (**b**) Platform-switching rehabilitation with a tapered profile (functional) abutment. This kind of restoration provides space around the rehabilitation for the blood clot to form and stabilize

16.4.1.2 Stability of the Blood Clot

The second important point during the hemostatic phase is to promote the stability of the blood clot from the very beginning of the healing. If the flap collapses into the chamber or excessive shrinkage of the coagulum occurs, this may jeopardize the success of connective tissue repair [32]. The placement of the temporary crown at the time of abutment placement may enhance the clot stability (Fig. 16.6). Furthermore, a non-disconnection abutment protocol is mandatory to get such clot stability.

16.4.2 The Inflammatory Phase (First Days): The Stage Responsible for Removing the Debris, Bacterial Contamination, and Promoting the Proliferative Phase

Only 10 min after the wound, and for the next 4–7 days, the inflammatory phase takes place. The blood clot is infiltrated by several polymorphonuclears within a dense fiber network [34]. The endotoxins and exotoxins released by the bacteria and the effect of activation of the systemic and local immune response will cause important peri-implant tissue damage. The inflammatory phase, although being necessary,

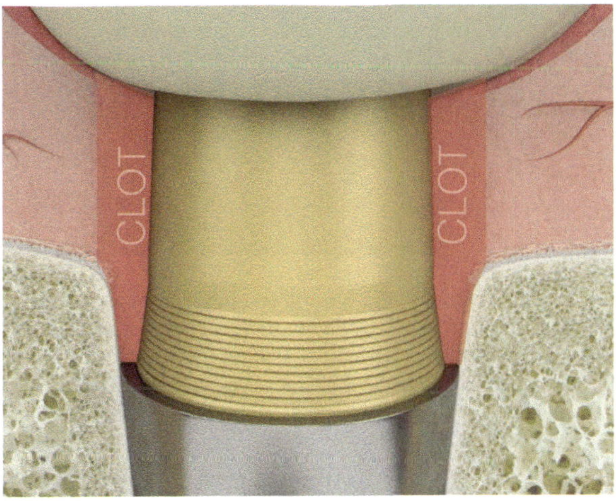

Fig. 16.6 Implant rehabilitation with a tapered abutment and provisional crown. The areas where the clot is preserved are shown. This would be the chamber effect [33]

always causes some peri-implant tissues destruction. The inflammatory phase is inevitable, but it should be as short as possible to minimize the tissue damage and bring about the proliferative phase [24]. Therefore the use of *antibiotic and anti-inflammatory therapy* is suggested.

16.4.3 The Proliferative Phase (First Month): The Phase Responsible for Repairing the Tissues Which Provide Structural Cells and Blood Supply

The proliferative phase ranges from a few days to a few weeks. This is the most transcendent phase of healing. The three-dimensional scaffold formed by the clot during the first minutes will be the scaffold where the tissues will grow. Stimulated by fibroblast grow factors from macrophages, fibroblasts from the surrounding healthy tissue migrate by amoeboid movement into the blood clot. The fibroblasts will grow and fill the room provided by the provisional restoration, and new blood vessels will come with them in their growth, encircling the abutment [31] (Fig. 16.7).

The organization of the collagen fibers is like a ring of collagen fibers around the abutment, and ultimately the stability of the soft tissue depends on them [14, 18, 35].

In this way, the tissues surrounding the tapered abutment will be thicker than the tissues surrounding the anatomical abutment due to the lack of clot space in the latter (Fig. 16.8).

Nevertheless, the most important effect of the tapered abutments isn't related to the room they created, but the effect which promotes myofibroblast contraction. The tissue healing surrounding the implant restoration heals by second intention. The main characteristic of the second intention wound healing is the capability of

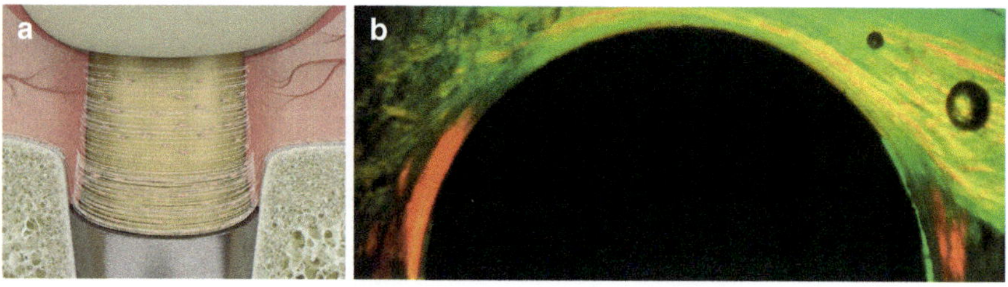

Fig. 16.7 Circular fibers: (**a**) Sketch of a tapered abutment in the proliferation phase is represented. Circular fibers, fibroblasts, and myofibroblasts following the abutment surface are shown. (**b**) Histologic sample harvested from an animal study (hematoxylin-eosin stain under polarize light microscope). Transversal cut at the abutment level is shown. The circular arrangement of the connective tissue fibers must be highlighted (yellow and orange fibers)

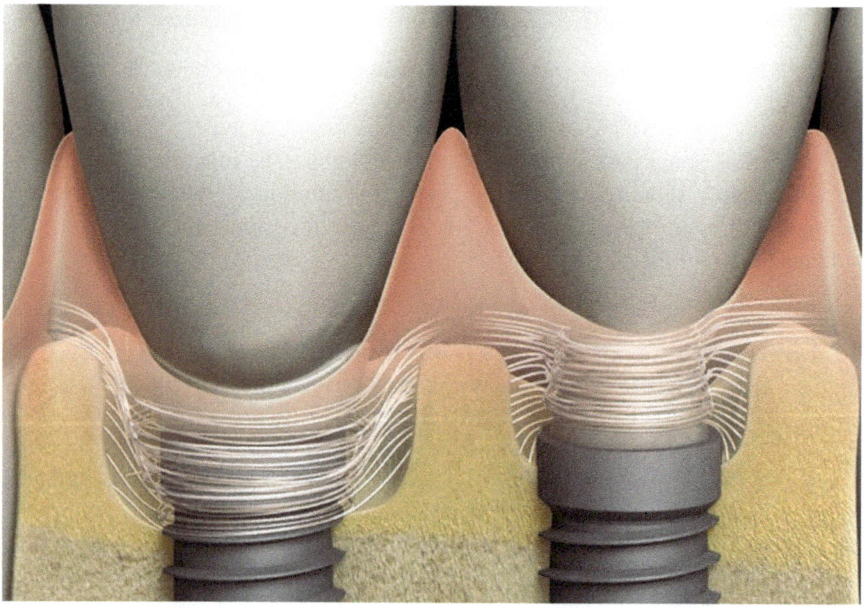

Fig. 16.8 Sketch of the connective tissue fibers arrangement around standard matched implant restorations with anatomical abutments (left) and platform-switching restoration with a tapered abutment. Circular connective tissue fibers are apically stopped by the rehabilitation macrodesign

contracting [36]. This feature is mediated by the myofibroblasts. Within 6–15 days some fibroblasts turn to myofibroblast, and these will shrink and contract to close the two sides of the wound. After 15 days, about 70% of fibroblasts in granulation tissue express alpha-smooth muscle actin [36] (Fig. 16.9).

The use of abutments with a tapered profile will promote soft tissue migration coronally, instead of apically into the bone [18]. The contraction of the myofibroblasts will produce a soft tissue migration from the wider diameter area of the tapered abutment (bottom) to the narrower diameter area of the abutment (coronal)

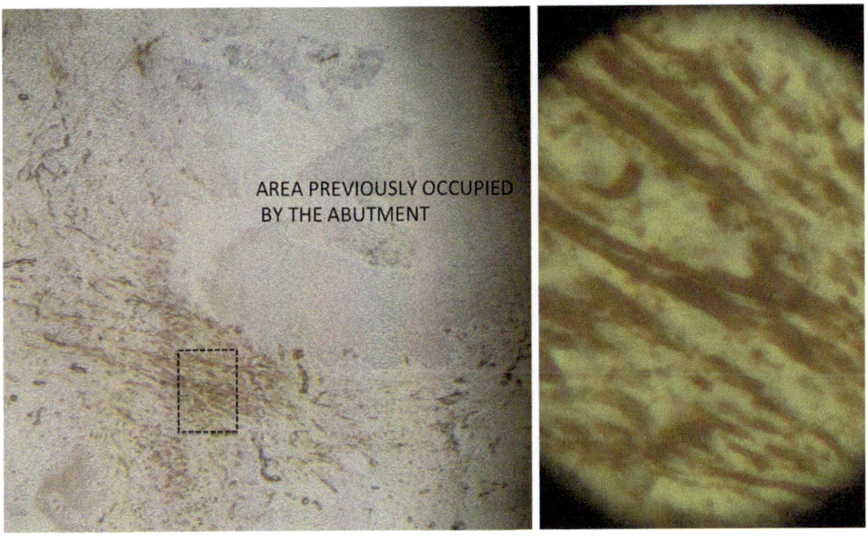

Fig. 16.9 (alpha-smooth muscle actin stain) Left picture: transversal cut of human gingiva after 3 weeks of healing (×10). It is noted that the long axis direction of the myofibroblast is parallel to the circular abutment area, which means in circular fashion. Thus, changes in the abutment diameter promote migration of the soft tissues during the myofibroblast contraction. Right picture: detail of the myofibroblast area

[18]. At the same time, the presence of a narrow abutment will provide space for a thicker band of soft tissue. In short, it could be said that during the proliferative phase, the tissues will grow and fill the free spaces, after which the tissues will shrink around the rehabilitation, and finally stabilize upon the rehabilitation. The epithelial cells will also proliferate down to the area where the connective tissue fibers stabilize on the restoration. The connective tissue and the granulation tissue have the ability to stop the apical migration of the epithelium [3]. By means of using tapered abutments, the epithelium will attach at the level to the crown surface through hemidesmosomes.

The threat of the apical collapse during the proliferative phase has led to the development of various abutments designs and surface modifications. Though we understand that the macrodesign of the abutment (shape and profile) exerts the greatest influence on the tissues behavior, it may also be that the abutment surfaces influence the tissue reaction [37, 38].

Among the different surface treatments, "contact guidance" must be highlighted. This is a microgrooved surface of the abutment: micromachined grooves of appropriate dimensions may improve connective tissue ingrowth and inhibit epithelial downgrowth [39, 40] (Fig. 16.10).

It has been described that the biologic width around a tooth is located at a supracrestal level and it is the main barrier responsible for preventing apical migration of the epithelium. Long sulcus length has been related to periodontal pockets and poor

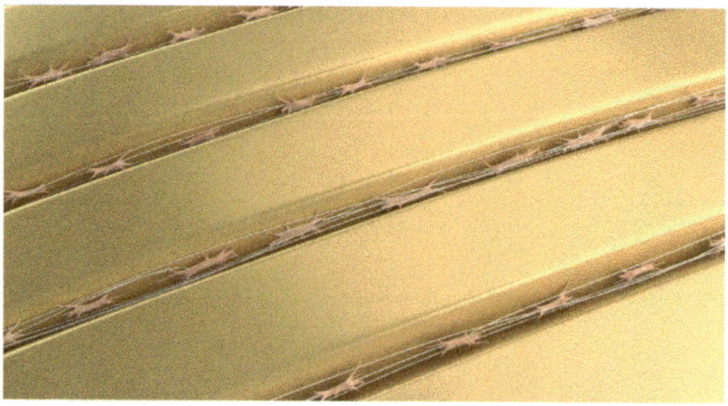

Fig. 16.10 Microthreads at the bottom of the abutment are represented. The myofibroblasts fit into the grooves as shown. The elongated fibroblasts are supposed to enhance early adhesion and activation, which may be critical for the formation of a biologic seal and promote tissue integration [40]

aesthetic results [6]. The presence of short sulcus length is advantageous for aesthetics, to prevent bacterial infection, and bone preservation [6].

Therefore a *microthreaded area at the bottom of the abutment* may enhance and promote the formation of a biological seal and tissue integration.

16.4.4 The Remodeling Phase: The One Responsible for Tissue Maturation, Collagen Realignment, and Tissue Growth as a Result of Homeostasis

The remodeling process is the final healing phase. The remodeling phase is often overlooked in terms of its importance in repairing the bone and soft tissues. It is neither swift nor highly reactive, but it does result in an organized, functional scar capable of behaving in a similar way to the parent tissue. The remodeling phase starts approximately 6 weeks after the exposure of the implant to the oral environment and continues indefinitely. During the remodeling phase, the collagen fibers are realigned in a parallel fashion which will increase the tissue strength. This phase involves remodeling of collagen fibers from type III to type I. Cellular activity decreases, along with the number of blood vessels in the wounded area [41]. The remodeling phase is no longer a simple event in the light of ever-increasing knowledge in the healing field.

The ideal rehabilitation should be one which improves the tissues response over time. Despite achieving successful results, the tissues around implant rehabilitations may worsen over time. There are numerous reports demonstrating early and late bone resorption, along with the gingival recession [42–45]. However, it must be taken into account that some implant systems have shown not only crestal bone level preservation but crestal bone gain after the insertion of the definitive restorations over time [21, 46, 47]. The question to be answered is the reason why the tapered shape implant restorations result in a soft and hard tissue growth in coronal direction, instead of apically as has been described around traditional implant restorations [42, 44] (Fig. 16.11).

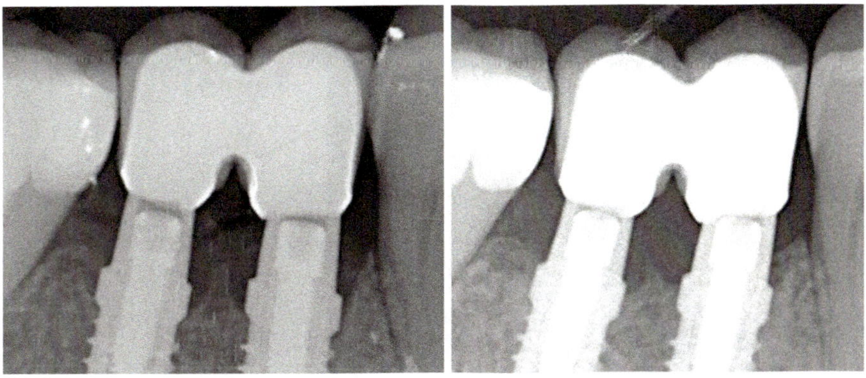

Fig. 16.11 Tapered abutment rehabilitation at the time of the bridge placement (left) and after 3 years of function (right). The coronal migration of the bone level is noted

Regarding soft tissues, it has been suggested that overcontoured implant crowns increase gingival thickness [23]. The authors called this term "gull-wing." The gingival increase is related to the tension produced by the negative pressure (mechanotransduction) at the area confined by the gingival margin, the buccal face of the implant crown, and the internal mucosa of the lip. At the same time, the combination of the tissue regenerative stimuli combined with the tapered abutment shape will promote coronal migration of the soft tissue. In summary, the narrow contour of the tapered abutment and the ovoid crown will promote coronal migration of the gingiva. The key factor which will drive this bone growth as the time goes on will be the intimate contact with the periosteum. Periosteum is the tissue which drives the bone growth. Despite the importance of the periosteum, it has received little attention in the literature in recent years [48]. This tissue has a major role in bone growth and bone repair and has an impact on the blood supply to the bone and muscle. Periosteum has two distinct layers, an outer fibrous layer and an inner layer that has significant osteoblastic potential.

Fibers that emerge from the outer layer of the periosteum end up in the connective tissue of the gingiva, inserted into the cementum along the tooth neck or surrounding the implant abutment (Fig. 16.12).

The fibers inserted in the cementum are the ones that pull the bone along as the tooth is erupting or during extrusive orthodontic movements. This may suggest that fibers which end up in the tooth neck cementum pull out the periosteum and the osteoblastic cells as strings pull puppets. So it could be understood promoting the coronal migration of the soft tissues as the time goes on. The periosteum will follow the connective tissue. That is why the greater improvements regarding the fBIC may be achieved by means of changes primarily in the abutment design and not on the implant surface. The existence of the tapered shape at the level of the transmucosal interface will easily allow soft tissue migration to the area with lesser diameter (coronal) and also the area with less pressure. This may be due to a strain on the connective tissue

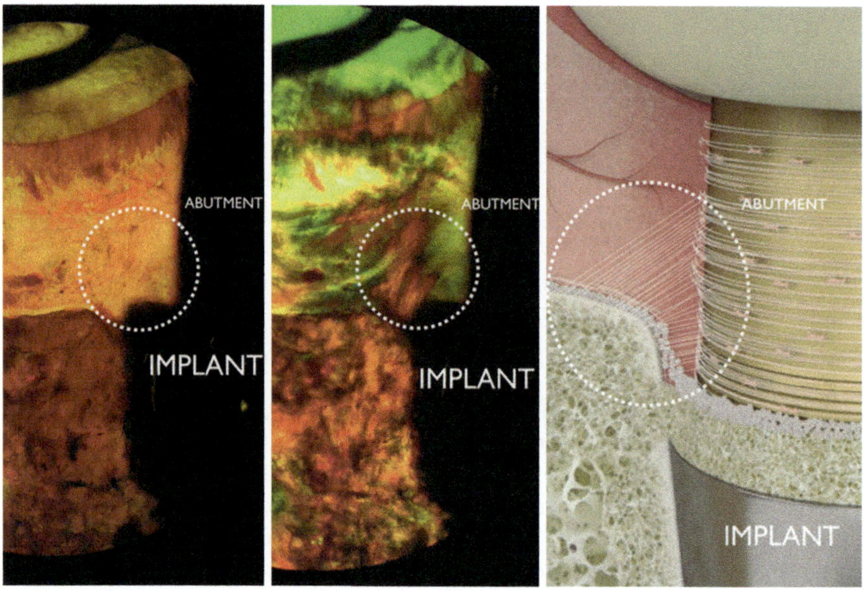

Fig. 16.12 Animal histologic sample under microscope light ×10. The directions of the connective tissue fibers are not noted. Middle: same sample under polarized light. The direction of the connective tissue fibers is shown. Those fibers go from the periosteum to the abutment area. Right: figure of the histologic sample showing the connective tissue fibers originated from the periosteum and trapped by the tapered abutment. The tapered abutment in the remodeling phase is represented. The periosteum's coronal migration is evident

fibers from the periosteum that stimulates cell proliferation (mechanotransduction) and osteoblastic migration to the coronal area. Fibroblasts sense changes in physical parameters in their extracellular matrix environment, transduce mechanical into chemical information, and integrate these signals with growth factor-derived stimuli to achieve specific changes in gene expression [49]. Mechanical stress influences cell proliferation and the survival of oral fibroblasts. Cyclic strain, tension, or negative pressure delivers anti-apoptotic and proliferative signals to gingival fibroblasts [50].

Therefore *tapered abutments could enhance the hard tissue growth* during the endless phase of remodeling (Fig. 16.13).

Conclusions

Aesthetic results depend primarily on the soft tissue stabilization, not only from a clinical point of view but also from a physiologic point of view.

The objective of implant rehabilitation is the replacement of the hopeless tooth in appearance but also in the biologic function of the neck area of the natural tooth. Furthermore, the ideal implant rehabilitation should be guided by the behavior of the surrounding tissues, and its shape should enhance the tissue behavior over time.

On implant restorations, the connective tissue fibers are retained at the first point where the rehabilitation turns from narrow to wider diameter. Apical to the

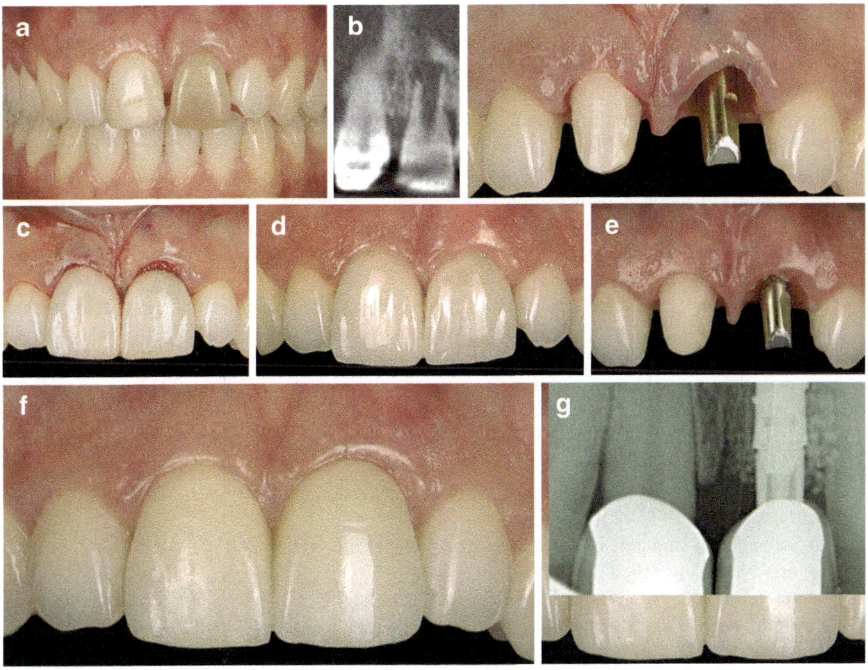

Fig. 16.13 Clinical case of implant restoration by means of the implant placement and restoration with tapered abutment. Picture (**a**), failed central incisor is shown. Picture (**b**), x-ray shows a resorbed root. Picture (**c**), immediate implant placement with the definitive tapered marginless abutment is shown. The room for the clot is noted. Picture (**c**), the provisional crown the day of the surgery. Pictures (**d** and **e**), the soft tissues aspect after 3 months of function are shown. Picture (**f**), the final result after 12 months of implant placement. Picture (**g**), x-ray showed a good crestal bone preservation

stabilized connective tissue, the internal area is isolated and consequently, the bone better preserved.

The use of a platform-switched implant design with narrow, conical abutments, placed once and never removed, and the use of biocompatible materials is the ideal method for tooth replacement in the aesthetic zone. If the clinical approach and material selection respect the soft tissue, the results will inevitably be more aesthetic and predictable.

References

1. Schroeder HE, Listgarten MA. The gingival tissues: the architecture of periodontal protection. Periodontology. 1997;2000(13):91–120. https://doi.org/10.1111/j.1600-0757.1997.tb00097.x.
2. Fürhauser R, Florescu D, Benesch T, Haas R, Mailath G, Watzek G. Evaluation of soft tissue around single-tooth implant crowns: the pink esthetic score. Clin Oral Implants Res. 2005;16(6):639–44. https://doi.org/10.1111/j.1600-0501.2005.01193.x.

3. Rompen E, Domken O, Degidi M, Pontes AEP, Piattelli A. The effect of material characteristics, of surface topography and of implant components and connections on soft tissue integration: a literature review. Clin Oral Implants Res. 2006;17(Suppl 2):55–67. https://doi.org/10.1111/j.1600-0501.2006.01367.x.
4. Abrahamsson I, Berglundh T, Lindhe J. The mucosal barrier following abutment dis/reconnection. An experimental study in dogs. J Clin Periodontol. 1997;24(8):568–72. https://doi.org/10.1111/j.1600-051X.1997.tb00230.x.
5. Berglundh T, Lindhe J. Dimension of the periimplant mucosa. Biological width revisited. J Clin Periodontol. 1996;23(10):971–3. https://doi.org/10.1111/j.1600-051X.1996.tb00520.x.
6. Spear FM. Interdisciplinary esthetic management anterior gingival embrasures. Adv Esthet Interdiscip Dent. 2006;2(2):20–8.
7. Pavasant P, Yongchaitrakul T. Role of mechanical stress on the function of periodontal ligament cells. Periodontol. 2011;56(1):154–65. https://doi.org/10.1111/j.1600-0757.2010.00374.x.
8. Johal A, Katsaros C, Kuijpers-Jagtman AM. State of the science on controversial topics: missing maxillary lateral incisors--a report of the Angle Society of Europe 2012 meeting. Prog Orthod. 2013;14(1):20. https://doi.org/10.1186/2196-1042-14-20.
9. Ahmad I. Anterior dental aesthetics: dental perspective. Br Dent J. 2005;199(3):135–41.; quiz 174. https://doi.org/10.1038/sj.bdj.4812534.
10. Hall WB. Present status of soft tissue grafting. J Periodontol. 1977;48(9):587–97. https://doi.org/10.1902/jop.1977.48.9.587.
11. Al-Sabbagh M. Implants in the esthetic zone. Dent Clin N Am. 2006;50(3):391–407. https://doi.org/10.1016/j.cden.2006.03.007.
12. Lemongello GJ. Customized provisional abutment and provisional restorations for an immediately-placed implant. Pract Proced Aesthet Dent. 2014;20(1 Neurology of Pregnancy):9–10. https://doi.org/10.1212/01.CON.0000443830.87636.9a.
13. Isidor F. Influence of forces on peri-implant bone. Clin Oral Implants Res. 2006;17(Suppl 2):8–18.
14. Rodríguez X, Vela X, Calvo-Guirado JL, Nart J, Stappert CFJ. Effect of platform switching on collagen fiber orientation and bone resorption around dental implants: a preliminary histologic animal study. Int J Oral Maxillofac Implants. 2012;27(5):1116–22.
15. Davarpanah M, Martinez H, Tecucianu JF. Apical-coronal implant position: recent surgical proposals. Technical note. Int J Oral Maxillofac Implants. 2000;15:865–72.
16. De Bruyn H, Vandeweghe S, Ruyffelaert C, Cosyn J, Sennerby L. Radiographic evaluation of modern oral implants with emphasis on crestal bone level and relevance to peri-implant health. Periodontol. 2013;62(1):256–70. https://doi.org/10.1111/prd.12004.
17. Östman PO, Hellman M, Sennerby L. Ten years later: results from a prospective single-centre clinical study on 121 oxidized (TiUnite™) Brånemark implants in 46 patients. Clin Implant Dent Relat Res. 2012;14(6):852–60. https://doi.org/10.1111/j.1708-8208.2012.00453.x.
18. Rodríguez X, Navajas Acedo Á, Vela X, Fortuño À, Jiménez García J, Nevins M. Arrangement of peri-implant connective tissue fibers around platform-switching implants with conical abutments and its relationship to the underlying bone: a human histologic study. Int J Periodontics Restorative Dent. 2016;36(4):533–40. https://doi.org/10.11607/prd.2580.
19. Saadoun AP, Touati B. Soft tissue recession around implants: is it still unavoidable?- part II. Pract Proced Aesthet Dent. 2007;19(2):81–7.
20. Vela-Nebot X, Rodríguez-Ciurana X, Rodado-Alonso C, Segalà-Torres M. Benefits of an implant platform modification technique to reduce crestal bone resorption. Implant Dent. 2006;15(3):313–20. https://doi.org/10.1097/01.id.0000226788.19742.32.
21. Braun E, Iacono V. Guest editorial tapered tips to think about. Int J Periodontics Restorative Dent. 2006;26(1):7–93.
22. Abrahamsson I, Berglundh T, Sekino S, Lindhe J. Tissue reactions to abutment shift: an experimental study in dogs. Clin Implant Dent Relat Res. 2003;5(2):82–8. https://doi.org/10.1111/j.1708-8208.2003.tb00188.x.
23. Loi I, Di Felice A. Biologically oriented preparation technique (BOPT): a new approach for prosthetic restoration of periodontically healthy teeth. Eur J Esthet Dent. 2013;8(1):10–23.

http://search.ebscohost.com/login.aspx?direct=true&AuthType=cookie,ip,cpid&custid=ns083137&db=ddh&AN=90073645&site=ehost-live
24. Terheyden H, Lang NP, Bierbaum S, Stadlinger B. Osseointegration - communication of cells. Clin Oral Implants Res. 2012;23(10):1127–35. https://doi.org/10.1111/j.1600-0501.2011.02327.x.
25. Finelle G, Papadimitriou DEV, Souza AB, Katebi N, Gallucci GO, Araújo MG. Peri-implant soft tissue and marginal bone adaptation on implant with non-matching healing abutments: micro-CT analysis. Clin Oral Implants Res. 2015;26(4):e42–6. https://doi.org/10.1111/clr.12328.
26. Gamborena I, Lee J, Fiorini T, Wenzel BA, Schüpbach P, Wikesjö UME, Susin C. Effect of platform shift/switch and concave abutments on crestal bone levels and mucosal profile following flap and flapless implant surgery. Clin Implant Dent Relat Res. 2015;17(5):908–16. https://doi.org/10.1111/cid.12208.
27. Lazzara RJ, Porter SS. Platform switching: a new concept in implant dentistry for controlling postrestorative crestal bone levels. Int J Periodontics Restorative Dent. 2006;26:9–17.
28. Redemagni M, Cremonesi S, Garlini G, Maiorana C. Soft tissue stability with immediate implants and concave abutments. Eur J Esthet Dent. 2009;4(4):328–37.
29. Rompen E, Raepsaet N, Domken O, Touati B, Van Dooren E. Soft tissue stability at the facial aspect of gingivally converging abutments in the esthetic zone: a pilot clinical study. J Prosthet Dent. 2007;97(6 Suppl):S119–25. https://doi.org/10.1016/S0022-3913(07)60015-8.
30. Atieh M a, Ibrahim HM, Atieh AH. Platform switching for marginal bone preservation around dental implants: a systematic review and meta-analysis. J Periodontol. 2010;81(10):1350–66. https://doi.org/10.1902/jop.2010.100232.
31. Makigusa K. Histologic comparison of biologic width around teeth versus implant: the effect on bone preservation. J Implant Reconstr Dent. 2009;12(6):20–4. http://www.moderndentistrymedia.com/nov_dec2010/makigusa.pdf
32. Wikesjö UM, Nilvéus RE, Selvig K a. Significance of early healing events on periodontal repair: a review. J Periodontol. 1992;63(3):158–65. https://doi.org/10.1902/jop.1992.63.3.158.
33. Degidi M, Daprile G, Nardi D, Piattelli A. Immediate provisionalization of implants placed in fresh extraction sockets using a definitive abutment: the chamber concept. Int J Periodontics Restorative Dent. 2013;33(5):559–66. https://doi.org/10.11607/prd.1795.
34. Berglundh T, Abrahamsson I, Welander M, Lang NP, Lindhe J. Morphogenesis of the peri-implant mucosa: an experimental study in dogs. Clin Oral Implants Res. 2007;18(1):1–8. https://doi.org/10.1111/j.1600-0501.2006.01380.x.
35. Schierano G, Ramieri G, Cortese M, Aimetti M, Preti G. Organization of the connective tissue barrier around long-term loaded implant abutments in man. Clin Oral Implants Res. 2002;13(5):460–4.
36. HÄKkinen L, Uitto V-J, Larjava H. Cell biology of gingival wound healing. Periodontology. 2000;24(1):127–52. https://doi.org/10.1034/j.1600-0757.2000.2240107.x.
37. do Nascimento C, Pita MS, Fernandes FHNC, Pedrazzi V, de Albuquerque Junior RF, Ribeiro RF. Bacterial adhesion on the titanium and zirconia abutment surfaces. Clin Oral Implants Res. 2014;25(3):337–43. https://doi.org/10.1111/clr.12093.
38. Wennerberg A, Sennerby L, Kultje C, Lekholm U. Some soft tissue characteristics at implant abutments with different surface topography. A study in humans. J Clin Periodontol. 2003;30(1):88–94. https://doi.org/10.1034/j.1600-051X.2003.10026.x.
39. Brunette DM, Chehroudi B. The effects of the surface topography of micromachined titanium substrata on cell behavior in vitro and in vivo. J Biomech Eng. 1999;121(1):49–57. https://doi.org/10.1115/1.2798042.
40. Guillem-Marti J, Delgado L, Godoy-Gallardo M, Pegueroles M, Herrero M, Gil FJ. Fibroblast adhesion and activation onto micro-machined titanium surfaces. Clin Oral Implants Res. 2013;24(7):770–80. https://doi.org/10.1111/j.1600-0501.2012.02451.x.
41. Schreml S, Szeimies R-M, Prantl L, Landthaler M, Babilas P. Wound healing in the 21st century. J Am Acad Dermatol. 2010;63(5):866–81. https://doi.org/10.1016/j.jaad.2009.10.048.
42. Apse P, Zarb GA, Schmitt A, Lewis DW. The longitudinal effectiveness of ossointegrated dental implants. The Toronto study: peri-implant mucosal response. Int J Periodontics Restorative Dent. 1991;11(2):94–111.

43. Chaytor DV, Zarb GA, Schmitt A, Lewis DW. The longitudinal effectiveness of osseointegrated dental implants. The Toronto study: bone level changes. Int J Periodontics Restorative Dent. 1991;11:112–25.
44. Cosyn J, Eghbali A, Hermans A, Vervaeke S, De Bruyn H, Cleymaet R. A 5-year prospective study on single immediate implants in the aesthetic zone. J Clin Periodontol. 2016;43(8):702–9. https://doi.org/10.1111/jcpe.12571.
45. Oh T-J, Yoon J, Misch CE, Wang H-L. The causes of early implant bone loss: myth or science? J Periodontol. 2002;73(3):322–33. https://doi.org/10.1902/jop.2002.73.3.322.
46. Ganeles J, Zöllner A, Jackowski J, Ten Bruggenkate C, Beagle J, Guerra F. Immediate and early loading of Straumann implants with a chemically modified surface (SLActive) in the posterior mandible and maxilla: 1-year results from a prospective multicenter study. Clin Oral Implants Res. 2008;19(11):1119–28. https://doi.org/10.1111/j.1600-0501.2008.01626.x.
47. Urdaneta RA, Seemann R, Dragan I-F, Lubelski W, Leary J, Chuang S-K. A retrospective radiographic study on the effect of natural tooth-implant proximity and an introduction to the concept of a bone-loading platform switch. Int J Oral Maxillofac Implants. 2014;29(6):1412–24. https://doi.org/10.11607/jomi.3699.
48. Dwek JR. The periosteum: what is it, where is it, and what mimics it in its absence? Skelet Radiol. 2010;39(4):319–23. https://doi.org/10.1007/s00256-009-0849-9.
49. Chiquet M, Gelman L, Lutz R, Maier S. From mechanotransduction to extracellular matrix gene expression in fibroblasts. Biochim Biophys Acta. 2009;1793(5):911–20. https://doi.org/10.1016/j.bbamcr.2009.01.012.
50. Danciu TE, Gagari E, Adam RM, Damoulis PD, Freeman MR. Mechanical strain delivers anti-apoptotic and proliferative signals to gingival fibroblasts. J Dent Res. 2004;83(8):596–601. https://doi.org/10.1177/154405910408300803.

9783319726007